Additional Praise for *Strategies in Biomedical Data Science: Driving Force for Innovation*

"The allure of data analytics is in knowing what is currently unknowable by identifying patterns in apparent chaos. If these insights could be applied in the healthcare field to individualized patient care, the improvement in outcomes could be profound indeed. This type of research and innovation right here in Tempe (ASU) demonstrates why ASU is ranked as the number one most innovative university in the nation.

"Industry analysts expect there will be three to four connected Internet of Things (IoT) devices for every person on the planet by 2020. Healthcare can and is leading the way in IoT adoption. To prepare for the coming deluge of IoT data, healthcare IT organizations should be investing in data analytics capability to convert that raw data flood into actionable information that delivers better healthcare outcomes."

—Steve Phillips
Senior Vice President and Chief Information Officer, Avnet, Inc.
Twitter: @Avnet

"I think it is really great that Jim Etchings is working on this; the dearth of information for dealing with large, complex biomedical data sets makes building systems capable of supporting precision medicine very challenging. I would say that we are not yet at the "blueprint" stage, but we certainly can use help in getting the right people thinking about this, so we can build the recipes going forward. While true clinical application at scale is still not here, we are rapidly approaching that event horizon, and as we have learned in biomedical research, the infrastructure challenges alone require careful planning and very deliberate applications of the proper technologies to deal with the vast amount of data that is generated. The algorithms to automate things such as true clinical decision guidance have yet to be written, and although some approaches such as neuro-linguistic programming or machine learning look promising, actually creating a "doc in a box" is probably many years off. This does not mean we should not be striving to move forward as rapidly as possible, because the impact that can be had on a patient's life is truly inspirational and that should always be remembered. This is not building systems to showcase technology or how smart we are, it is to help propel a truly world changing methodology of how medicine is practiced."

—James Lowey, CIO
TGen, The Translational Genomics Research Institute
Twitter: @loweyj, @Tgen

"The journey to precision medicine will require the confluence and analysis of enormous amounts of data from genomics, clinical and fundamental research, clinical care, and environmental and lifestyle data, including connected health data from the "Internet of Medical Things." The entire healthcare ecosystem needs to work together, along with the information and communications technology ecosystems, to collect, transport, analyze, and leverage the vast amount of data that can be honed to develop insights and recommendations for precision medicine. The opportunity to improve healthcare is compelling, the data is vast and will continue to grow, and we need to work together to realize improved outcomes. We need to build the technology and process-enabled capabilities to protect the data and the people. The need for increased TIPPSS—trust, identity, privacy, protection, safety, and security—mechanisms is critical to the success and safety in our ongoing healthcare journey."

—Florence D. Hudson
Senior Vice President and Chief Innovation Officer, Internet2
Twitter: @FloInternet2

"In the last decade, the wave of data coming off modern sequencing instruments is transforming bioscience into a digital science. Not only are the data sets enormous, the need to work through them quickly to have a real-time impact on therapy is crucial, requiring all of the elements of high-performance computing: fast compute, storage and networking, sophisticated data management, and highly parallel application codes.

The ability to quickly crunch massive amounts of disease and patient data is at the heart of precision medicine. While much of the promise of precision medicine is still on the horizon, advances have already led to life-saving treatments for children and adults with lethal cancers and genetic diseases. At the Center for Pediatric Genomic Medicine (CPGM) at Children's Mercy Hospital in Kansas City, MO, researchers used 25 hours of supercomputer time to decode the genetic variants of an infant suffering from liver failure. Thanks to the fast genomic diagnosis, doctors were able to proceed with the most effective treatment and the baby is alive and well."

—Tiffany Trader
Managing Editor, *HPCwire*

Strategies in Biomedical Data Science

Wiley & SAS Business Series

The Wiley & SAS Business Series presents books that help senior-level managers with their critical management decisions.

Titles in the Wiley & SAS Business Series include:

Analytics in a Big Data World: The Essential Guide to Data Science and Its Applications by Bart Baesens

Bank Fraud: Using Technology to Combat Losses by Revathi Subramanian

Big Data Analytics: Turning Big Data into Big Money by Frank Ohlhorst

Big Data, Big Innovation: Enabling Competitive Differentiation through Business Analytics by Evan Stubbs

Business Analytics for Customer Intelligence by Gert Laursen

Business Intelligence Applied: Implementing an Effective Information and Communications Technology Infrastructure by Michael Gendron

Business Intelligence and the Cloud: Strategic Implementation Guide by Michael S. Gendron

Business Transformation: A Roadmap for Maximizing Organizational Insights by Aiman Zeid

Connecting Organizational Silos: Taking Knowledge Flow Management to the Next Level with Social Media by Frank Leistner

Data-Driven Healthcare: How Analytics and BI Are Transforming the Industry by Laura Madsen

Delivering Business Analytics: Practical Guidelines for Best Practice by Evan Stubbs

Demand-Driven Forecasting: A Structured Approach to Forecasting, Second Edition by Charles Chase

Demand-Driven Inventory Optimization and Replenishment: Creating a More Efficient Supply Chain by Robert A. Davis

Developing Human Capital: Using Analytics to Plan and Optimize Your Learning and Development Investments by Gene Pease, Barbara Beresford, and Lew Walker

Economic and Business Forecasting: Analyzing and Interpreting Econometric Results by John Silvia, Azhar Iqbal, Kaylyn Swankoski, Sarah Watt, and Sam Bullard

Foreign Currency Financial Reporting from Euros to Yen to Yuan: A Guide to Fundamental Concepts and Practical Applications by Robert Rowan

Harness Oil and Gas Big Data with Analytics: Optimize Exploration and Production with Data Driven Models by Keith Holdaway

Health Analytics: Gaining the Insights to Transform Health Care by Jason Burke

Heuristics in Analytics: A Practical Perspective of What Influences Our Analytical World by Carlos Andre Reis Pinheiro and Fiona McNeill

Human Capital Analytics: How to Harness the Potential of Your Organization's Greatest Asset by Gene Pease, Boyce Byerly, and Jac Fitz-enz

Implement, Improve and Expand Your Statewide Longitudinal Data System: Creating a Culture of Data in Education by Jamie McQuiggan and Armistead Sapp

Killer Analytics: Top 20 Metrics Missing from Your Balance Sheet by Mark Brown

Predictive Analytics for Human Resources by Jac Fitz-enz and John Mattox II

Predictive Business Analytics: Forward-Looking Capabilities to Improve Business Performance by Lawrence Maisel and Gary Cokins

Retail Analytics: The Secret Weapon by Emmett Cox

Social Network Analysis in Telecommunications by Carlos Andre Reis Pinheiro

Statistical Thinking: Improving Business Performance, Second Edition by Roger W. Hoerl and Ronald D. Snee

Style and Statistics: The Art of Retail Analytics by Brittany Bullard

Taming the Big Data Tidal Wave: Finding Opportunities in Huge Data Streams with Advanced Analytics by Bill Franks

The Analytic Hospitality Executive: Implementing Data Analytics in Hotels and Casinos by Kelly A. McGuire

The Executive's Guide to Enterprise Social Media Strategy: How Social Networks Are Radically Transforming Your Business by David Thomas and Mike Barlow

The Value of Business Analytics: Identifying the Path to Profitability by Evan Stubbs

The Visual Organization: Data Visualization, Big Data, and the Quest for Better Decisions by Phil Simon

Too Big to Ignore: The Business Case for Big Data by Phil Simon

Using Big Data Analytics: Turning Big Data into Big Money by Jared Dean

Win with Advanced Business Analytics: Creating Business Value from Your Data by Jean Paul Isson and Jesse Harriott

For more information on any of the above titles, please visit www.wiley.com.

Strategies in Biomedical Data Science

Driving Force for Innovation

Jay Etchings

WILEY

Cover image: DNA strand © Don Bishop/Getty Images, Inc.
Cover design: Wiley

Published by John Wiley & Sons, Inc., Hoboken, New Jersey.

Published simultaneously in Canada.

Library of Congress Cataloging-in-Publication Data:

Names: Etchings, Jay, 1966– author. | SAS Institute, issuing body.
Title: Strategies in biomedical data science : driving force for innovation / Jay Etchings.
Other titles: Wiley and SAS business series.
Description: Hoboken, New Jersey : John Wiley & Sons, Inc., [2017] | Series: Wiley & SAS business series | Includes bibliographical references and index.
Identifiers: LCCN 2016036794 (print) | LCCN 2016037346 (ebook) | ISBN 978-1-119-23219-3 (hardcover) | ISBN 978-1-119-25597-0 (ePub) | ISBN 978-1-119-25618-2 (ePDF)
Subjects: | MESH: Medical Informatics | Computational Biology—methods | Cybernetics—methods
Classification: LCC R859.7.A78 (print) | LCC R859.7.A78 (ebook) | NLM W 26.5 | DDC 610.285—dc23
LC record available at https://lccn.loc.gov/2016036794

Printed in the United States of America

10 9 8 7 6 5 4 3

Contents

Foreword xi

Acknowledgments xv

Introduction 1
- Who Should Read This Book? 3
- What's in This Book? 4
- How to Contact Us 6

Chapter 1 Healthcare, History, and Heartbreak 7
- Top Issues in Healthcare 9
- Data Management 16
- Biosimilars, Drug Pricing, and Pharmaceutical Compounding 18
- Promising Areas of Innovation 19
- Conclusion 25
- Notes 25

Chapter 2 Genome Sequencing: Know Thyself, One Base Pair at a Time 27

Content contributed by Sheetal Shetty and Jacob Brill
- Challenges of Genomic Analysis 29
- The Language of Life 30
- A Brief History of DNA Sequencing 31
- DNA Sequencing and the Human Genome Project 35
- Select Tools for Genomic Analysis 38
- Conclusion 47
- Notes 48

Chapter 3 Data Management 53

Content contributed by Joe Arnold
- Bits about Data 54
- Data Types 56
- Data Security and Compliance 59
- Data Storage 66
- SwiftStack 70
- OpenStack Swift Architecture 78
- Conclusion 94
- Notes 94

Chapter 4 Designing a Data-Ready Network Infrastructure 105
Research Networks: A Primer 108
ESnet at 30: Evolving toward Exascale and Raising Expectations 109
Internet2 Innovation Platform 111
Advances in Networking 113
InfiniBand and Microsecond Latency 114
The Future of High-Performance Fabrics 117
Network Function Virtualization 119
Software-Defined Networking 121
OpenDaylight 122
Conclusion 157
Notes 157

Chapter 5 Data-Intensive Compute Infrastructures 163
Content contributed by Dijiang Huang, Yuli Deng, Jay Etchings, Zhiyuan Ma, and Guangchun Luo
Big Data Applications in Health Informatics 166
Sources of Big Data in Health Informatics 168
Infrastructure for Big Data Analytics 171
Fundamental System Properties 186
GPU-Accelerated Computing and Biomedical Informatics 187
Conclusion 190
Notes 191

Chapter 6 Cloud Computing and Emerging Architectures 211
Cloud Basics 213
Challenges Facing Cloud Computing Applications in Biomedicine 215
Hybrid Campus Clouds 216
Research as a Service 217
Federated Access Web Portals 219
Cluster Homogeneity 220
Emerging Architectures (Zeta Architecture) 221
Conclusion 229
Notes 229

Chapter 7 Data Science 235
NoSQL Approaches to Biomedical Data Science 237
Using Splunk for Data Analytics 244
Statistical Analysis of Genomic Data with Hadoop 250
Extracting and Transforming Genomic Data 253
Processing eQTL Data 256
Generating Master SNP Files for Cases and Controls 259
Generating Gene Expression Files for Cases and Controls 260
Cleaning Raw Data Using MapReduce 261
Transpose Data Using Python 263
Statistical Analysis Using Spark 264
Hive Tables with Partitions 268
Conclusion 270
Notes 270

Appendix: A Brief Statistics Primer 290
Content Contributed by Daniel Peñaherrera

Chapter 8 Next-Generation Cyberinfrastructures 307
Next-Generation Cyber Capability 308
NGCC Design and Infrastructure 310
Conclusion 327
Note 330

Conclusion 335

Appendix A The Research Data Management Survey: From Concepts to Practice 337
Brandon Mikkelsen and Jay Etchings

Appendix B Central IT and Research Support 353
Gregory D. Palmer

Appendix C HPC Working Example: Using Parallelization Programs Such as GNU Parallel and OpenMP with Serial Tools 377

Appendix D HPC and Hadoop: Bridging HPC to Hadoop 385

Appendix E Bioinformatics + Docker: Simplifying Bioinformatics Tools Delivery with Docker Containers 391

Glossary 399

About the Author 419

About the Contributors 421

Index 427

Foreword

The emergence of data science is radically transforming the biomedical knowledge generation paradigm. While modern biomedicine has been a pioneer in evidence-based science, its approach for decades has largely followed a well-worn path of experimental design, data collection, analysis, and interpretation. Data science introduces an alternative pathway—one that starts with the vast collections of diverse digital data increasingly accessible to the community.

While the data science evidence generation concept has many birth parents, Jim Gray of Microsoft best described the unique opportunity afforded by this new paradigm. In a 2007 address to the U.S. National Research Council, Gray argued: "With an exaflood of unexamined data and teraflops of cheap computing power, we should be able to make many valuable discoveries simply by searching all that information for unexpected patterns" [1]. Gray coined the phrase "data-intensive scientific discovery." Notably, he broke with the high-performance computing "high priests" and advocated the adoption of new models of computing. Following Gray's untimely death shortly after his address, his colleagues captured this concept in a collection of essays ultimately published as *The Fourth Paradigm: Data-Intensive Scientific Discovery* [2]. It was within these essays that the term "big data" was introduced.

"Data science" and "big data" are now overburdened terms with many meanings. The most useful definitions are operational in nature. One of the most colorful comes from John Myles of Facebook, who indicates that big data is any problem "so large that traditional approaches to data analysis are doomed to failure" [3]. I find the definition of the chief architect of Data.gov, Philip Ashlock, most elucidating: "Analysis that can help you find patterns, anomalies, or new structures amidst otherwise chaotic or complex data points" [3].

Data science remains controversial in biomedicine. Jeff Drazen, the editor in chief of the *New England Journal of Medicine*, has described data science practitioners as "research parasites" [4]. More subtly, Robert Weinberg openly questions whether such approaches have any potential to generate real insight in his article describing an emerging crisis in understanding cancer, "Coming Full Circle—From Endless Complexity to Simplicity and Back Again" [5].

I have been an eyewitness and co-conspirator in the data science transformation occurring in biomedicine. I grew up with the Human Genome Project and the rapid accumulation of large volumes of big data it generates. I have made contributions through the "Discovery Science" paradigm that the Genome Project made acceptable in biomedicine. For example, with my colleagues at the Cooperative Human Linkage Center, we were early adopters of computational science and the Internet (then NSFnet) in our efforts to construct the map of human inheritance [6]. For us at the time, big data topped out at a gigabyte! While serving as the founding director of the National Institutes of Health's National Cancer Institute's Center for Biomedical Informatics and Information Technology, I was tasked with helping bring data science to the cancer community. The charge was broad—including basic science, clinical research, and health encounter data. It was technologically challenging—predating many technology paradigms now taken for granted as standard in data science. Through these pioneering efforts, I experienced the aforementioned controversial nature of data science and the second of Arthur C. Clarke's laws: "The only way of discovering the limits of the possible is to venture a little way past them into the impossible" [7].

Strategies in Biomedical Data Science is an ambitious attempt to look at "the limits of the possible" for data science in biomedicine. Unique in its scope, it takes a comprehensive look at all aspects of data science. Work in the sciences is routinely compartmentalized and segregated among specialists. This segregation is particularly true in biomedicine as it wrestles with the integration of data science and its underpinning in information technology. While such specialization is essential for progress within disciplines, the failure to have cross-cutting discussions results in lost opportunities. This book is significant in that it purposely embraces the "transdisciplinary" nature of biomedical data science. Transdisciplinary research (a foundational aspect of Arizona State University's "New American University") brings together different disciplines to create innovations that are beyond the capacity of any single specialty. Data science is definitionally transdisciplinary and somewhat ironically is discipline-agnostic.

Strategies in Biomedical Data Science unapologetically mixes biology, analytics, and information technology. Its transdisciplinary topics cover diverse data types—genomic, clinical encounter, personal monitoring devices—and the data science opportunities (and challenges) in each. Within each of these topics, it provides insights into the software capabilities that are used to wrangle Gray's "exaflood" of data and to find his "unexpected patterns." It provides insightful discussions of the underpinning computational and network infrastructure necessary to realize the potential of data science. More specifically, it provides practical blueprints that translate Gray's suggested alternative to traditional high-performance computing paradigms into reality. Within each of these, it provides case studies written by experts that transition the topics from concept to real-world examples. Importantly, these case studies are provided by both academics and industry sources, demonstrating the importance of both to the biomedical data science progress as well as the need to blend these often-adversarial communities.

I have had the opportunity to know the author, Jay Etchings, for over three years. Jay is a true computational renaissance man, as reflected in the breadth of topics facilely presented in *Strategies in Biomedical Data Science*. I was first introduced to Jay when he was an architect for Dell. Jay translated ASU's vision for a first-generation, purpose-built data science research platform into the operational Next Generation Cyber Capability (NGCC) described in the book. The NGCC is a physical instantiation of what Gray envisioned. Now at ASU as the director of Research Computing Operations, Jay and his team deliver biomedical data science to a diverse collection of international scientists.

Jay brings a fresh perspective and a diverse pedigree of work experiences to biomedical data science. He has been at the forefront of developing and deploying big data capabilities throughout his career. For example, Jay was on the leading edge in bringing big data infrastructure to the gaming industry—a community that is always an early adopter of breakthrough technology. Jay has hands-on experience in the complexities of biomedical data from his efforts to provide support for the Centers for Medicare and Medicaid Services. Jay's commercial background brings with it a can-do approach to problems and a low tolerance for the arcane consternation that often paralyzes academics. This fresh perspective and his enthusiasm for biomedicine pervade his writing. *Strategies in Biomedical Data Science* is a one-stop shop of data science essentials and is likely to serve as the go-to resource for years to come.

Ken Buetow, Ph.D.,
Professor, Arizona State University
Director, Computational Science and Informatics Core Program
Director, Complex Adaptive Systems Initiative

NOTES

1. David Snyder. 2016. "The Big Picture of Big Data—IEEE—The Institute." http://theinstitute.ieee.org/ieee-roundup/members/achievements/the-big-picture-of-big-data.
2. Anthony J. G. Hey, ed. 2009. *The Fourth Paradigm: Data-Intensive Scientific Discovery*. Redmond, WA: Microsoft Research.
3. Jennifer Dutcher. 2014. "What Is Big Data?" September 3. https://datascience.berkeley.edu/what-is-big-data/.
4. Dan L. Longo and Jeffrey M. Drazen. 2016. "Data Sharing." *New England Journal of Medicine* 374, no. 3: 276–277. doi: 10.1056/NEJMe1516564.
5. Robert A. Weinberg. 2014. "Coming Full Circle—From Endless Complexity to Simplicity and Back Again." *Cell* 157 (1): 267–71. doi: 10.1016/j.cell.2014.03.004.
6. J. C. Murray, K. H. Buetow, J. L. Weber, S. Ludwigsen, T. Scherpbier-Heddema, F. Manion, et al. 1994. "A Comprehensive Human Linkage Map with Centimorgan Density. Cooperative Human Linkage Center (CHLC)." *Science* 265, no. 5181: 2049–2054.
7. Arthur C. Clarke. 1962. "Hazards of Prophecy: The Failure of Imagination" In *Profiles of the Future: An Inquiry into the Limits of the Possible*. New York: Harper & Row.

Acknowledgments

Most broadly, this book has been inspired by the need for a collaborative and multidisciplinary approach to solving the intricate puzzle that is cancer. Cancer poses a complex adaptive challenge that reaches across all domains: medicine, biology, technology, and the social sciences. Transdisciplinary collaboration is the only true path to the future. Ubiquitous research computing in support of "open science" and open big data has an essential role to play in this collaborative process.

More specifically, this book is dedicated to Sue Stigler and the family she leaves behind. Her three-and-a-half-year battle with cancer came to a close on December 7, 2015. Sue's kindness and devotion, and her endless support for others even while ill, were remarkable; her selflessness will always be remembered. If you would like to donate to the Stigler family college fund, please visit their GoFundMe page, https://www.gofundme.com/bpebavas.

Author proceeds support childhood brain cancer research through an ASU Foundation account supporting Dr. Joshua LaBaer's work in the Biodesign Institute. Dr LaBaer is conducting cutting-edge research on pediatric low-grade astrocytomas (PLGAs), which are the most common cancers of the brain in children.

In the research and discovery leading to this book, I have worked with more amazing and committed individuals than I could have ever imagined. My mentor and friend Ken Buetow is fond of saying, "If you're the smartest person in the room, you are in the wrong room." Time and again I have been in the right room. I am able to count some of the smartest people on the planet as colleagues and friends. Publication of this book was made a reality by their support and example.

A very special thanks to my good friend Phil Simon for convincing me to put thoughts, concepts, and theory on paper and share it with the world.

At Arizona State University I would like to thank Gordon Wishon, Dr. Elizabeth Cantwell, and Dr. Sethuraman Panchanathan ("Panch") for giving me the opportunity to drive innovation at the university.

I would also like to recognize the dedication of our Research Computing team at Arizona State University for the continued commitment to our "commander's intent" and to Christopher Myhill for sharing the commander's intent with me while at Dell Enterprise.

Tremendous thanks to the teamwork of Jon McNally, Johnathan "Jr." Lee, Lee Reynolds, Ram Polur, Daniel Penaherrera, Sheetal Shetty, James Napier, Tiffany Marin, Deborah Whitten, Curtis Thompson, Srinivasa Mathkur, Marisa

Brazil, and of course Carol Schumacher, arguably the best administrative assistant alive. Special thanks also to Wendy "DigDug" Cegielski for her editing hours and continued motivation; next year you will be Dr. Wendy.

In no specific order I also would like to thank this list of super-smart and generous folks as well as our many terrific and invaluable partners: NimbleStorage, Brocade, Internet2, ESNET, Penguin Computing, TGEN, SwiftStack, MarkLogic, the Open Daylight Foundation, the Linux Foundation, Open Networking Foundation, IT Partners, friends at University of Arizona, Northern Arizona University, Dell Enterprise, University of Massachusetts-Lowell, Baylor University, Washington State University, Georgia Tech, Broad Institute of MIT and Harvard, University of Nevada Las Vegas, and the College of Southern Nevada (formally CCSN), and thanks for the support and mentorship from domain professionals both public and private like Mark "Pup" Roberts, Brandon Mikkelsen, Sean Dudley, Joel Dudley, James Lowey, Todd Decker, Jeff Creighton, Jim Scott, Gregory Palmer, Neela Jacques, Al Ritacco, and of course my engineer stepbrother Pedro Victor Gomes.

Last but certainly not least, I would like to recognize my awesome team of Jacob, Dixon, and Annika for their enduring patience throughout the never-ending collecting of the data and experience that comprises this text.

Heather, though you have departed from my arms, there is always a place for you in my heart.

Introduction

Never let the future disturb you.

You will meet it, if you have to, with the same weapons of reason which today arm you against the present.

—Marcus Aurelius

Some time ago, while I was engaged as a consultant, it became painfully obvious that the approaches to healthcare data management and overall infrastructure architecture were stuck in the Stone Age. While data and information technology (IT) professionals sprinted to remain on the cutting edge of top tech trends, much of the healthcare system remained a technical backwater. The many explanations for this include compliance controls, challenges associated with the rapid proliferation of data, and reliance on old systems with proprietary code where porting was more painful than the day-to-day operations. This state of affairs has been frustrating for all involved. But beyond the very real frustrations, there are far more important negative impacts. Technical inefficiencies increase costs, lead to a loss of research productivity, and hurt clinical outcomes. In other words, everyone suffers. When I talk to people about data management and IT support within the healthcare field, a recurring theme is that much is "lost in translation" between the various stakeholders: IT professionals, researchers, doctors, clinicians, and administrators.

Over the past 20 years, much of my time has been spent in medical and technical fields. I have held positions with two large insurance payer providers and have worked with the Centers for Medicare & Medicaid Services (CMS) as a recovery audit contractor. I have even worked clinically as an emergency medical technician with a strong background in exercise physiology. Seeking greater challenges led me to Las Vegas, Nevada, where I was fortunate to work on the first cloud-enabled centrally deterministic (Class 2) gaming systems for the state lottery. This was well before the term "cloud" had even arrived. At the close of the project, I returned to the medical field, joining a Fortune 50 payer provider ingesting targeted acquisitions.

My wide-ranging work experiences have showed me that medical and research professionals are usually not technology experts, and most do not desire to be. At the same time, computer scientists and infrastructure experts are not biologists, doctors, or researchers. This longtime disconnect paves the way for high-paid consultants to act as intermediaries brought in to work between IT and biomedical staff.

Not surprisingly, this does not work terribly well, neither does it best serve the medical and research communities. Consultants typically demand high compensation and often are not able to perform the sort of knowledge transfer necessary to make a meaningful and sustainable impact. There are many different permutations and possible explanations for this. But, in the end, I think it is at heart a failure to adequately translate or bridge biomedicine and IT.

The primary motivation for this book is to begin to create a sustainable and readily accessible bridge between IT and data technologists, on one hand, and the community of clinicians, researchers, and academics who deliver and advance healthcare, on the other hand. This book is thus a translational text that will hopefully work both ways. It can help IT staff learn more about clinical and research needs within biomedicine. It also can help doctors and researchers learn more about data and other technical tools that are potentially at their disposal.

My experience in healthcare has shown me that both IT professionals and biologists tend to become isolated or siloed in their professional worlds. This isolation hurts us all: IT staff, biologists, doctors, and patients alike. This is not to suggest that IT staff and data managers should get master's degrees in biology or epidemiology. Rather, I am suggesting that as IT staff and data managers learn more about the biomedical context of their work, they will be able to work better and more efficiently. Furthermore, as biomedicine becomes ever more dependent on computing and big data, there is more and more domain-specific technical knowledge to assimilate.

As IT and biomedicine innovate with increasing rapidity, I predict that we will see more and more hybrid job titles, such as health technologist and bioinformatician. In order to stay current, both IT professionals and biomedical professionals will need to become less isolated. This book begins to bring together these two fields that are so dependent on each other and have so much to offer each other. It is my sincere hope that this work will narrow the gap between those engaged in use-inspired research and those supporting that research from an infrastructure delivery perspective.

In the interest of creating as accessible a bridge text as possible between IT staff and biomedical personnel, this book is relatively nontechnical. For the most part, the aim is to offer a conceptual introduction to key topics in data management for the biomedical sciences. While a certain familiarity with IT, networking, and applications is assumed, you will find very little in the way of code examples. The goal is to equip you with some foundational concepts that will leave you prepared to seek out whatever additional information you and your institution might need.

I have worked in IT for over 20 years, but I am most inspired by how computing technologies can be used to solve human problems. I certainly appreciate elegant code and innovative technical solutions. But at the end of the day, it is the prospect of improving patient outcomes that keeps me engaged and driven to learn and continually extend the boundaries of the possible. One area of biomedical research that I find particularly inspiring is the potential to use targeted therapies to more effectively treat pediatric low-grade astrocytomas (PLGAs). PLGAs are by far the most common cancer of the brain among children. They are often fatal, and current chemotherapies frequently have lifelong side effects, including neurocognitive impairment. Dr. Joshua LaBaer, interim director of the Biodesign Institute at Arizona State University, is working to develop effective targeted therapies that reduce harmful effects on normal cells. Proceeds from this book support the ASU Research Foundation and the work of Dr. Joshua LaBaer, Director, The Biodesign Institute, Personalized Diagnostics and Virginia G. Piper Chair in Personalized Medicine.

In reflecting on the important roles to be played by humans and by computing, I am reminded of a frequently cited quote by Leo M. Cherne, an American economist and public servant, that is often inaccurately attributed to Albert Einstein: "The computer is incredibly fast, accurate, and stupid. Man is unbelievably slow, inaccurate, and brilliant. The marriage of the two is a force beyond calculation." As our capabilities to gather, analyze, and archive data dramatically improve, computing is likely to be increasingly valuable to biomedical research and clinical medicine. Yet let us always remember the need for humans, slow and inaccurate as we usually are.

WHO SHOULD READ THIS BOOK?

Strategies in Biomedical Data Science is designed to help anyone who works with biomedical data. This certainly includes IT staff and systems administrators. These readers will hopefully gain a deeper understanding of particular challenges and solutions for biomedical data management. The target audience also includes bioscience researchers and clinical staff. While persons in these roles are not typically directly responsible for data management, they are most certainly concerned with and affected by how data is created, used, and archived. I hope these readers will gain a deeper understanding of how IT staff tend to approach systems architecture and data management. Quite frequently we focus on research academic and other public research institutions. Such institutions are tremendously important for cutting-edge research and collaboration. Most of the best practices and scenarios presented in the book are, however, equally applicable to private-sector use cases.

All readers are welcome to work through this book in whatever order best suits their particular interests and needs.

WHAT'S IN THIS BOOK?

Strategies in Biomedical Data Science offers a relatively high-level introduction to the cutting-edge and rapidly changing field of biomedical data. It provides biomedical IT professionals with much-needed guidance toward managing the increasing deluge of healthcare data. This book demonstrates ways in which both technological development and more effective use of current resources can better serve both patient and payer. The discussion explores the aggregation of disparate data sources, current analytics and tool sets, the growing necessity of smart bioinformatics, and more as data science and biomedical science grow increasingly intertwined. Real-world use cases and clear examples are featured throughout, and coverage of data sources, problems, and potential mitigation provides necessary insight for forward-looking healthcare professionals.

The book begins with an overview of current technical challenges in healthcare and then moves into topics in biomedical data management, including network infrastructure, compute infrastructure, cloud architecture, and finally next-generation cyberinfrastructures.

Many of the chapters include use cases and/or case studies. Use cases examine a general use case and typically focus on one application or technology. Case studies are more particular examinations of how a company or institution has used an application or technology to meet an operational need. One of our objectives is to shine a light into the black box that is the emerging realm of precision medicine. Much of the case study data has been compiled over the past few years and has been updated to include as much current data as available. Please be aware that some case study materials have been anonymized at the request of the institution providing the information. Case studies appear after chapters, while use cases are presented within the chapters.

Strategies in Biomedical Data Science has benefited tremendously from the many wonderful experts who have generously contributed content. Contributors are acknowledged throughout the book, alongside their contributions, and you can find their biographies in the "About the Contributors" section.

Chapter 1, "Healthcare, History, and Heartbreak," examines some of the current top issues in healthcare that pertain to data and IT. There are great challenges but also tremendous opportunities for innovation in IT and data science. Chapter 1 also presents some promising areas for innovation, including the Internet of Things, cloud computing, and dramatic advances in data storage. Chapter 2, "Genome Sequencing," recaps the remarkable history of how scientists deciphered the central dogma, the deceptively simple model that explains the molecular basis of biological life. We then review the history of genomic sequencing from its origins to next-generation sequencing (NGS) and recount its startling price drop. Perhaps most important, we survey some common genomics tools and resources for analyzing and working with genomics data in silico. Following this chapter you will find a case study presenting a dramatic example of exome sequencing leading to clinical diagnosis.

Chapter 3, "Data Management," explores challenges and solutions for managing large quantities of biomedical data. The chapter begins with an overview of different types of data and moves on to issues of security and compliance in biomedical research. We offer a general research data life cycle to help you plan and anticipate potential problems. Particular storage technologies covered include iRODS, OpenStack Swift, SwiftStack, and NimbleStorage, a performance storage array. Following this chapter you will find three case studies. The first considers the data demands of genetic sequencing. The second offers specification for HudsonAlpha's SwiftStack storage cluster. The third focuses on the use of NimbleStorage's predictive flash storage at ASU.

Chapter 4, "Designing a Data-Ready Network Infrastructure," offers a brief history of computer networking before examining research networks and some advances in networking. We also share a model that can be used to deliver secure and regulated data storage and services so that institutions can comply with security standards. Networking advances discussed include InfiniBand, a computer-networking communications standard used in high-performance computing, which features very high throughput and very low latency; network function virtualization (NFV); and software-defined networking (SDN). The bulk of this chapter is a detailed guide to OpenDaylight, an open source SDN platform.

Chapter 5, "Data-Intensive Compute Infrastructures," is all about big data. It starts with a brief survey of the current state of big data efforts in healthcare and biomedicine. We consider big data applications as well as data sources. From there we dive into infrastructure for big data analytics, first examining service-oriented architecture and cloud computing. We then focus on hierarchical system structures and discuss the following layers: sensing, data storage and management, data computing and application services, and application services. We end by presenting graphics processing unit (GPU) accelerated computing. Following the chapter you will find two case studies. The first reports on how computational modeling and scientific computing can model treatment options for vascular disease. The second presents how GPU was used to model the molecular dynamics of antibiotic resistance.

Chapter 6, "Cloud Computing and Emerging Architectures," begins with an overview of cloud computing, including service and deployment models as well as challenges. After this we examine Research as a Service (RaaS) and cluster homogeneity, key components of some versions of cloud computing, and we also consider federated access. The second half of the chapter dives into Zeta Architecture, an emergent architecture that is used by Google and that offers better hardware utilization, fewer moving parts, and greater responsiveness and flexibility. Zeta and other emerging architectures are catalyzed by limitations on one-size-fits-all enterprise architectures. Following this chapter is a case study on using on-demand computing for biomedical research on ventricular tachycardia.

Chapter 7, "Data Science," focuses on the tools and techniques demanded by this exciting and rapidly growing field. First we examine some basic statistical concepts as these are the foundation of much data science. From there we explore some NoSQL database offerings and Splunk, and offer a detailed example of genomic analysis (eQTL), which entails Apache Spark and Hive tables. Following this chapter you will find two case studies: one on UC Irvine Health's Hortonworks Data Platform and the second on subclonal variations and the computing and data science strategies used to study these.

Chapter 8, "Next-Generation Cyberinfrastructures," brings together many of the central strands of this book. It reports on the Next-Generation Cyber Capability (NGCC), which is Arizona State University's approach to meeting compute and data needs for its research community and key collaborators. Following this chapter is a case study on one of the first NGCC projects, the National Biomarker Development Alliance.

A brief conclusion reviews the book's goals and invites feedback and suggestions.

In addition to the case studies, *Strategies in Biomedical Data Science* contains five appendixes and a glossary.

Appendix A reports on a survey about research management. Appendix B reports on a survey about the current state and desired capabilities for IT resources at research universities. Appendix C offers some high-performance computing working examples. Appendix D details how to bridge high-performance computing to Hadoop. Finally, Appendix E discusses using Docker for bioinformatics.

Thanks for reading!

Should this book inspire the reader to dig deeper into research computing or the research itself, we will consider it a win. If you find this book to be of little value, please leave it on your next flight, bus ride, or at a homeless shelter for some other reader to find and take to their next job interview.

HOW TO CONTACT US

As you use this book and work with biomedical data, we welcome your comments and feedback. In the hybrid and rapidly evolving field of biomedical data, collaboration and exchange are truly essential. We hope there will be a second edition of this book, and I would value comments and feedback to help improve this material.

You can reach Jay at Jay@JayEtchings.com or Jay.Etchings@asu.edu.

CHAPTER 1

Healthcare, History, and Heartbreak

Over the past decade, we have unlocked many of the mysteries about DNA and RNA. This knowledge isn't just sitting in books on the shelf nor is it confined to the workbenches of laboratories. We have used these research findings to pinpoint the causes of many diseases. Moreover, scientists have translated this genetic knowledge into several treatments and therapies prompting a bridge between the laboratory bench and the patient's bedside.

—Barack Obama on the Genomics and Personalized Medicine Act (S. 976), March 23, 2007

While we are surely poised to continue to make tremendous medical advances—notably in personalized medicine, pharmacogenomics, and precision medicine—we are also facing substantial challenges. The challenges facing healthcare today are many, and if we do not adequately address them we risk missing opportunities, pushing the cost of care up, and slowing the pace of biomedical innovation. In briefly surveying the state of healthcare, it is not my intention to offer a political diagnosis or solution. Rather, it is my intention to use our current technical knowledge to point the way to practical solutions. For example, a long-theorized solution to health records management would be a single cloud-based system where healthcare information sharing exists universally. But if I were to present this as the best technical solution, it would not be my intention to also advocate for a shift to a single-payer healthcare system. As much as possible this book and the discussions in this chapter aim to avoid politics.

After decades of technological lag, biomedicine has started to embrace new technologies with increasing rapidity. Next-generation sequencing, mobile technologies, wearable sensors, three-dimensional medical imaging, and advances in analytic software now make it possible to capture vast amounts of information. Yet we still struggle with the collection, management, security, and thoughtful interpretation of all this information. At the same time, healthcare is changing quickly as the field grapples with new technologies and is transformed by mergers and new partnerships. As a complex adaptive system, healthcare is more than the sum of its parts, and it is always difficult to predict the future. But we do know that as the post–Affordable Care Act healthcare landscape takes shape, the industry is shifting toward digitally enabled, consumer-focused care models. Given these trends, technology will be granted many opportunities to improve patient care.

At the outset of this book it is worth surveying some of the top issues in healthcare. For many of you, these will be quite familiar. Whether you're an expert or not, you should feel free to skip ahead if you like. But it is my sincere hope that the background material will be of real value in bridging the gap between healthcare and biomedicine, on the one hand, and information technology (IT) and data management, on the other. Just as doctors in an age of increasing specialization can benefit from attending to the whole patient, it is very valuable for IT staff to have a more holistic and systemic understanding of healthcare.

TOP ISSUES IN HEALTHCARE

There are many, many sources that comment on the state of healthcare and biomedicine more broadly. Although I worked as a contractor for two of the country's largest Medicare/Medicaid contract holders, I am not a policy expert. But I have come to appreciate the importance of taking in the bigger picture. My admittedly incomplete survey of top healthcare issues is drawn from PwC's *Top Health Industry Issues of 2016* and PwC's *Top Health Industry Issues of 2015* [1]. These two brief reports offer compelling syntheses and analyses of current trends. In rereading these reports and reflecting on my own experiences in the field, I was struck by the number of top issues that are substantially or in part data or IT issues. Many of the top healthcare issues are centrally concerned with the storage, security, sharing, and analysis of data. In other words, IT and data management will be called on to make major contributions to advancing the dynamic healthcare field. Next I explore nine key issues impacting healthcare.

Mergers and Partnerships

As the health sector continues to change in response to the Affordable Care Act (2010), we are seeing many mergers and partnerships. "The ACA's emphasis on value and outcomes has sent ripples through the $3.2 trillion health sector, spreading and shifting risk in its wake. At the same time, capital is inexpensive, thanks to sustained low interest rates. Industry's response? Go big" [2]. Mergers between large insurance providers are consolidating the insurance market. In 2015, the second largest U.S. insurer, Anthem, made a $48.4 billion offer for health and life insurance provider Cigna. Mergers have also been common in the pharmaceutical field, including Pfizer's whopping $160 billion deal for specialty pharmaceutical star Allergan. While these deals are still awaiting regulatory approval, 2016 and 2017 will likely see more mergers and acquisitions. Many new partnerships are also being formed between pharmaceutical, life sciences, software, pharmacy, healthcare providers, and engineering companies, among others.

Mergers, acquisitions, and partnerships are driven by a number of larger market forces. Sometimes predicted lower IT or data costs drive consolidation. More often it is simply that IT and data will need to be able to respond nimbly to these changes. One of the largest challenges is postacquisition data management.

Many providers in the healthcare space have grown through organic means and have survived on shoestring budgets. When compliance moved to the forefront, many chief information officers were granted grace periods to meet compliance and conducted internal audits, patching together existing components to meet the objectives. This expenditure had the systemic impact of preventing the distribution of funds toward infrastructure improvements. The maintenance of many legacy systems resulted, leaving organizations with out-of-date, proprietary, inflexible systems that were simply not designed to interoperate on the larger scale. Now when that smaller provider, which potentially maintains a large collection of Medicare/Medicaid accounts, is acquired by a larger entity, the most significant challenge is the integration of those legacy systems without impacting operational activities. The challenge of migrating years of patient data records into a system from an out-of-date platform encumbered by complex and tangled spaghetti code and created by a resource long since departed is substantial. The need to do so while maintaining business continuity drives many a large entity to maintain the down-level system for years following the acquisition.

Cybersecurity and Data Security

As more and more patient data is stored and shared, security is an increasing concern. Patient data typically contains individualized information. If that data is stolen, the risks of identity theft are substantial, and there exists a thriving black market for stolen health records. Data security breaches are relatively common. "During the summer of 2014, more than 5 million patients had their personal data compromised" [1]. These breaches are often costly for companies. Medical devices themselves can also be hacked. For example, in 2015 the government warned that "an infusion pump . . . could be modified to deliver a fatal dose of medication" [2].

The needs for elastic scalability, rapid provisioning, resource orchestration, high availability, and storage efficiency have contributed to the explosion in cloud providers and niche service offerings. However, this explosion has also opened holes in known security elements that were once sealed. Cloud security challenges can range from the innocuous VM sprawl, where virtual machines are orphaned in an on/off state and fall outside of the domain security policy for things as basic as patching and maintenance [3]. On the other end of the spectrum there would be virtualization hacking, where an adversary gains access to a host (a larger component [server] that houses multiple guests). Hypervisors or virtual machine monitors (VMMs) have been hardened over the years; however, they are only as fortified as their caretakers determine. One key determinant is the organizational structure or culture. A company that owned 100 bare-metal servers in a medium-size data center may have had 10 employees assigned to manage the environment and provide operational support. With the advent of virtualization, workforce reductions have taken place and the distribution ratio of humans to servers has changed. Between 1991 and 2006, a ratio of 1:100 was typical for a large company that provided operational support like a web hosting company [4]. These numbers do not include application specialists and development staff. In today's cloud and highly virtualized environments you could see 1:1,000 ratio of humans (admins) to guest (virtual machines/computers). Efficient providers like Rackspace.com and GoDaddy.com may have 10 to 20 times that ratio [5, 6].

A key component that supports that exponential ratio is robust resource orchestration, which supplies the common ecosystem bits such as backups, network routing, addressing, domain name space management, and availability. Years ago these elements had unique humans as designees owning the responsibility.

Now we can understand how an environment could grow organically, leading to VM sprawl that opens up security gaps. What can be done with orphaned guests long since forgotten by their caretakers?

Adversaries compromise vulnerable virtual machines and enlist armies of botnets or zombie computers assigned to unified tasks [7]. The best-known tasks are distributed denial-of-service (DDoS) attacks aimed at larger public targets, like universities or public businesses. Such large-scale attacks were described in the 11th Annual Worldwide Infrastructure Security Report [8]. Let us also remember that small-scale orphans, like zombies, can still make efficient spam servers, darknet servers, hubs for the distribution of pirated software, and so on. These examples of nefarious computing are familiar to administrators and have just moved to the cloud, where watchful eyes lack the granularity once associated with higher human-to-machine ratios. The relative anonymity behind these expansive and sometimes liberal usage models provides spammers, malicious code authors, and hacktivists opportunities to conduct their activities with relative impunity [9]. Private/public cloud Platform as a Service (PaaS) installations are typically the low-hanging fruit for these breaches, although recent evidence shows hackers targeting some larger Infrastructure as a Service (IaaS) vendors [10]. Hacking of PaaS or IaaS can be referred to more accurately as virtualization hijacking rather than hacking, as the virtual machines are hijacked and enlisted to perform some nefarious task.

Securing Multitenant Hosts

Cloud computing has a key characteristic, the virtualization layer. However, all virtualized systems and cloud systems have underlying components building up the infrastructure (e.g., network, storage, central processing unit, graphics processing unit, etc.) that were not dedicated or optimized specifically for virtualization until recently. The delivery of strong isolation capability in a multitenant environment is typically the first identified gap in security audits. What does it matter if security exists at the guest level if the underlying host can be exploited with a known UNIX kernel exploit? Addressing this security vulnerability can be accomplished through means that are beyond the scope of this text. The suggested reference materials align the host with Defense Information Systems Agency Security Technical Implementation Guide (DISA-STIG) guidelines [11].

Insider Threats

The threat of a malicious insider is a well-known constant to most organizations. This threat is controlled through authentication, authorization, access, and audit mechanisms. Internal or trusted users pose the most significant threat in the form of data leakage. The larger percentage of these potential incidents are managed through policy and audit mechanisms. Users will tend to navigate systems they have access to, whereas the average casual attacker will look for unsecured data and/or servers where a crime of opportunity may present itself. Strategies such as microsegmentation of domains can protect not only against the casual opportunist but also effectively minimize the attack footprint during a breach from an external adversary.

Data Integrity

Data integrity through policy-driven storage management should be central to any cloud, public or private. Accidental or intentional deletion or alteration of records without a backup of the original content can pose a serious security issue in the cloud. Mature organizations have determined classification of data types, which drive access-specific policies that dictate storage parameters and provide audit trails as well. The management policy must securely guarantee that unauthorized or unauthenticated entities are prevented from accessing private data. Exposure to data compromise increases exponentially in the cloud due to the number of transactions and interoperation between private and public cloud edges. Chapter 3 on data management discusses these principles at greater depth.

Encryption

Wide-area network (WAN) traffic is often the target for malicious access. In this section we will not address potential WAN attack vectors. In the previous section we touched on DDoS. But why settle for simple denial of service when you can instead steal a victim's traffic, take a few milliseconds to inspect or modify it, then pass it along to the intended recipient? As evidence, about 1,500 individual Internet Protocol (IP) blocks were hijacked in 2013 [12]. These events last from minutes to days, by attackers working from various countries. Current levels of encryption are often vulnerable to attack from persons with access to supercomputers. Current-generation Suite B encryption (AES 128–256 bit) modalities are gaining popularity and soon will become the standard, as will encryption of L2 extended tunnels (virtual local area networks or VLANs), or what now is being termed Encryption as a Service through public cloud providers. And automated certificate management for identity validation for intercloud connectivity will become standard.

As with many difficult issues, cybersecurity and data security is a question of balance. In particular: What is the right balance between privacy, on the one hand, and convenience and innovation, on the other? Likely this balance will continue to be dynamic. Strong security measures could be a competitive advantage.

In the past, many collaborative efforts have been met with insurmountable security parameters set into place years earlier prior to when many technologies emerged. A simple example would be the inability to share network ports on a device between development groups and production groups years after the VLANs technology was prevalent and accepted by many respected security and compliance professionals. A change to this policy came about in 2013. Centers for Medicare & Medicaid Services regulatory guidelines and DISA-STIG models reflect the update, but bear in mind that VLAN segmentation has been in wide use since 1985 as defined in IEEE 802.1Q. The DISA-STIGs comprise a library of documents that explain very specifically how computing devices should be configured to maximize security. Currently, there are over 400 STIGs, each describing how a specific application, operating system, network device, or smartphone should be configured. The DISA-STIGs represent the best practices in security but also are in the late majority or oftentimes laggards group when it comes to acceptance of new technologies. The consumer demand for innovative healthcare aims to find a balance between required security elements and the delivery of patient-focused healthcare [3].

Homomorphic Encryption

Homomorphic encryption allows for instant-read operations and/or calculations on encrypted information without the need for decryption prior to the read operation. The potential for a reliable model for homomorphic encryption exponentially increases security in cloud computing by facilitating encryption at rest with dual-factor authentication modes for intercloud data transfer or something as simple as computation supplied in the public cloud working on data in the private cloud [13, 14].

The Proliferation of Devices and Apps

Rapid growth in the use of smartphones and medical devices offers great opportunities to innovate how medical care is delivered. The shift toward handheld or "do-it-yourself" medicine is being driven both by a push to lower costs and by customers' desire for convenience. Improved cellular networks mean that consumers spend most of their time in areas with access to high-speed networks. This enables consumers to use apps and connected devices and, increasingly, to share this data in near real time with their medical providers.

From just 2013 to 2015 the percentage of consumers with at least one health or fitness app on their mobile device grew from 16% to 32%. According to one source, "86% of clinicians believe that mobile apps will become important to physicians for patient health management in the next 5 years" [1].

All these devices and apps can seamlessly collect data, but this means more and more data to analyze and archive. This also brings with it challenges around data integration and management.

From the perspective of the patient, there is not too much excitement in standing in line overnight at Best Buy or the Apple Store to get the latest and greatest glucose monitor or heart rate monitor; however, the mobile devices we all know and love may soon have these Internet of Things (IoT)–type features integrated into their hardware and software platforms, allowing for relationship analysis, precision medicine, and whole-life healthcare, where healthcare and condition management becomes fashionable.

A glucose meter that not only measures blood sugar but also tracks it over time will not only help the patient but the industry as well. Imagine if the integration extended to smart devices that tracked diet and exercise, building them into the "whole health" metric and providing exercise, dosing schedule, and dietary guidance to users. This is where the IoT becomes a game changer. Precision medicine can only be as precise as the data it measures or has access to. The ability to collect data from an array of sources will give new freedom to patients on managed care routines that previously could not exist.

Conversely, the challenge in this grand opportunity relates to the tenets of security in the cloud that we discuss throughout the book. There is a very real potential for an adversary to steal data from unsuspecting patients to use in nefariously. This very same deficiency is prevalent in public networked systems now where a power grid or water supply could be taken offline or suffer some type of service interruption. Suite B encryption components and/or emerging encryption techniques for securing network transmissions or data at rest or in flight will need to stay ahead of the would-be attacker. Homomorphic encryption and dynamic certificate services in theory offer next-generation protection.

New Sources of Data Both Public and Private

"High hopes surrounding big data investments in healthcare have been dampened by the challenge of converting large and diverse datasets into practical insights. In 2016, the health industry will begin to use these data in new ways, thanks to high-tech, so-called 'non-relational' databases" [1].

The term "nonrelational database" should be considered synonymous with NoSQL, which for clarification is not no SQL. In fact, NoSQL is short for "not only SQL," meaning *supporting* SQL and more. NoSQL represents a database that does not incorporate the table/key model that relational database management systems (RDBMSs) are built on.

Nonrelational databases are targeted for workloads that need data manipulation techniques and processes designed to provide solutions to data-intensive/big data challenges within the enterprise. Again, the nonrelational model is best known as NoSQL, but there are multiple flavors, all with their own strengths and weaknesses, and all should be considered prior to settling on a database model for your enterprise.

Now let's consider whether a nonrelational database might be a good fit for your use case. If you have designed an application that dynamically creates, harvests, or stores rapidly changing data that spans multiple data types from standard structured, semistructured, and unstructured at large volume and or velocity, you have a strong use case. If your application is intolerant of the 12- to 18-month waterfall development cycle and requires research-style agility in the form of agile sprints, iterating quickly and pushing code weekly, daily, or even multiple times a day, then you may desire this database model. In past well-known database management system (DBMS) models, something as simple as adding a schema extension to an existing database could require a herculean effort where paid service engagements were the only way to ensure success. Perhaps your application was once siloed, serving a finite audience, but is now delivered as a service requiring high availability (always on), global access, and it must have in-built flexibility to be accessible from a host of devices that did not exist a few years ago. This is another situation in which a nonrelational database might work well. And last and possibly most significant, research institutions are adopting scale-out architectures deployed on commodity X86 hardware and largely are vendor agnostic in their open source movement toward distributed cloud computing models.

The mainframe style of large monolithic servers, storage area networks, and locked-in vendor-driven infrastructures are simply not producing competitive results any longer.

These new ways of using data depend on consumers and organizations sharing data. One area where data access promises to improve is clinical trial data. In Europe, clinical trial data for approved drugs is publicly available. "As of October 2014, 520 organizations—including physician groups, patient advocates, government regulatory bodies and one large pharmaceutical company, GlaxoSmithKline—had signed the AllTrials petition, which calls for 'all trials registered, all results reported'" [1].

DATA MANAGEMENT

Another key area is research data management, which has become the number one topic discussed between vice presidents of research and CIOs at the university level. In its simplest terms, research data management amounts to the organization of data throughout its life cycle in your organization. The research life cycle could begin with a data download, generation of de novo artifacts through to the research process, publication and dissemination, and ending with the archiving of valuable results for inclusion in future research initiatives.

It is important to understand that research data management is a key component of the research process and should be as seamless, nonintrusive, and efficient as possible to meet the expectations and requirements of the researcher, the institution/university, funding organization, and legislation. It is also critical that a human within the organization owns the process. One of the hottest new job roles in almost any organization is the director of data management or director of research data management in the case of the university. A quick look at ZipRecruiter shows 1,129 director of data management jobs in Wilmington, Delaware, alone [15]. On a personal note, Arizona State University recently appointed a director of research data management after a 15-month search and recruitment process.

For researchers, research data management should be seamless and nonintrusive to the actual science objectives of that research. The policy of maintaining data artifacts throughout the life span of the funding opportunity has been extended indefinitely, mainly due to the advent of nonrelational database storage. The results from research today that fell short of its objective may be highly useful in discoveries of public value in future years. NoSQL implementations, such as MongoDB, that can store massive amounts of diverse data while keeping the data "warm" and readily available to search queries and perhaps machine learning mechanisms of the future. Be prepared to hear the term "deep learning" as machine learning crawlers continually index data in these massive online collections. The topic of research data management is discussed in depth in chapters 3 and 4 and should be considered central to sustainability in research institutions.

A 2011 white paper further explains the importance and changing conventions of research date management:

> The scientific process is enhanced by managing and sharing research data. Good research data management practice allows reliable verification of results and permits new and innovative research built on existing information. This is important if the full value of public investment in research is to be realized. These principles have been recognized by key stakeholders: most Research Councils now have policies in place which encourage or mandate the creation of a research data management plan and the deposit of research data in a recognized data center where such exist. Many leading journals require underlying datasets also to be published or made accessible as part of the essential evidence base of a scholarly article. [16]

The Precision Medicine Initiative

In 2015 President Barack Obama launched the Precision Medicine Initiative. Its mission is "To enable a new era of medicine through research, technology, and policies that empower patients, researchers, and providers to work together toward development of individualized care" [17].

The White House's website explains further:

> The future of precision medicine will enable health care providers to tailor treatment and prevention strategies to people's unique characteristics, including their genome sequence, microbiome composition, health history, lifestyle, and diet. To get there, we need to incorporate many different types of data, from metabolomics (the chemicals in the body at a certain point in time), the microbiome (the collection of microorganisms in or on the body), and data about the patient collected by health care providers and the patients themselves. Success will require that health data is portable, that it can be easily shared between providers, researchers, and most importantly, patients and research participants. [17]

In March 2015, Dr. Francis Collins, director of the National Institutes of Health, tasked a Working Group of his Advisory Committee to the Director to develop a plan for creating and managing a large research cohort. On September 17, 2015, Dr. Collins accepted the framework outlined in the Working Group report and began building the infrastructure so that participants can begin enrolling in the cohort in 2016 [18].

Research institutions have long understood that the more we learn, the less we know or the more we realize we do not know. The idea had been that once the code of the genome was decoded, we would have the insight to eradicate many disease conditions once and for all. However, this great discovery in modern science served to illuminate how much we really did not know about how gene signaling and biomarkers interoperate. There is a huge demand now for greater insights into the biological, environmental, and behavioral factors that influence disease conditions. A staggering number of diseases lack any reliable and reproducible treatments. Precision medicine offers the best approach for disease prevention and treatment. The science of evaluating individual variability in genes, hereditary factors, lifestyle, and environment factors for each unique patient promises to unlock targeted treatments that will be breakthroughs in the coming years. Evaluation of epigenetics for changes in organisms caused by modification of gene expression rather than alteration of the genetic code itself is just one of the emerging areas directly related to precision medicine. Over the past 10 years we have witnessed significant advances in precision medicine; however, there is quite a bit of work to be done at the federal, public institution, and private industry level to realize precision medicine's full value. In this author's opinion, we are still at a point where we know only a minuscule amount of what precision medicine holds for the future of medicine.

BIOSIMILARS, DRUG PRICING, AND PHARMACEUTICAL COMPOUNDING

Biosimilars, drug pricing, and pharmaceutical compounding are key drivers and benefits of precision medicine initiatives. They pave the road for pharmacogenomics. Biosimilars are often created using genetic technology and made from sugars, proteins, or engineered cells and/or tissues. It is worth clarifying that not all biosimilars are made from genetic technology. Two popular and well-known biologics are adalimumab (Humira) for rheumatoid arthritis and trastuzumab (Herceptin) for breast cancer. Due to the complex research required to engineer these treatments, they can be expensive; biologics can run $50,000 a year or more. It is no easy feat to create a biosimilar drug; it is far more challenging than creating the generic version of a brand-name drug, which typically just re-creates the same chemical recipe in a different preparation. Most common drugs are made from chemicals having a known chemical structure. Biosimilar and biologic drugs are far more complex.

Biosimilar drugs, while similar to the biologic drugs in target and purpose, have "allowable differences because they are made from living organisms," according to the FDA [19]. The FDA keeps a watchful eye on this emerging science, which again is another product of pharmacogenomics. Recently the FDA has gained the authority to approve biosimilar products under a provision of the Affordable Care Act.

PROMISING AREAS OF INNOVATION

The top issues in healthcare, discussed earlier, will be met at least in part by advances in data management, IT, and other technical innovations. While these innovations will likely occur in somewhat surprising ways and cut across numerous fields, I see six areas as particularly promising and worth a relatively high-level discussion.

The Internet of Things

Goldman Sachs, in a 2014 equity research report, listed the Internet of Things as a megatrend, explaining:

> The Internet of Things (IoT) is emerging as the third wave in the development of the Internet. The 1990s' fixed Internet wave connected 1 billion users while the 2000s' mobile wave connected another 2 billion. The IoT has the potential to connect 10X as many (28 billion) "things" to the Internet by 2020, ranging from bracelets to cars. [20]

Cisco Internet Business Solutions Group, as shown in Figure 1.1, places the number of interconnected devices even higher: at 50 billion by 2020.

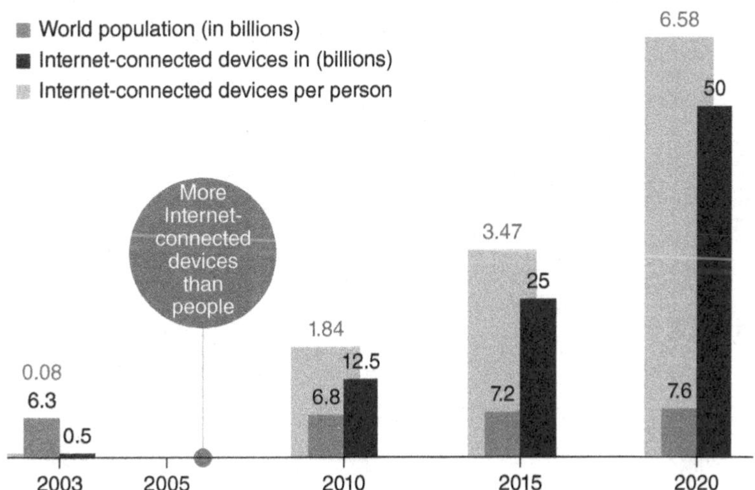

Figure 1.1 Growth in Internet-Connected Devices by 2020
Cisco IBSG, April 2011

Now is a terrific time for biomedicine to jump onboard IoT as sensor prices have dropped by 50% in the past 10 years and processing also has dropped as raw computational cycles have dropped 50 times in price per floating-point operation per second (FLOP). Wireless networks are ubiquitous, with the price of Internet bandwidth declining as much as 40 times over the past 10 years; smartphones are ever more common and increasingly incorporated into automobiles; and Internet Protocol version 6 (IPv6) is in wide deployment across large-scale provider networks. Software-defined networking (SDN) is prevalent on provider backbones, and of course big data analysis is on the minds of many software development firms readying for the volumes of data that will be produced by the IoT.

Figure 1.2 shows many of the companies currently developing IoT projects. There is no shortage of investor interest; some analysts estimate that as much as $5 billion in mergers, acquisitions, and venture capital will be raised in 2016. There are certainly infrastructure challenges to the collection and aggregation of data; however, the question remains: Can wearables (IoT) improve healthcare? As we continue to learn in the realm of big data analysis, the challenge lies in interpreting the data and creating applications that make the data actionable. We already know that wearables can collect wide varieties of data. For example, exercise and activity levels, sleep quality measurements, heart-rate

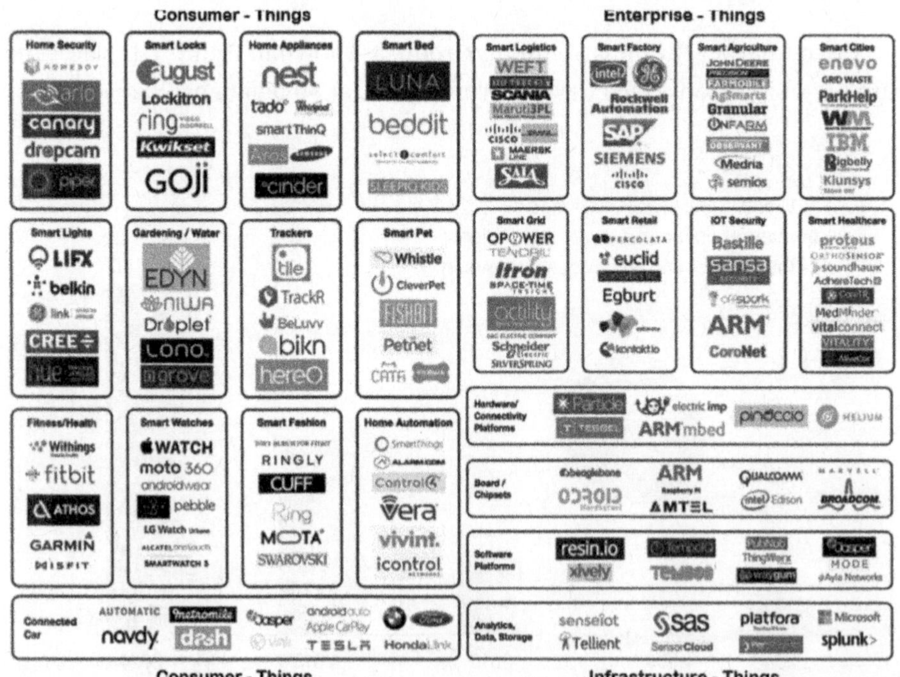

Figure 1.2 Brands in the IoT Realm

values, and blood sugar readings can benefit patients with risk factors for congestive heart failure, diabetes, and arrhythmias. In the next year we expect these devices to collect even more biometric data, including: detection of galvanic skin response through noninvasive methods, which can be critical in monitoring and understanding the stress response; blood glucose levels, which have the potential to reduce the cost and burden of managing diabetes; and tracking of pulse transit time to monitor blood pressure in real time.

Continued innovation in this realm aims to make healthcare devices ubiquitous. There are only two main potential roadblocks to widespread adoption. The first pertains to how device data will be treated by FDA regulatory guidelines for delivery of clinical care. Many conditions require close monitoring from FDA-listed devices, and this should remain standard practice. However, even when treating these conditions, and certainly when monitoring less critical patients, wearable devices can provide contextual, continuous data that helps connect the dots between regulated medical device readings and provider encounters.

The FDA's role continues to grow and evolve as it races to keep pace with emerging technologies. The FDA works to protect consumers while attempting to not inhibit discoveries of public value. This challenge extends to the IoT and medical devices. The FDA, in collaboration with the National Health Information Sharing Analysis Center, the Department of Health and Human Services, and the Department of Homeland Security, hosted a public workshop titled "Moving Forward: Collaborative Approaches to Medical Device Cybersecurity" in 2016. [21]. Such collaborations will likely become more common in the coming years.

The second challenge area is security. Insecure software/firmware, inability to provide physical security, potential identity theft, other unforeseen privacy concerns, insecure network access methods, weak encryption or lack thereof, and insufficient authentication/authorization all come to mind as both challenges and potential opportunities as the IoT continues to grow. The IoT faces all the same security challenges as, and perhaps more than, other types of networking and data sharing.

Data Visualization and Imaging

One path to understanding data is by seeing it. Data visualizations can be key to unlocking the path from data to information to knowledge. The ability to collect and explore complex data leads to an inevitable desire to see the data for interpretative analysis through the next generation of tools. According to Suhale Kapoor, the cofounder and executive vice president of Absolutdata Analytics: "Visuals will come to rule: The power of pictures over words is not a new phenomenon—the human brain has been hardwired to favour charts and graphs over reading a pile of staid spreadsheets. This fact has hit data engineers who are readily welcoming visualization softwares that enable them to see analytical conclusions in a pictorial format" [22]. Tools that present information in complex data as visual representations have matured and continue to grow in adoption.

Visualization leverages knowledge from data, driving more adaptive and dynamic visualization tools. The charts and graphs of the past are still compelling in their own right, although they are static and lack the real-time feel of the adaptive nature of "live data." Data visualization tools will continue to move beyond graphs and dynamically open new windows into the potential of simulations for every science domain imaginable. Dynamic dashboards, three-dimensional simulations, and automated diagnostic systems populated by incoming data sources reflecting up-to-the-minute fluctuations reveal hidden insights that would otherwise go unnoticed. These are perhaps some of the most exciting opportunities for biomedicine on the horizon.

Visualization has undergone a recent refresh as the advent of big data required a translational tool to become "human readable." Looking at human genomic data, which for the most part is a collection of base pairs, tells even the most astute researcher little. However, with the right visualization tool, that same data becomes more than coordinates; it becomes a map, or perhaps the Google Earth of life sciences. It should be noted that although we can sequence a human genome for $1,000, this does not include any analysis. The most significant costs are in the postprocess and analytics phases.

We know there are 3 billion diploid base pairs but 6 billion haploid sequences (because half come from your mother and half from your father). Discoveries mined from this extensive collection of data can be examined in postprocess pipelines in genome browsers with relative ease, comparatively speaking, when considering the enormity of the collection. Numerous methods have been developed to automate the analysis of genomic data. Nonetheless, the visual exploration of alterations in cancer genomes, epigenomes, and transcriptomes in multidimensional data sets and of the relationships among these alterations presents specific challenges. Schroeder, Gonzalez-Perez, and Lopez-Bigas's paper details the many offerings of targeted tool sets for genomics visualization [23].

Data Storage

The race is on to capture your data. The big cloud players, including Amazon Web Services, Dropbox, BOX, and Microsoft Azure, are in a heated competition to become the one-stop shop for institutions everywhere to move their data to. These providers are planning for the future and are not simply after flat file, unstructured, typical internal data assets. They are also planning for the storage of research data, web platform data, structured data from various

RDBM systems, and mobile device and sensor data gathered in emerging IoT efforts. About 85% of IoT data at this point is of no use to the companies that collect it. However, someday it may be, and that makes it worth retaining. The challenge now for institutions is determining which approach is sustainable over the long haul from compliance, financial, and availability perspectives. Is Hadoop, either in the cloud (Amazon Elastic MapReduce) or on premises, a viable solution? Should we still look toward an infrastructure of large-scale storage area networks that have evolved into data management platforms in many cases? Is a distributed server–based storage system (ephemeral) the best method to ensure robust scalability? In the coming chapters we take a deeper look at these options, share our experiences, and allow readers to determine which option or options will best meet their enterprise requirements.

Data Analytics

Data scientists, statisticians, and analysts are quickly moving to the forefront of many environments. Enterprises now expect that data scientists will be able to wrangle data, mine valuable insights, build complex models, identify difficult to discern patterns and relationships, and use data to predict future outcomes. Researchers and senior leaders recognize that uncovering insights that are locked away in the vast amounts of data is critical. Prescriptive analytics have replaced descriptive analysis or sentiment analysis, and statistical testing is now more commonplace in research sciences. Enabling the personalized medicine revolution will require a diverse collection of analytic tools including R, Apache Mahout, and Spark as well as custom tools to fuel novel genomic analysis and the integration of multidimensional molecular and clinical data.

The challenges of big data are well understood, while the benefits at this point are only imagined. Due to architected deployment options, our ability to gain insights from diverse forms of data previously considered difficult data types and formats is now much greater. With the democratization of big data, deep data analysis is nearly limitless in its scope.

Compute Capabilities

Data-intensive (big data) analytic frameworks and traditional high-performance computing (HPC) have evolved along diverse paths over the past 10 years. However, they are slowly converging again as institutions begin to find target workloads for each. Hadoop is certainly not the magic bullet, and the traditional "big iron" community cluster does not meet all aspects of many mature research pipelines. Typically, Hadoop (big data) is regarded to be about "data" and HPC clusters are about "computational compute." The current confluence of big data, computation, and analytics is driving "data-intensive compute" with the goal of solving the grand challenges. Solving these grand challenges will require a fundamental redesign of enterprise infrastructures as well as legacy thought processes. Thoughtful choreography of a diverse collection of physical and logical capabilities that perform as an integrated whole will attempt to overcome the physical limitations of Moore's Law. Delivery, open access, and support of these diverse environments will enable tomorrow's brilliant researchers to reveal new horizons in deep machine learning, artificial intelligence, cryptography, and complexity sciences, continuing to push the boundaries of emergent architectures toward realized quantum computing.

Cloud

The cloud is ubiquitous, and widespread adoption at extreme volumes will continue as cloud offerings right-size their consumption models for greater efficiency and competitiveness. Data is the driver for much of the public cloud's growth, and the cloud is becoming more useful as it expands from PaaS offerings to IaaS and raw compute (bare metal nodes versus virtual nodes). Analytic tools are also on the rise as Microsoft Analytics (which utilizes Hortonworks for its underlying Hadoop distribution), Amazon Redshift, and Google BigQuery gain ground and customer footprint.

Playing it safe in your cloud adoption is no longer considered a progressive strategy. The most prevalent strategy from 2016 to 2020 will be to determine which components to maintain in the on-premises portion of your hybrid cloud and which to farm out to public providers, and how to remain cloud vendor agnostic with a high availability, elastic, and dynamically mobile public presence. When one public provider fails to meet the desired service-level workloads, enterprises will adaptively relocate to another provider or to the on-premises capacity without service interruption. Cloud solutions and services will continue to innovate to support this model.

Emerging compliance models, legacy applications, and laggards will hold a portion of the IT roadmap landlocked on premise. But make no mistake: A paradigm shift is under way in how organizations understand and approach cloud adoption. As touched on earlier, not every aspect of research technology will be cloud ready in 2017 or perhaps even 2020; quite candidly, research institutions represent a relatively small customer base and therefore will be a bit behind public enterprise adoption. The current trend will continue as elements continue to move into the cloud. As we work through the remainder of the text, one specific aim is to inspire thought around hybrid-cloud architectures, highlighting achievable outcomes through integration of on-premises and public cloud-based resources.

CONCLUSION

Healthcare and biomedical research are incredibly dynamic sectors. Healthcare is still adapting to the mandates and policies of the Affordable Care Act, while biomedical research is expanding into precision medicine, the IoT, and advanced computational modeling (to name just a few innovative directions). There are many substantial challenges facing healthcare and biomedical research. Notable for this book is the fact that many of these challenges have substantial data or IT components. In other words, many will be solved, at least in part, by advances in data storage, analytics, network, and systems architecture. The chapters that follow explore these and other topics.

NOTES

1. Health Research Institute. December 2014. "Top Health Industry Issues of 2015." https://www.pwc.com/us/en/health-industries/top-health-industry-issues/assets/pwc-hri-top-healthcare-issues-2015.pdf.
2. Health Research Institute. December 2015. "Top Health Industry Issues of 2016." https://www.pwc.com/us/en/health-industries/top-health-industry-issues/assets/2016-us-hri-top-issues.pdf.
3. Steven Warren. December 9, 2008. "What Is Your Best Definition of VM Sprawl?" *TechRepublic.* http://www.techrepublic.com/blog/virtualization-coach/what-is-your-best-definition-of-vm-sprawl/.
4. Mark Verber. 2008. "How Many Administrators Are Enough?" Updated December 1. http://www.verber.com/mark/sysadm/how-many-admins.html.
5. Rackspace Hosting. "Rackspace: Managed Dedicated & Cloud Computing Services." https://www.rackspace.com/.
6. GoDaddy. "Domain Names | The World's Largest Domain Name Registrar—GoDaddy." https://www.godaddy.com/.
7. Imperva Incapsula. "Botnet DDoS Attacks." https://www.incapsula.com/ddos/ddos-attacks/botnet-ddos.html.
8. Arbor Networks. 2016. *Worldwide Infrastructure Security Report.* https://www.arbornetworks.com/images/documents/WISR2016_EN_Web.pdf.
9. SearchSecurity. "Definition: What Is Hacktivism?" http://searchsecurity.techtarget.com/definition/hacktivism.
10. Kevin Kell. November 11, 2013. "EC2 Security Revisited." Learning Tree Blog EC2 Security Revisited Comments. http://blog.learningtree.com/en/ec2-security-revisited/.
11. IASE. "Security Technical Implementation Guides (STIGs)." http://iase.disa.mil/stigs/Pages/index.aspx.
12. Dyn Research. November 19, 2013. "The New Threat: Targeted Internet Traffic Misdirection." http://research.dyn.com/2013/11/mitm-internet-hijacking/.
13. Craig Gentry. September 2009. *A Fully Homomorphic Encryption Scheme.* PhD Thesis. https://crypto.stanford.edu/craig/craig-thesis.pdf.
14. Andy Greenberg. November 3, 2014. "Hacker Lexicon: What Is Homomorphic Encryption?" Wired.com. https://www.wired.com/2014/11/hacker-lexicon-homomorphic-encryption/.
15. ZipRecruiter. "1,129 Director Data Management Jobs in Wilmington, Delaware." https://www.ziprecruiter.com/jobs/delaware/wilmington/director-data-management.
16. A. Whyte and J. Tedds. September 1, 2011. "Making the Case for Research Data Management." Digital Curation Centre. http://www.dcc.ac.uk/resources/briefing-papers/making-case-rdm.
17. White House. "White House Precision Medicine Initiative." https://www.whitehouse.gov/precision-medicine.

18. National Institutes of Health. "Precision Medicine Initiative Cohort Program." https://www.nih.gov/precision-medicine-initiative-cohort-program.
19. U.S. Food and Drug Administration. Updated August 2015. "Information for Consumers (Biosimilars)." http://www.fda.gov/Drugs/DevelopmentApprovalProcess/HowDrugsareDevelopedandApproved/ApprovalApplications/TherapeuticBiologicApplications/Biosimilars/ucm241718.htm.
20. Goldman Sachs. September 3, 2014. "Internet of Things Primer." http://www.goldmansachs.com/our-thinking/outlook/internet-of-things/iot-report.pdf.
21. U.S. Food and Drug Administration. 2016. "Moving Forward: Collaborative Approaches to Medical Device Cybersecurity," Public workshop, January 20–21. http://www.fda.gov/MedicalDevices/NewsEvents/WorkshopsConferences/ucm474752.htm.
22. Quoted in Bruce Robbins, "5 Predictions for 2016 on Data, Analytics and Machine Learning." January 3, 2016. Data Science Central. http://www.datasciencecentral.com/profiles/blogs/5-predictions-for-2016-on-data-analytics-and-machine-learning.
23. M. Schroeder, A. Gonzalez-Perez, and N. Lopez-Bigas. 2013. "Visualizing Multidimensional Cancer Genomics Data." *Genome Medicine* 5, no. 9, https://genomemedicine.biomedcentral.com/articles/10.1186/gm413.

CHAPTER 2

Genome Sequencing

Know Thyself, One Base Pair at a Time

Content contributed by Sheetal Shetty and Jacob Brill

Dr. Joel Dudley, the coauthor of the groundbreaking 2013 textbook *Exploring Personal Genomics*, has stated that you can now "know thyself, one base pair at a time" [1]. Dudley is a leader in biomedical informatics and the director of Biomedical Informatics at the Icahn School of Medicine at Mount Sinai. *Exploring Personal Genomics* appeared at a time of extremely rapid advances in sequencing technologies and techniques for analyzing all that newly available information.

We've seen genomic sequencing costs drop astronomically. The Human Genome Project took 13 years and cost US$3 billion. Now author Peter White of Nationwide Children's Hospital notes that "even the smallest research groups can complete genomic sequencing in a matter of days" and at a cost of around $1,000 [2, 3]. During a speaking trip to Phoenix in October 2014, Google Cloud Genomics evangelist Dr. Allen Day went so far as to say that "DNA sequencing is well on its way to being free." [4] This sentiment is shared throughout the omics community, and now the magic and the challenge lie in what the end product has to tell us, what secrets remain tightly locked in the code.

Increasingly the chokepoints lie in the steps following sequencing, which involve calibrating and analyzing the billions of generated data points for genetic variants that could lead to diseases. These steps require time, expense, and expertise. While research budgets are generally not increasing, analytic tools and computing speed are.

With clinical and research medicine using genomics data at greatly increasing rates, we will gradually—or not so gradually—move toward a future in which computer science and biology become ever more intertwined. This intertwining should open avenues to address large-scale, multistakeholder, transdisciplinary research initiatives. And if this is done in line with the Reference Model of Open Distributed Processing systems architecture (ISO/IEC 10746), we will ensure that our systems are open and flexible, able to meet grand challenges.

While an inspiring vision for the future is essential, we are getting rather ahead of ourselves. In this chapter we explore at a conceptual level the computational and logistical challenges of genomic analysis. After this brief examination we take a step back and offer a primer on DNA, RNA, and protein synthesis. From there we move to a history of DNA sequencing that will take us up to the present moment of next-generation sequencing. Finally, we present a number of common tools for genomic sequence analysis.

This chapter is not a definitive guide to genomic computation nor is it a substitute for a deep understanding of biology. Rather, we offer a primer so that systems architects, administrators, programmers, and enthusiasts can understand many of the data types, tools, processing engines, and approaches to omics science and research. If you would like a definitive guide, we suggest these publications:

- Stuart M. Brown, ed., *Next-Generation DNA Sequencing Informatics.* Cold Spring Harbor, NY: Cold Spring Harbor Press, 2013.
- Joel T. Dudley and Konrad J. Karczewski, *Exploring Personal Genomics.* Oxford: Oxford University Press, 2013.

CHALLENGES OF GENOMIC ANALYSIS

To begin to understand the scope of the challenges that we face in genomic analysis, let's turn to a popular metaphor. Imagine that I ask you to find the sequence of numbers "5247" in 100 different telephone books. It would probably take you years, right? But let's think through how we might accelerate this and how this might create new challenges.

- **Scale out.** What if there were 1,000 of you ripping out a page at a time?
- **Administration.** You'd need someone to coordinate the effort and collect results.
- **Communication.** You'd need a standard method to let everyone know when you found a match.
- **Interconnect.** You'd need a quick way of contacting everyone (a blackboard? e-mail? text message?).
- **Shared storage for input/output.** Everyone would need quick, easy, and coordinated access to the telephone books. The administrator would need to copy all matching pages, collate them into one document, then put them into a folder shared by many groups doing the same thing. Could get busy, eh?

How do these steps mirror the steps of the genomics process? Well, scaling out would be the multiple labs generating their sequence data for their own analysis on whichever organism they need to be examining. Even data from nonhuman species can be crucial to finding insight. Administration is taking this data and changing the format to a usable file type that all parties can read and work with—for example, a BAM or SAM file. Publications and supplementary data are great ways of communicating your findings to the world, and web repositories for journals can be a great way of interconnecting. The next step would be shared storage of genomics data. Genbank at the National Center for Biotechnology Information (NCBI) and Ensembl at the European Bioinformatics Institute are examples of data sharing so that labs have the ability to upload their sequences for other parties to work with in a genomics environment. Data from these repositories is just as valuable as generating data on first principle for bioinformaticians.

THE LANGUAGE OF LIFE

Dr. Francis Collins, best known for his leadership of the Human Genome Project, has stated that "DNA is the language, the blueprint for all living things." And former president Bill Clinton described the Human Genome Project as "Without a doubt, . . . the most important, most wondrous map ever produced by humankind" [4]. Many readers are no doubt deeply familiar with how DNA and RNA and genes work (and if this is you, feel free to skip ahead). But for those of you who are less familiar, we have included an encapsulated crash course on genetics. Our aim is to supply you with the needed vocabulary to work with biologists and researchers alike.

There is no better place to begin than with what is known as the central dogma. The central dogma explains how genetic information flows within a biological system. The basics are that "DNA codes for RNA, which codes for proteins. DNA is the molecule of heredity that passes from parents to offspring. It contains the instructions for building RNA and proteins, which make up the structure of the body and carry out most of its functions" [5].

- **DNA replication** is the process by which the two strands of a DNA molecule are duplicated to generate two exact copies of the original DNA molecule.
- **Transcription** is the process of synthesizing RNA using a DNA template. The product is a single-stranded RNA molecule that is the complement of the DNA template.
- **Translation** is the process of synthesizing new proteins according to the directions of messenger RNA (mRNA). The net result is the translation of nucleic acid information into protein information.

To recap:

1. DNA is *transcribed* into RNA in the process of *transcription*.
2. RNA is *translated* into protein in the process of *translation*.

Now that we are somewhat familiar with the general life process as explained by Francis Crick's central dogma, let's look at the building blocks and process in more detail.

Deoxyribonucleic acid (DNA) carries genetic information and is structured as a double helix composed of two strands of nucleic acid. The DNA (or genome) for an individual is a sequence of about a billion values from an alphabet of size 4 (A, C, T, G). A, C, T, and G stand for adenine, cytosine, thymine, and guanine, which are the four molecules, also known as nucleotides or bases, that make up DNA. These bases are linked together into a strand of nucleic acid by a phosphodiester backbone and are bound to a complementary strand by hydrogen bonds. The sequences are complementary because each C in one strand is complemented by a G on the complementary strand [6]. These pairs, A-T and C-G, are often referred to as *base pairs*. The two complementary strands of DNA spiral around each other, creating the well-known double helix.

Genes are special subsequences of base pairs interspersed throughout the genome that are responsible for encoding traits inherited from our ancestors. When activated, genes produce RNA and protein, which are the workhorses of cells and carry out the "instructions" of the DNA. RNA is a single-stranded nucleic acid similar to DNA, but with thymine (T) replaced by uracil (U). Inside the nucleus of cells, genes are "transcribed" into RNA, and in most cases, the RNA transcript is then "translated" into protein. It is important to mention here that protein does not carry genetic information. Each sequence of three bases in the RNA represents one of 20 different amino acids, the building blocks of protein.

Biologists have identified about 20,000 different genes in the human genome that encode such protein. Researchers originally thought that there were millions of genes, but much of the human genome is composed of noncoding regions. In fact, over 98% of the human genome is non–protein coding. It is also important to note that not every gene is transcribed and translated into protein in every cell. In reality, some genes are active and create high volumes of RNA and protein, while other genes are less active. Which genes are active at any given time varies by cell type. For example, genes responsible for cell growth are likely to be more active in cancer cells than in normal cells. Likewise, genes responsible for producing the oxygen-carrying protein hemoglobin will be more active in blood cells than in skin cells. Even though almost all cells in the human body contain the entire genetic code, only a subset of genes are actually active at any given time in any given cell. The level of activity, or "expression," of a gene can be almost as important as the gene itself for determining phenotype (the physical manifestation of a gene). As a result, mechanisms for regulating the expression of certain genes are an active area of research. Microarray technology supports the measurement of the expression level of thousands of genes at the same time with a single chip. For example, Affymetrix sells quartz chips containing tens of thousands of microscopic probes designed to detect the presence and relative amount of specific segments (subsequences) of RNA. Biologists often collect microarray data for thousands of tissue samples from different patients in order to perform some sort of statistical analysis. This data collection results in a large, dense matrix of floating point values, in which the columns correspond to different genes and the rows correspond to tissue samples of different patients.

A BRIEF HISTORY OF DNA SEQUENCING

DNA was discovered and isolated by Friedrich Miescher in 1869. He named the new substance "nuclein" since it was found in the nucleus. Miescher speculated widely about the possible roles it played, from a storage unit for phosphorus to providing mobility to sperm [7]. Although some of his speculations pointed toward nuclein playing a role in transmitting hereditary information, he was not very convinced himself. It was not until the early 20th century with Fred Griffith's discovery of the "transforming principle" that our understanding of how hereditary material is transmitted started to take shape. Griffith studied pneumococcal bacterial strains, and his experiments on nonvirulent (nonharmful) pneumococcal bacteria strains showed that these bacteria could change their profile to become virulent (harmful) by being grown in the same plate as a virulent strain. These bacteria changed while they were reproducing, and this change could be transmitted to future generations. The groundbreaking 1944 experiment of Avery, Macleod, and McCarty proved the "transforming principle" to be predominantly DNA by completely degrading any proteins and carbohydrates in the bacterial cell and observing that the cell maintained its transformative property [8].

The wider acceptance of DNA as the hereditary material in the scientific community finally came with Alfred Hershey and Martha Chase's experiments in 1952 with bacteriophages, viruses infected with bacteria. By radioactively labeling the DNA and protein parts of the viruses, they were able to demonstrate that it was the DNA, and not the protein, that got transmitted within the bacteria. These experiments conclusively laid to rest the then-prevailing concept that DNA was too scarce to carry genetic information and hold the genetic blueprint to life and that proteins carried this information due to their abundance in the cells.

Following on Avery, McCarty, and MacLeod's work, biochemist Erwin Chargaff studied the ratio of nucleotides adenine, cytosine, thymine, and guanine in various species. He found that though this ratio varied among species, the amount of adenine and thymine was identical, as was the amount of cytosine and guanine [9]. Later, scientists would discover that this was because adenine always bonds with thymine and cytosine always bonds with guanine. This and X-ray crystallographic work done by Rosalind Franklin and Maurice Wilkins laid the foundation for James Watson and Francis Crick to finally decipher the structure of DNA.

Watson and Crick discovered and forwarded the now widely known double-helix model of DNA, which depicts the DNA strand being constructed by two strands of nucleotides coiled together and linked by hydrogen bonds in the well-known spiral configuration. Each strand was theorized to be composed of four complementary nucleotides. The configuration of adenine, cytosine, thymine, and guanine made up the master organism, reconstructing cells and passing genetic information between generations.

In 1956 Francis Crick published the central dogma, pictured in Figure 2.1 [10]. The central dogma states that DNA contains the code for the building blocks of life (proteins), which is transcribed by RNA and finally translated into proteins.

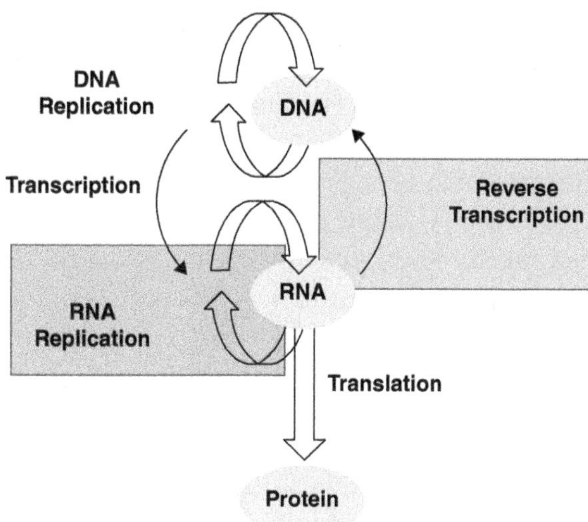

Figure 2.1 The central dogma of molecular biology

The key principles are:

1. DNA is *transcribed* into RNA (transcription).
2. RNA is *translated* into protein (translation).

DNA is double stranded and has a very specific base pairing. Adenine always pairs with thymine, and cytosine always pairs with guanine. DNA replication is the process by which the two strands of a DNA molecule are duplicated to generate two accurate copies of the original DNA molecule. The double-stranded DNA separates into single strands and is replicated by the process of complementary base pairing following the rule stated above. Replication from the parental DNA produces two daughter copies, with a single strand of the original parental copy serving as a template to generate the complementary newly synthesized strand, thus creating two identical double-stranded daughter DNA strands. This is known as the semiconservation method of replication, and was demonstrated experimentally by Matthew Meselson and Franklin Stahl in 1958 [9].

Transcription is the process of synthesizing RNA using the original DNA template. The information contained within the DNA is transcribed onto single-stranded RNA molecules known as messenger RNA (mRNA). mRNA undergoes further editing to remove pieces of information called introns, which have been transcribed from the DNA, and keep only the parts called exons, which contain the code to make proteins. Then mRNA travels into the cytoplasm and is finally translated into new proteins according to directions coded in the mRNA.

The genetic code was cracked in the 1960s through the combined efforts of Marshall Nirenberg, Heinrich Matthaei, H. Gobind Khorana, and Severo Ochoa, who discovered the basic code for each of the 22 amino acids that form the building blocks of proteins [9]. The links among DNA, RNA, and proteins, and finally to the genetic code, are the most important pieces of information needed to understand life at the molecular level. Sequences of three nucleotides, called codons, code for each amino acid. These amino acid sequences strung together form proteins. Genes code for proteins, which get transcribed onto the mRNA and finally travel out of the nucleus into the cytoplasm to get translated to proteins. These proteins are required for the functioning of our various cellular systems. Figure 2.2 shows the codon table for RNA.

Second Position

First Position [5' end]	U	C	A	G	Third Position [3' end]
U	UUU] Phe UUC UUA] Lev UUG	UCU UCC] Ser UCA UCG	UAU] Tyr UAC UAA *Stop* UAG *Stop*	UGU] Cys UGC UGA *Stop* UGG Trp	U C A G
C	CUU CUC] Lev CUA CUG	CCU CCC] Pro CCA CCG	CAU] His CAC CAA] Gln CAG	CGU CGC] Arg CGA CGG	U C A G
A	AUU AUC] Ile AUA AUG Mel	ACU ACC] Thr ACA ACG	AAU] Asn AAC AAA] Lys AAG	AGU] Ser AGC AGA] Arg AGG	U C A G
G	GUU GUC] Val GUA GUG	GCU GCC] Alo GCA GCG	GAU] Asp GAC GAA] Glu GAG	GGU GGC] Gly GGA GGG	U C A G

Figure 2.2 RNA Codon Table
Bree, "What's the Big Deal? Proteins," The Poached Egg, August 3, 2011, http://www.thepoachedegg.net/the-poached-egg/2011/08/proteins-whats-the-big-deal.html.

There are two main types of RNA:

1. **Coding RNA:** messenger RNA (mRNA)
2. **Noncoding RNA:** transfer RNA (tRNA) and ribosomal RNA (rRNA)

Other categories of noncoding RNA, such as small nuclear RNA (snRNA) and small interfering RNA (siRNA), are areas of active research.

RNA also has the same helical shape as DNA but is single stranded, unlike DNA. It has the same nucleotide bases as DNA, but uracil replaces thymine.

Thus the three major forms of RNA seen within cells are:

1. **mRNA,** which copies information from genes (DNA), which code for specific proteins;
2. **tRNA,** which attaches to specific amino acid bases on mRNA coding during protein synthesis; and
3. **rRNA,** which helps in stringing together amino acids to form long polypeptide protein chains.

DNA SEQUENCING AND THE HUMAN GENOME PROJECT

Several new methods for DNA sequencing were developed in the mid- to late 1990s and were implemented in commercial DNA sequencers by the year 2000. A list of the breakthroughs is briefly summarized next.

DNA sequencing is the decoding of genetic information locked in the DNA through machine translation of the nucleotide sequence, which makes up the 3 billion bases of human genetic code. Fred Sanger introduced the chain-termination method for base determination, which gained wide acceptance as the preferred method for sequencing [11]. Although another method, by Allan Maxam and Walter Gilbert using base-specific chemical degradation, was introduced at the same time, the Sanger method became more popular due to its ease of use [12, 13].

DNA sequencing can be broadly divided into four steps:

1. Reaction
2. Separation
3. Detection
4. Data analysis [13]

The reaction step is specific to the type of method being used. Broadly, double-stranded DNA is broken mechanically or chemically into single-stranded DNA, and mixed with a DNA polymerase, DNA primer, and the four nucleotide bases (adenine, guanine, thymine, and cytosine) along with a chemical called dideoxynucleotide (ddNTP), which when incorporated during the polymerase reaction stops the lengthening of the DNA chain. Each type of radioactively or fluorescently labeled ddNTP (ddATP, ddTTP, ddCTP, and ddGTP) is aliquoted, or divided, into a separate reaction.

The separation step involves separating the DNA fragments obtained from the reaction step based on size. Earlier methods used polyacrylamide gels. The DNA fragments traveled vertically through the gel and settled at locations based on size. Currently, this separation process is done by the capillary-based system, where the samples are run through a very fine capillary. The samples can be read simultaneously by the detector as the DNA sample travels through the capillary.

The detection step formerly involved exposing the separated sample to X-rays when using radioactive labeling. This is, however, not done anymore. The current method is the use of fluorescently labeled ddNTPs exposed to laser light, which is simultaneously detected by the detecting machine. The analysis step compiles all this information into a single continuous sequence of As, Ts, Cs, and Gs.

The automation of the Sanger sequencing method led to the ambitious Human Genome Project, with its aim of sequencing the entire human genome. The project was completed in 2001, much earlier than expected [9]. The sequencing was done using the method just described together with shotgun assembly.

In the shotgun assembly process, the entire genome is broken into random smaller pieces. These pieces are first amplified by cloning in bacterial cells (plasmids/bacterial artificial clones). These pieces are then further amplified through a polymerase chain reaction (PCR) [14].

These PCR products have known fragment sizes (insert sizes). The major contribution of the Sanger sequencing group was the development of mate-pair reading methods. Different-size libraries of these inserts were created and clonally amplified. Multiple clonally amplified fragments of circularized DNA sequences from each library were cut into linear pieces and read from both ends of the pieces. Finally these were put together to form sets of overlapping DNA segments, known as contigs, with unread gaps in between. These contigs were finally assembled together bioinformatically into overlapping scaffolds in the analysis step [9]. The size of the gap can be estimated with reasonable confidence based on the segment length of the DNA library (the insert size). This mate-pair sequencing and assembly method was a major step in the direction of high-throughput analysis. This was a huge achievement; the entire human genome was decoded and made publicly available through NCBI. The expectation from this outcome was determining the exact genomic etiology for most disease. This step was far from easy.

Technology for faster sequencing has improved over the years, and the cost of the sequencing process has dropped drastically due to these new sequencing methods. These newer-generation sequencing technologies are collectively called next-generation sequencing (NGS). The most commonly used technologies are from Roche/454, Illumina/Solexa, Life/APG, and Helicos BioSciences and are reviewed by Metzker [15]. The flow of steps is more or less the same as with Sanger sequencing and includes template preparation, sequencing, viewing, and data analysis. The major improvements are in template preparation and sequencing.

Template preparation has seen major advances in NGS methods. There has been a shift from bacterial artificial chromosomes (BACs), which had problems with loss of genomic material in the BACs during cell replication and introduction of replication errors introduced through human error during the mapping process [16, 17]. The two major types of template preparation in NGS technology are clonally amplified templates and single-molecule templates [15].

Clonally amplified templates use a single-stranded DNA molecule with a universal primer attached to beads. These PCR-amplified beads can then be placed on a glass slide for the NGS sequence reading.

Solid-phase amplification or bridge amplification is another method where the primers are attached to a glass slide and DNA fragments plus polymerase are added to the slide to produce spatially separated clones of amplified DNA fragments. The single-molecule template has a major advantage as it does not require PCR amplification; therefore, errors are reduced. There is no need for clonal amplification in this method, and therefore this method is more representative of the original sample. The results are read in real time. The next step in the process is sequencing the single-stranded DNA and reading it using imaging of fluorescent probes attached to the nucleotides. Currently four methods are used for sequencing [15]:

1. Cyclic reversible termination
2. Sequencing by ligation
3. Single-nucleotide addition/pyrosequencing
4. Real-time sequencing

Cyclic reversible termination uses the cyclical process of incorporating fluorescent nucleotides, imaging, and termination of process using ddNTP. Each step of a single nucleotide incorporation, termination, imaging, and washing an unbound nucleotide is repeated until the entire template is read. This process is most commonly used in clonally amplified templates. This method relies on the use of modified ddNTPs with more efficient cleavage of the fluorescent labels compared to Sanger sequencing.

Sequencing by ligation uses DNA ligase attached to fluorescent dye-labeled probes, washing extra probes away, and reading by imaging in a cyclical way. The pyrosequencing method uses sulfurylase and luciferase to detect bioluminescence instead of fluorescently labeled nucleotides. Real-time sequencing is the most advanced of these technologies, as it does not require any terminators to stop the process of sequencing. DNA polymerases are attached to the glass slides; therefore, the sequencing can be processed without the need to terminate, with release of fluorescence from the nucleotide being read in real time by imaging. Technological advances are constantly improving these NGS technologies, with the goal of reducing errors introduced during the sequencing process.

NGS has led to dramatically lower sequencing costs. The costs of genomic sequencing, as shown in Figure 2.3, are now falling faster that the cost of storage.

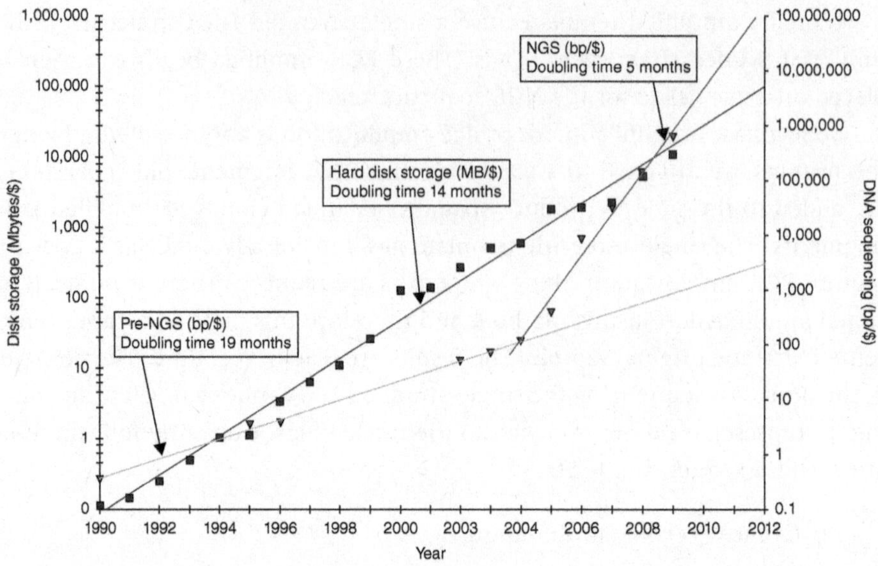

Figure 2.3 Sequencing Costs Compared to Storage Costs

Now that we know a bit more about the data and processes of genomic analysis, we should briefly discuss what can be done with this highly unique code. Next we discuss some tools for genomic analysis.

SELECT TOOLS FOR GENOMIC ANALYSIS*

We have selected a handful of common tools and provided explanations and screenshots to further understanding. The short section is by no means all-inclusive, but it offers an introduction to many common and useful tools.

Genbank

Genbank at the NCBI is the National Institutes of Health's open access genetic sequence database and tool set for sequence analysis. The NCBI database exchanges annotated collections of publicly available DNA with other members of the International Nucleotide Sequence Database Collaboration. More simply put, Genbank is a genome browser and its repository and tools have become a cornerstone in omics and bioinformatics research. Large swaths of data can be gathered and processed right from Genbank using the Basic Local Alignment Search Tool (BLAST). BLAST and the Genbank database have become standard tools for any biotechnologist or informatics specialist.

*Content contributed by Jacob Brill.

BLAST is based on the Smith-Waterman algorithm, which puts the search for maximally similar segments on a mathematically rigorous basis but can be efficiently and simply programmed on a computer [18]. BLAST uses a modified version of this algorithm to give a more heuristic approach that allows much faster queries and alignments against larger databases while retaining relatively high accuracy.

This algorithm's specific approach to maintaining this balance of speed and accuracy consists of three steps:

1. Filter out low-complexity/repeat regions, as these are the types of sequences that would confuse the program.
2. Create "word" lists of the sequence and then score them against the possible matching words [19]. Figure 2.4 shows a BLAST word list.
3. Score the matches based on the algorithm parameters set by the user and then repeat the process. Scoring is based on a percent accepted mutations (PAM) or Blocks substitution (BLOSUM) matrix. Figure 2.5 shows the BLAST scoring phase.

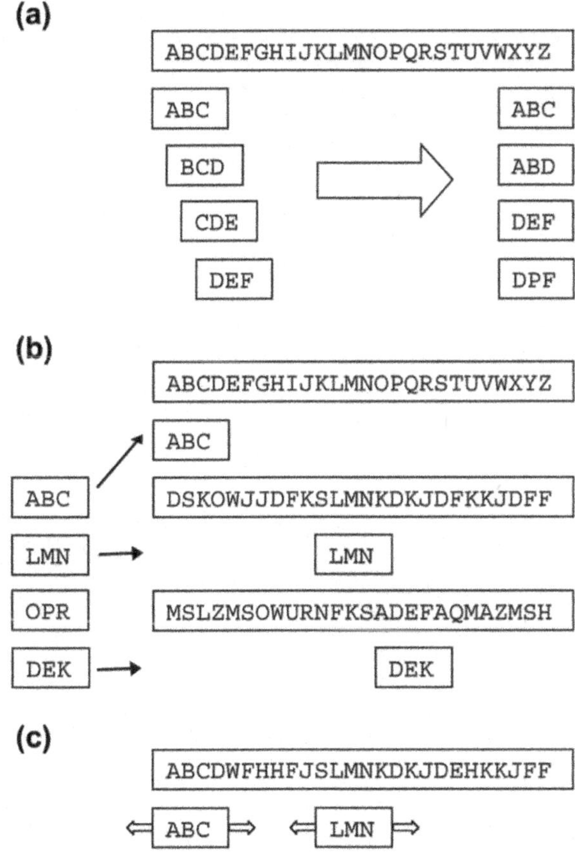

Figure 2.4 BLAST Word List

BLAST word list from a query of length L; word length is 3 for amino acid sequences and 11 for nucleotides.

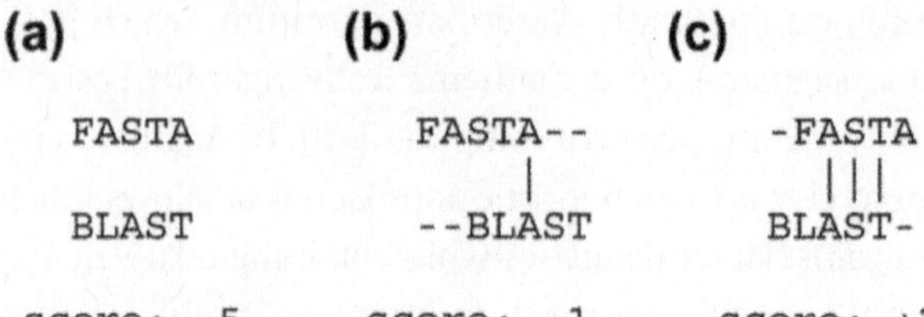

Figure 2.5 BLAST Scoring Phase
The quality of an alignment for the queried sequences determines how well the algorithm can score the sequence.

A fantastic feature of BLAST and Genbank is that usage is free, and you don't even need to create an account with the NCBI to use its tools. The tool set is open source, which has led to a wide variety of different BLAST tools to create more specialized alignments. While there are multitudes of offshoot BLAST-like projects available on the web, Table 2.1 shows the NCBI-supported features and their functions.

Table 2.1 Basic Blast Category and Database Queries

Search Page	Query and Database Combination	Alignment Type	Programs and Functions (default program in bold)
nucleotide blast	nucleotide vs. nucleotide	nucleotide vs. nucleotide	**megablast**: For sequence identification, intraspecies comparison discontiguous megablast: For cross-species comparison, searching with coding sequences blastn: For searching with shorter queries, cross-species comparison
protein blast	protein vs. protein	protein vs. protein	**blastp**: General sequence identification and similarity searches DELTA-BLAST: Protein similarity search with higher sensitivity than blastp PSI-BLAST: Iterative search for position-specific score matrix construction or identification of distant relatives for a protein family PHI-BLAST: Protein alignment with input pattern as anchor/constraint
Blastx	nucleotide (translated) vs. protein	protein vs. protein	blastx: For identifying potential protein products encoded by a nucleotide query
Tblastn	protein vs. nucleotide (translated)	protein vs. protein	tblastn: For identifying database sequences encoding proteins similar to the query
Tblastx	nucleotide (translated) vs. nucleotide (translated)	protein vs. protein	tblastx: For identifying nucleotide sequences similar to the query based on their coding potential

Completed BLASTs output a graphical summary, significant sequence alignment descriptions, and plain alignments. A good starting point for interoperating the data is to look for the expect (e-values) under the alignment descriptions tab. The lower the e-value, the less likely it is that the alignment is due to random chance; this gives the user more confidence in the accuracy of the selected alignment. Following the hyperlink from the e-value will display the selected sequence alignment in plain text.

With all this dynamically generated data from Genbank, there is now the task of determining how this data is helpful for use or advancement of the bioinformatics field. Biologists will see this type of sequence analysis data and use it to determine relationships or maybe even construct a phylogeny; the usefulness of the data for them is that it can be used to answer questions. Not every biologist is going to understand the details of how or why this type of approach to data generation works, but all should be confident that the data generated is accurate and that their labs can independently generate high quantities of sequence data and then subsequent alignments. Bioinformatics tools like Genbank are wonderful not just in their direct data generation but also in their ability to mitigate the time and cost that this research would have incurred previously.

The R Project

R is a statistical computing language and software environment developed by the R Development Core Team. R's design is influenced by Rick Becker, John Chambers, and Alan Wilkis's "S" and Gerald Sussman's "Scheme." R's interpreted computing language allows for branching, looping, and modular programming functions to create a stable environment for statistical analysis and graphical representation. The participation of R in GNU, a free software system, has allowed for the development of a multitude of open source modules to help specialized data collection and interpretation. R has been made available in precompiled binary distributions for Windows, Mac, Linux, and a source code release for all platforms. More recent versions of the program have also allowed for combinations with specialized packages to let R use cluster computing and other parallel processing options. Now a fundamental tool in the bioinformatics field, R simplifies the process of statistical analysis and aiding in the creation of accurate models and graphs.

R is an interpreted language that can also function as an object oriented, or procedural programming language. It is designed to work with complete data sets on a single machine to create publication-quality statistical solutions and graphs. Recent iterations of the program allow for parallel computing with Hadoop, to link to other forms of resource management and batch processing. An R session is capable of performing extensive calculations, from simple arithmetic to matrix computation directly in the working space. However, R works best when importing data files from Excel, Open Office, Minitab, Matlab, and other file and program types to perform highly accurate large-scale statistical analysis on the data. GPU-accelerated computing is capable of increased performance gains for analysis of larger data sets or creation of graphically intensive representations of the data.

In addition to the base systems of R, the program hosts a suite of packages that are collections of R functions, compiled code, and some data. These packages assist in streamlining the process of data analysis or allow for R to interface with other types of data or systems. Currently the Comprehensive R Archive Network's package repository hosts 7,738 available packages, and all available packages are tested on machines where R is available (cran.r-project.org). Some notable packages are rJava, which allows low-level R to interface with Java, and plyr, which is a tool for splitting and combining data. Since 2011, RStudio has been a free and open source–integrated development environment for R that gives users an integrated console, a syntax editor, and code execution.

As with many other informatics tool sets, the R Project is completely free, and is an invaluable tool for anyone in the data sciences field. The strengh of R's programming environment and simple facilitation of packages have allowed R to give users the access to professional-level analysis and data visualization with minimal stress on the user.

Genome Analysis Toolkit

The Genome Analysis Toolkit (GATK) is a software package for analysis of NGS data. GATK has become a standard tool in recent years for identifying single nucleotide polymorphisms and insertion/deletions (indels) from germline and RNAseq data. GATK is a pipeline, a sequential set of data processing elements connected in a series so that an output from one element becomes the input of the next one. GATK in particular has been designed to process exomes (the exon portion of the genome) and whole genome sequences generated by Ilumina machines.

GATK was designed with Java. It runs as a Java app on Linux or POSIX-compatible platforms and comes with a suite of methods and algorithms predefined within the tool set. Many bioinformatics tools work through a command line instead of a graphical user interface (GUI), and GATK is one of those. GATK's site at the Broad Institute has lists of each argument and detailed summaries of the purpose and which specific tool they will work for. Figure 2.6 shows the terminal structure for the GATK interface.

The GATK pipeline follows the NGS reads that have been converted into FASTQ, uBAM, or other raw read files for the next set of processing which is their "Best Practices" step, as shown in Figure 2.7.

```
Terminal — bash — 126×27
Last login: Tue Jul 17 21:14:27 on ttys003
ggimac:~ GG$ cd /Users/GG/codespace/GATK/release/resources
ggimac:resources GG$ java -jar GenomeAnalysisTK.jar -T CountReads -R exampleFASTA.fasta -I exampleBAM.bam
INFO  21:15:02,020 HelpFormatter - --------------------------------------------------------------------------------
INFO  21:15:02,022 HelpFormatter - The Genome Analysis Toolkit (GATK) v1.5-30-g27e7e17, Compiled 2012/04/13 12:17:15
INFO  21:15:02,022 HelpFormatter - Copyright (c) 2010 The Broad Institute
INFO  21:15:02,023 HelpFormatter - Please view our documentation at http://www.broadinstitute.org/gsa/wiki
INFO  21:15:02,023 HelpFormatter - For support, please view our support site at http://getsatisfaction.com/gsa
INFO  21:15:02,024 HelpFormatter - Program Args: -T CountReads -R exampleFASTA.fasta -I exampleBAM.bam
INFO  21:15:02,024 HelpFormatter - Date/Time: 2012/07/17 21:15:02
INFO  21:15:02,024 HelpFormatter - --------------------------------------------------------------------------------
INFO  21:15:02,024 HelpFormatter - --------------------------------------------------------------------------------
INFO  21:15:02,029 GenomeAnalysisEngine - Strictness is SILENT
INFO  21:15:02,077 SAMDataSource$SAMReaders - Initializing SAMRecords in serial
INFO  21:15:02,094 SAMDataSource$SAMReaders - Done initializing BAM readers: total time 0.02
INFO  21:15:02,199 TraversalEngine - [INITIALIZATION COMPLETE; TRAVERSAL STARTING]
INFO  21:15:02,199 TraversalEngine -        Location processed.reads  runtime per.1M.reads completed total.runtime remaining
INFO  21:15:02,200 Walker - [REDUCE RESULT] Traversal result is: 33
INFO  21:15:02,201 TraversalEngine - Total runtime 0.01 secs, 0.00 min, 0.00 hours
INFO  21:15:02,223 TraversalEngine - 0 reads were filtered out during traversal out of 33 total (0.00%)
INFO  21:15:03,821 GATKRunReport - Uploaded run statistics report to AWS S3
ggimac:resources GG$
```

Figure 2.6 Terminal Structure for GATK Interface
Broad Institute, https://software.broadinstitute.org/gatk.

Break it down
We currently have two separate workflows for Germline DNA and for RNAseq, and we are developing a workflow for Somatic DNA. All of them are divided into three sequential phases:

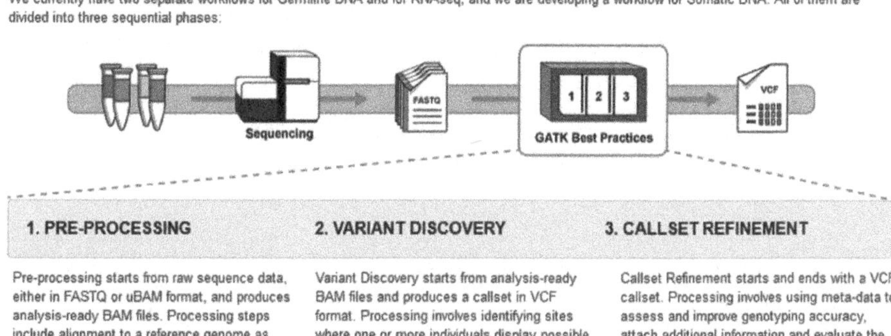

Pre-processing starts from raw sequence data, either in FASTQ or uBAM format, and produces analysis-ready BAM files. Processing steps include alignment to a reference genome as well as some data cleanup operations to correct for technical biases and make the data suitable for analysis.

Variant Discovery starts from analysis-ready BAM files and produces a callset in VCF format. Processing involves identifying sites where one or more individuals display possible genomic variation, and applying filtering methods appropriate to the experimental design.

Callset Refinement starts and ends with a VCF callset. Processing involves using meta-data to assess and improve genotyping accuracy, attach additional information and evaluate the overall quality of the callset.

Figure 2.7 Basic Steps for GATK
Broad Institute, https://software.broadinstitute.org/gatk.

The best practices workflow is the recommended stepwise procedure for discovering variants from the high-throughput data. This allows for the discovery of single nucleotide polymorphisms, structural variants, or copy number variants with careful regulation of workflow and resource management.

There have been many significant benefits from the adoption of GATK into the bioinformatics field. The tool set has seen an explosion in usage in research computing, especially with further advances in parallel processing and GATK's ability to utilize Queue scripts to increase data coverage. One of the methods used to determine transmissibility and prevalence in drug-resistant tuberculosis was GATK's ability to detect indel realignment [20]. GATK has also been very useful in the medical field, assisting physicians in diagnosing patients. According to one user: "We then adopted the GATK Best Practices pipeline to re-process the raw data and that's when we found the culprit: a frameshift mutation in *PROP1*, present in homozygous form in both siblings" [21].

Molecular Evolutionary Genetics Analysis

The Molecular Evolutionary Genetics Analysis kit (MEGA) is a tool created to conduct sequence alignments and to help researchers infer phylogenetic trees. These phylogenetic trees were originally constructed based on inferred heritability of traits based on morphology. Now phylogenies are constructed computationally, combining data science with biological methods to construct genetically based hypothetical trees. MEGA has been developed as a computational tool for biological sciences to aid in the construction of these trees by allowing the user to generate multiple phylogenies with a large data set, using multiple computational methods. Current iterations of MEGA have integrated tool sets for Windows and Mac operating systems, with a command-line interface version for high-performance computing.

MEGA software was developed for comparative analysis of DNA and protein sequences that are aimed at inferring the molecular evolutionary patterns of genes, genomes, and species over time [22]. To accurately construct a phylogeny, MEGA supports multiple models of evaluation to represent the data to be interpreted, as shown in Figure 2.8 [23].

Sequence alignments

- **DNA, codon, and protein alignments; both manual and automated alignments with trace file Editor. Built-in automated aligners: CLUSTALW and MUSCLE*.**

Major analyses (statistical approach in parentheses)

- **Models and parameters: Select Best-Fit Substitution Model* (ML); test pattern homogeneity; Estimate Substitution Pattern (MCL, ML*); Estimate Rate Variation Among Sites* (ML); Estimate Transition/Transversion Bias (MCL, ML*); Estimate Site-by-Site Rates* (ML).**
- **Infer phylogenies: Infer Phylogenetic Trees (NJ, ML*, ME, MP); Phylogeny Tests (Bootstrap and Branch-length tests); Branch-and-Bound Exact Search (MP); Heuristic Searches: Nearest-Neighbor-Interchange (NNI; ML*, ME, MP), Close-Neighbor-Interchange (CNI; ML*, ME, MP), and Max–Mini (MP)**
- **Compute distances: Pairwise and Diversity; Within- and Between-Group Distances; Bootstrap and Analytical Variances; separate distances by Site Degeneracy, Codon Sites; Separation of Distances in Transitions and Transversions; Separate Nonsynonymous and Synonymous Changes**
- **Tests of Selection: For Complete Sequences or Set of Codons; Sequence Pairs or Groups (Within and Between)**
- **Ancestral Sequences: Infer by ML with Relative Probabilities for bases or residues* or by MP (all parsimonious pathways)**
- **Molecular Clocks: Tajima's 3-Sequence Clock Test*; Likelihood Ratio Test (ML) for a Topology*; Estimate Branch Lengths under Clock***

Substitution models (+F = with empirical frequencies; REV = reversible)

- **DNA: General Time Reversible (GTR)*, Tamura–Nei, Hasegawa–Kishino–Yano*, Tamura Three-Parameter, Kimura Two-Parameter, Tajima–Nei, Jukes–Cantor**
- **Codons: Nei–Gojobori (original and modified), Li–Wu–Lou (original and modified)**
- **Protein: Poisson, Equal-Input, Dayhoff (+F), Jones–Taylor–Thornton (+F), Whelan and Goldman (+F)*, Mitochondrial REV (+F)*, Chloroplast REV (+F)*, Reverse Transcriptase REV (+F)***
- **Rate Variation and Base Compositions: Gamma rates (G) and Invariant sites (I)* models; Incorporate Compositional Heterogeneity.**

Figure 2.8 Supported Models in MEGA v5 and MEGA CC

Both the GUI and command-line versions of MEGA can parse sequence data directly from database repositories or sequence data in FastA or MEGA formatted files for computation. Phylogenies constructed in both MEGA and MEGA CC can be statistically tested by the bootstrap method and Bayesian analysis. Using the sequence alignment data and the created phylogenetic trees, the user may perform further analyses into the inference of ancestral sequences, tests of natural selection, molecular clock tests, and estimates of evolutionary rates [24].

As evolutionary and molecular biology evolve into larger fields, the creation of accurate phylogenies requires more powerful software with great computing abilities. MEGA provides the resources for small-scale and batch processing of sequence data for construction of publishable phylogenies that can be used to advance fields outside bioinformatics, such as evolutionary medicine and genomics. Figure 2.9 shows a sample phylogeny created using MEGA 4.0 [25]. While MEGA is a regularly updated resource, it continues to be distributed for free, with full documentation and version support, from megasoftware.net.

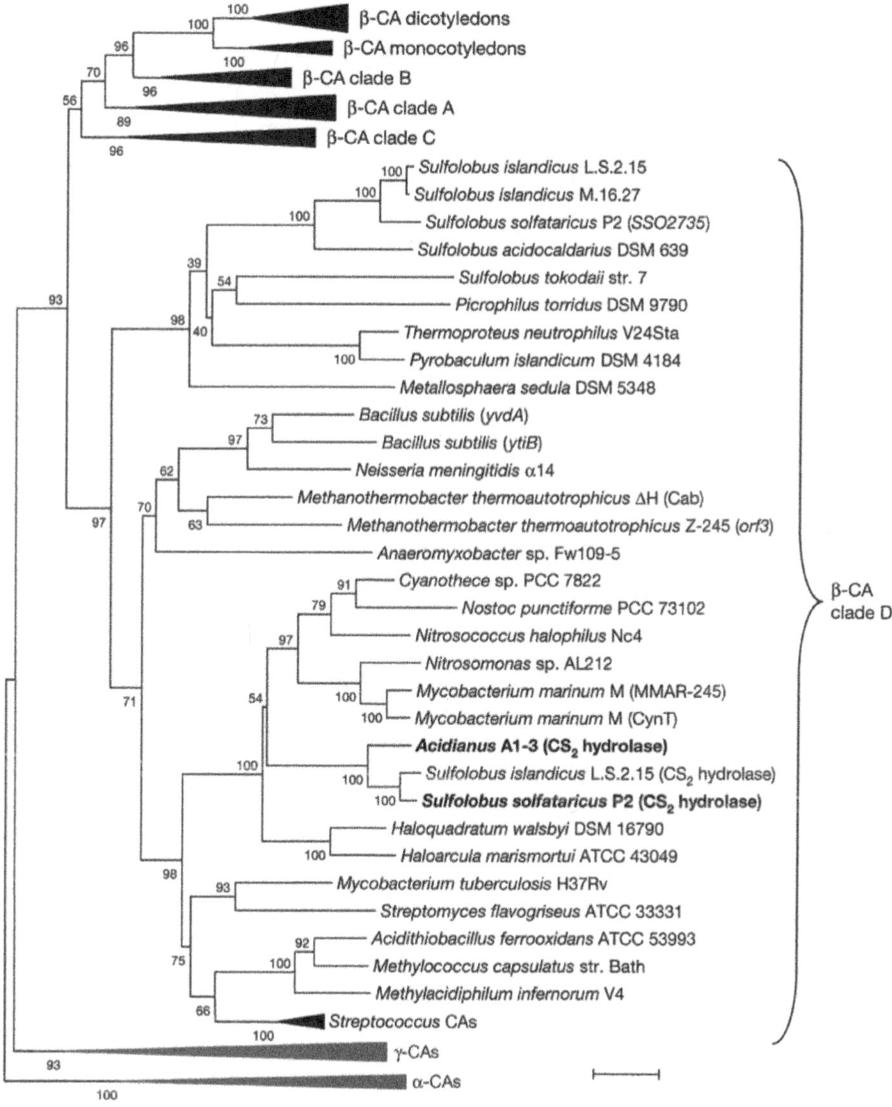

Figure 2.9 Sample Phylogeny Created Using MEGA 4.0

Bowtie

Bowtie is another tool for DNA sequence alignment, although it is a much more specialized tool than MEGA. Bowtie specializes in comparing large sets of short sequences or reads to large genomes. Bowtie is part of a suite of alignment, sequencing, and mapping tools intended to work with data sets of varying sizes in a quick and memory-efficient manner. Bowtie and its suite are available for 64-bit architecture of Windows, MacOS, and Linux, with source available for GNU-like environments (bowtie-bio.sourceforge.net). While it's available for these systems, Bowtie is run through a command line and graphical outputs are usually viewed through an interpreter, such as the Integrative Genome Viewer (IGV) and SAMtools.

Bowtie's inner workings are based on indexing the genome with a Burrows-Wheeler index, to keep the memory footprint small. This memory-saving strategy is one of the main reasons why Bowtie is effective as a bioinformatics tool. The Burrows-Wheeler transformation is a reversible permutation of characters in the text, which in Bowtie indexes the reference genome and allows for the human genome to fit into 2.2 gigabytes on disk with a memory footprint of 1.3 gigabytes during alignment [26]. Figure 2.10 shows a sample Burrows-Wheeler transformation.

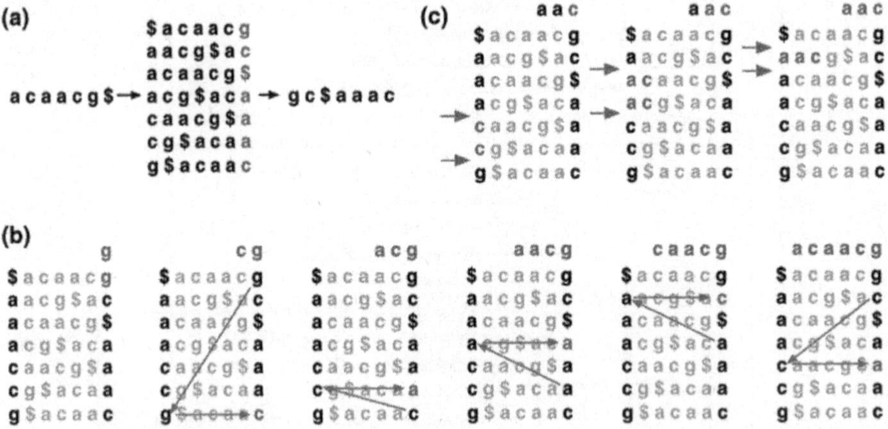

Figure 2.10 Sample of a Burrows-Wheeler Transformation

Completed alignments from Bowtie can be printed in the Sequence Alignment Map (SAM) format or left in the original Bowtie output format of one alignment per line. Sample workflow for Bowtie includes making a copy of the reference genome and indexing the short reads from the FASTA or FASTQ format. The finished sequence would be saved in SAM format to allow SAMtools for postdata processing. IGV renders the graphical output, as shown in Figure 2.11.

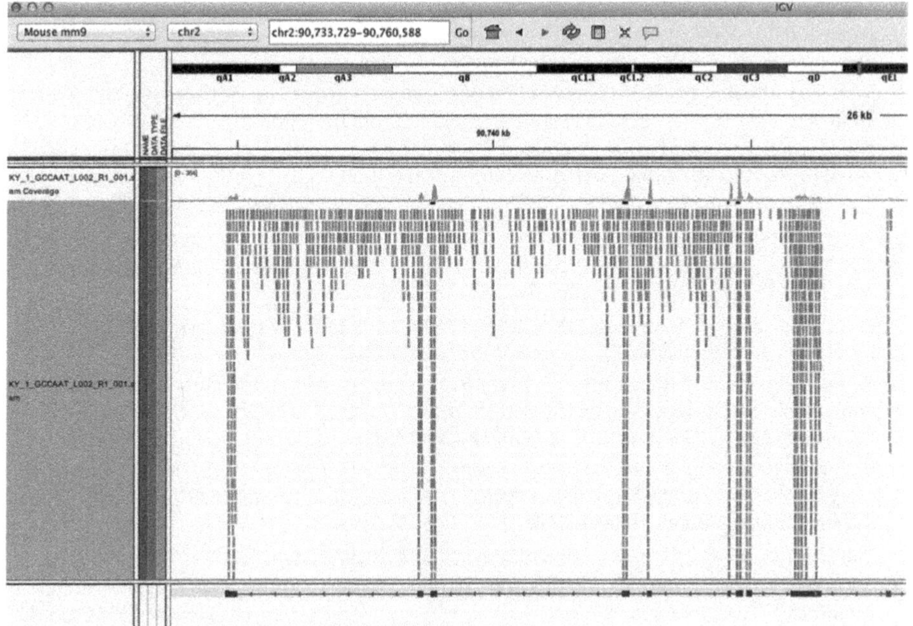

Figure 2.11 IGV Output from Bowtie and SAMtools
John B. Johnston, "Bowtie and IGV: A Mapping and Visualization Workflow." Bioinformatics Support—HPCC Wiki, 2013. https://wiki.hpcc.msu.edu/x/c4E2AQ.

Bowtie and its companion utilities are effective ways to rapidly create sequence alignments with low memory and minimal disk requirements. Bowtie's efficiency in short-read alignments makes it a valuable bioinformatics tool for users working with a single machine or batch processing on a cluster. Simplified workflow gives users of all practices the opportunity to work efficiently and produce publication-quality results. And like many other bioinformatics tools, Bowtie and its utilities are free to users.

CONCLUSION

Ours is a remarkable historic and scientific moment. With the central dogma deciphered and sequencing costs dramatically lower, genomics is poised to make great contributions. Genomics analytics are developing rapidly. Now that we have reviewed some of the basics of genetics and explored common genomics tools, we are ready to dive into data management and the other central concerns of this book. After this chapter you will find a case study detailing how exome sequencing was used in clinical diagnosis.

NOTES

1. Joel T. Dudley and Konrad J. Karczewski. 2013. *Exploring Personal Genomics.* Oxford: Oxford University Press.
2. Nationwide Children's. "Novel Software, Churchill, Allows for Full Analysis of 1,000 Genomes in One Week Using Cloud Resources." http://www.nationwidechildrens.org/medical-professional-publications/novel-software-churchill-allows-for-full-analysis-of-1000-genomes-in-one-week-using-cloud-resources?contentid = 138534.
3. Brian K. Nunnally, ed. 2005. *Analytical Techniques in DNA Sequencing.* Boca Raton, FL: Taylor & Francis.
4. DNA Learning Center. Completion of a draft of the human genome, Bill Clinton. https://www.dnalc.org/view/15073-Completion-of-a-draft-of-the-human-genome-Bill-Clinton.html.
5. Learn.genetics. "RNA's Role in the Central Dogma." http://learn.genetics.utah.edu/content/molecules/centraldogma/.
6. J. C. Venter, M. D. Adams, E. W. Myers, et al. 2001. "The Sequence of the Human Genome." *Science* 291 (5507): 1304–1351. doi: 10.1126/science.1058040.
7. Ralf Dahm. 2008. "Discovering DNA: Friedrich Miescher and the Early Years of Nucleic Acid Research." *Human Genetics* 122, no. 6: 565–581. doi: 10.1007/s00439–007–0433–0.
8. Klaus Eichmann and Richard M. Krause. 2013. "Fred Neufeld and Pneumococcal Serotypes: Foundations for the Discovery of the Transforming Principle." *Cellular and Molecular Life Sciences* 70, no. 13: 2225–2236. doi: 10.1007/s00018-013-1351-z.
9. P. Portin. 2014. "The Birth and Development of the DNA Theory of Inheritance: Sixty Years since the Discovery of the Structure of DNA." *Journal of Genetics* 93, no. 1: 293–302. http://www.ncbi.nlm.nih.gov/pubmed/24840850.
10. Francis Crick. 1970. "Central Dogma of Molecular Biology." *Nature* 227, no. 5258: 561–563.
11. F. Sanger, S. Nicklen, and A. R. Coulson. 1977. "DNA Sequencing with Chain-Terminating Inhibitors." *Proceedings of the National Academy of Sciences of the United States of America* 74, no. 12: 5463–5467. http://www.ncbi.nlm.nih.gov/pmc/articles/PMC431765/.
12. A. M. Maxam and W. Gilbert. 1977. "A New Method for Sequencing DNA." *Proceedings of the National Academy of Sciences* 74, no. 2: 560–564. http://www.pnas.org/content/74/2/560.
13. Brian K. Nunnally. 2005. "Introduction to DNA Sequencing: Sanger and Beyond." In B. Nunnally, ed., *Analytical Techniques in DNA Sequencing.* Boca Raton, FL: Taylor & Francis.
14. Sorin Istrail, Granger G. Sutton, Liliana Florea, et al. 2004. "Whole-Genome Shotgun Assembly and Comparison of Human Genome Assemblies." *Proceedings of the National Academy of Sciences of the United States of America* 101, no. 7: 1916–1921. doi: 10.1073/pnas.0307971100.
15. Michael L. Metzker. 2010. "Sequencing Technologies—The Next Generation." *Nature Reviews Genetics* 11, no. 1: 31–46. doi: 10.1038/nrg2626.
16. A. P. Monaco and Z. Larin. 1994. "YACs, BACs, PACs and MACs: Artificial Chromosomes as Research Tools." *Trends in Biotechnology* 12, no. 7: 280–286. doi: 10.1016/0167–7799(94)90140–6.
17. H. Shizuya and H. Kouros-Mehr. 2001. "The Development and Applications of the Bacterial Artificial Chromosome Cloning System." *Keio Journal of Medicine* 50, no. 1: 26–30.
18. T. F. Smith and M. S. Waterman. 1981. "Identification of Common Molecular Subsequences." *Journal of Molecular Biology* 147, no. 1: 195–197. doi: 10.1016/0022–2836(81)90087–5.
19. A. Pertsemlidis and J. Fondon. 2001. "Having a BLAST with Bioinformatics (and Avoiding BLASTphemy)." *Genome Biology* 2, no. 10. http://www.ncbi.nlm.nih.gov/pmc/articles/PMC138974/.
20. Nicola Casali, Vladyslav Nikolayevskyy, Yanina Balabanova, et al. 2014. "Evolution and Transmission of Drug-Resistant Tuberculosis in a Russian Population." *Nature Genetics* 46, no. 3: 279–286. doi: 10.1038/ng.2878.
21. "GATK | About." https://software.broadinstitute.org/gatk/.
22. Sudhir Kumar, Glen Stecher, Daniel Peterson, and Koichiro Tamura. 2012. "MEGA-CC: Computing Core of Molecular Evolutionary Genetics Analysis Program for Automated and Iterative Data Analysis." *Bioinformatics* 28, no. 20: 2685–2686. doi: 10.1093/bioinformatics/bts507.

23. K. Tamura, D. Peterson, N. Peterson, G. Stecher, M. Nei, and S. Kumar. 2011. "MEGA5: Molecular Evolutionary Genetics Analysis Using Maximum Likelihood, Evolutionary Distance, and Maximum Parsimony Methods." *Molecular Biology and Evolution* 28, no. 10: 2731–2739. doi: 10.1093/molbev/msr121.
24. Koichiro Tamura, Glen Stecher, Daniel Peterson, Alan Filipski, and Sudhir Kumar. 2013. "MEGA6: Molecular Evolutionary Genetics Analysis Version 6.0." *Molecular Biology and Evolution* 30, no. 12: 2725–2729. doi: 10.1093/molbev/mst197.
25. Marjan J. Smeulders, Thomas R. M. Barends, Arjan Pol, et al. 2011. "Evolution of a New Enzyme for Carbon Disulphide Conversion by an Acidothermophilic Archaeon." *Nature* 478, no. 7369: 412–416. doi: 10.1038/nature10464.
26. Ben Langmead, Cole Trapnell, Mihai Pop, and Steven L. Salzberg. 2009. "Ultrafast and Memory-Efficient Alignment of Short DNA Sequences to the Human Genome." *Genome Biology* 10: R25. doi: 10.1186/gb-2009-10-3-r25.

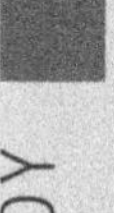

CASE STUDY 1: EXOME SEQUENCING IN CLINICAL DIAGNOSIS

CASE STUDY

Jay Etchings

"Whole-genome sequencing can determine the cause of undiagnosed diseases and can be done on a small scale," said Howard Jacob, PhD, from the Medical College of Wisconsin in Milwaukee, during the Future of Genomic Medicine VII conference in 2014.

As a consulting architect with Dell Enterprise, I often presented to research professionals and operations staff in the same sessions. There are challenges to explaining topics that have both biomedical and IT components to audiences of varied backgrounds. (These challenges are one of the main motivations for this book.)

One thing we can all understand is the unimaginable pain a family undergoes when their child is sick. The story of Nicholas Volker is one that I have told many times. Nicholas's story captivates audiences and shows very clearly the human stakes of biomedical innovation. It is also a story with a relatively happy ending [1].

In May 2007 the physicians at Children's Hospital of Wisconsin found that then four-year-old Nicholas had four fistulas and two or more fissures or tears in the lining of his rectum. These holes allowed waste in the form of feces to move into the tissue surrounding the anus and scrotum. As you can imagine, the potential for serious infection was great. This rare condition had been discovered when Nicholas was two. Between that time and 2007, Nicholas and his family had made more than 100 trips to doctors and the operating room. A component of the treatment was to divert the large intestine with a colostomy bag and stomata to stave off persistent infections and illness. However, this only treated a tertiary condition, while the root cause remained a mystery.

(*Continued*)

(*Continued*)

In the months following the May 2007 visit, Nicholas's condition worsened and became critical. Surgical wounds around the stomata refused to heal, additional fistulas established themselves, and feces once again leached into his skin. The tissue of his abdomen began to necrose, and he grew a sizable wound across his small body. Additionally, with his compromised digestive system, healing was delayed due to malnutrition. Hospital staff performed painful daily wound cleaning.

Early in 2009 doctors opted to remove Nicholas's scarred colon. Although his abdominal wounds had healed, the disease progressed internally from the rectum through the colon. An ileostomy now was required to remove waste from his body. (An ileostomy is a surgically made opening in the abdominal wall at the lowest end of the small intestine at the end of the ileum.) Waste could exit through this opening through a stoma placed on the lower right side of the abdomen. Nicholas required a placement higher than typical as much of his abdomen was previously damaged by infection.

The medical team considered a bone marrow transplant based on the belief that Nicholas's immune system had turned on itself and was killing off healthy cells. Given that bone marrow transplants are risky and often produce less than stellar results, the team opted against this.

Dr. James Verbsky, a pediatric rheumatologist with a strong background in microbiology and molecular genetics, was the immune disease specialist treating Nicholas. He and his colleagues had run every applicable test to rule out all possibilities. In July 2010 the medical team decided to sequence Nicholas's DNA. The hospital, however, had never sequenced a patient and was not even planning to implement the technology until 2014.

Sequencing Nicholas's DNA would cost around $2 million, and there was a good chance that it would only produce more questions rather than answers. Verbsky recalls: "I was skeptical when they said they were going to sequence him. I laughed, to be totally honest."

Humans have thousands of variations in our genetic code, and these differences define the uniqueness of our species. Perhaps 25,000 variations would be identified in Nicholas's genome. Verbsky and team worried that with the potential for so many variations, they might never determine which were responsible for the boy's illness. Seeking to identify the causative mutation(s), the team opted for exome sequencing versus whole-genome sequencing. This substantially reduced the cost to about $75,000—still hardly a trivial cost for the family. Exons carry instructions for protein encoding, and the failure to produce a protein is often causative in disease identification. Using this method, the team would target about 1% of Nicholas's genome.

Table CS2.1 outlines the types of available DNA-based tests.

Table CS2.1 Types of DNA-Based Tests

Type of DNA Testing	Description
DNA identification and profiling	Examines a scope of variable regions within DNA, determining the probability that the sample has a relationship to a known group or individual. This is the well-publicized process by which much forensic science is accomplished; however, this method is not utilized in disease probability or disease risk analysis.
Single gene	This test examines a specific region of a known disease-causing gene (e.g., a frequently mutated DNA nucleotide). Some gene-based tests sequence across the entire gene, including both exons and the intervening spaces known as introns. Several thousand nucleotides may be analyzed. Examples include HBB testing for the sickle cell mutation and sequencing the BRCA1 and BRCA2 genes for hereditary breast and ovarian cancer. Historically, these tests have involved older sequencing technologies, although a number of next-generation sequencing approaches are in development.
Exome	Selectively determines the sequence of exons, the coding regions of the genome. This represents only a small fraction of the entire genome, meaning less analysis and a lower cost.
Whole genome	Deciphers the complete sequence of an organism. Note: Some small portion of the genome (composed primarily of highly repetitive regions) resists sequencing, so the "whole" descriptor isn't quite accurate.

HudsonAlpha—Biotechnology

At the time, the Children's Hospital of Wisconsin only had one sequencer, and it was planning to do something not yet attempted by larger centers with far more resources. The team began by sequencing individual genes that were known candidates for irritable bowel syndrome (IBS) and Crohn's disease. Through this they were unable to identify mutations. Then the search expanded to include sequencing the exons of all the genes in Nicholas's genome. Nicholas's exons were sequenced extensively—an average of 34 times—to reduce the chance that a mutation might be overlooked. Soon after sequencing, the team identified 16,124 variants. Nicholas's sequences were compared against reference sequences generated by the Human Genome Project and its follow-on studies.

Additional analysis pointed to a novel genetic mutation in the inhibitor of the apoptosis gene. This mutation of the inhibitor of apoptosis was not previously associated with Crohn's disease but has a central role in the inflammatory response and bacterial sensing through the signaling pathway. The Sanger Institute confirmed the mutation in its clinical laboratory. Nicholas's cells had an increased susceptibility to activation-induced cell death due to this protein function in apoptosis.

(*Continued*)

(*Continued*)

CONCLUSION

> Based on his medical history, genetic and functional data, Nicholas Volker was diagnosed as having an X-linked inhibitor of apoptosis deficiency. Based on this finding, an allogeneic hematopoietic progenitor cell transplant was performed to prevent the development of life-threatening hemophagocytic lymphohistiocytosis, in concordance with the recommended treatment for X-linked inhibitor of apoptosis deficiency. At >42 days posttransplant, the child was able to eat and drink, and there has been no recurrence of gastrointestinal disease, suggesting this mutation also caused the gastrointestinal disease. This clinical research identified a novel cause of inflammatory bowel disease. Equally important, it demonstrates the power of exome sequencing to render a molecular diagnosis in an individual patient in the setting of a novel disease, after all standard diagnoses were exhausted, and illustrates how this technology can be used in a clinical setting [2].

This diagnosis enabled effective clinical treatment. The Volker family has since established the One in a Billion Foundation with the mission "to inspire the world to improve the quality of life for those with undiagnosed and rare disease by advancing the practice of personalized and genomic medicine" [3].

NOTES

1. "One in a Billion: A Boy's Life, a Medical Mystery." 2016. http://www.jsonline.com/news/health/111224104.html.
2. Worthey EA, Mayer AN, Syverson GD, et al. Making a definitive diagnosis: Successful clinical application of whole exome sequencing in a child with intractable inflammatory bowel disease. *Genetics in Medicine*. 2010;13(3):255–62. doi: 10.1097/gim.0b013e3182088158.
3. Amylynne Santiago Volker. 2016. One in a Billion Foundation Home page. http://www.oneinabillionic.com/.

CHAPTER 3

Data Management

Content contributed by Joe Arnold

In Francis Collins's 2015 keynote address at Datapalooza, the National Institutes of Health (NIH) director noted that the cost of full genome sequencing may drop to $1,000 by the end of that year [1].

With such dramatically lower sequencing costs, we are experiencing a tidal wave of data that is catalyzing exciting collaborative efforts to share and manage that data. The Global Alliance for Genomics & Health is working on a framework for sharing genomic and clinical data. Collins also mentioned PCORnet, the National Patient-Centered Clinical Research Network, which is focused on sharing large amounts of health data with the aim of making it faster, easier, and less costly to conduct clinical research. He described PCORnet as "an unprecedented network of networks" that lets you conduct observational trials almost for free. He also said NIH is working on a "data commons," explaining that "we ought to have a virtual place where people can find data not balkanized, but readily usable."

To be sure, there is much to be excited about, but these advances also pose new challenges in data management. Next-generation sequencing (NGS) has the capacity to generate data at rates that exceed the rate of growth of compute and storage, both in performance and in scale. Storing and analyzing genomics data has become a quintessential big data challenge due to the high cost of owning and maintaining adequate compute resources.

This chapter offers a brief overview of data, exploring some of the major types of data and examining how data now has a changed role in the scientific process. From there we move to considering how data is managed, covering issues of security and compliance, as well as more detailed treatments of object storage (iRODS and OpenStack Swift). Following the chapter are case studies on the data demands of genetic sequencing, a SwiftStack data cluster at HudsonAlpha, and NimbleStorage (predictive flash storage) at Arizona State University.

BITS ABOUT DATA

Data has grown greatly in complexity and scope. This chapter does not try to define data, and we devote only a bit of energy to a typology of data. Instead, we focus on the changed role that data, primarily digital data, plays in science and on the sheer scale of data produced by high-throughput genomics.

In a 2013 TEDMED presentation, Dr. Atul Butte, a professor at the University of California–San Francisco School of Medicine, declared that the scientific method is dead. "Who needs the scientific method? Vast stores of available data and outsourced research are simply waiting for the right questions" [2]. Butte's lab uses vast troves of genomic and other data to author advanced tools with the capacity to convert more than 400 trillion points of molecular, clinical, and epidemiological data collected by researchers and clinicians over the past decade (now colloquially known as big data) into diagnostics, therapeutics, and new insights into disease. According to Butte, big data has fundamentally changed the nature of science. Rather than beginning by defining a problem and asking questions, science can now begin with data, which in the past was gathered as the second phase of the scientific method. Table 3.1 offers a schematic representation of the scientific method. Regardless of whether you believe that the scientific method has been fundamentally changed, it is certain that big data is a huge resource that scientific research can and will draw on.

Table 3.1 The Scientific Method

Known Process (Simplified)	Related Activity	Emerging Process	Related Activity
1. Problem definition	Problem statement Desired outcome Ask a question	1. Information collection	Large-scale data repositories sit idle Collection not required
2. Information collection	Data collection (Information)	2. Problem definition	Problem statement Desired outcome Formulate a question
3. Formulate hypothesis	Educated guess	3. Formulate hypothesis	Educated guess
4. Test	Test	4. Test	Test
5. Conclusion	Conclusion/Retest Use results/Discard	5. Conclusion	Conclusion/Retest Use results/Discard

Historically, defining a problem and formulating a desired outcome led to the collection and identification of data for testing. Today there is much more data than resources to evaluate it, and the true challenges are around the questions and methodologies to extract actionable answers. In 2008, Chris Anderson, in an article titled "The End of Theory: The Data Deluge Makes the Scientific Method Obsolete," observed that viewing data through the lens of petascale was futuristic. In 2016 the challenge of *exascale* data is upon us [3]. With the Internet of Things (IoT) and countless sensors, cloud storage and processors, high-capacity imaging, high-throughput sequencing, numerous multipetabyte electronic medical records and electronic health repositories, and knowledge that all this data is potentially actionable, we find ourselves in a very different world—one in which we must struggle to generate the best questions to ask.

With the big data deluge we are only now coming to understand how different data sources interrelate in the realm of analysis of nonobvious relationships or Non-Obvious Relationship Awareness (NORA), a term coined by Jeff Jonas [4]. NORA is a technique originally designed to identify casino fraud and was funded by the Central Intelligence Agency; IBM acquired the technology in 2005. NORA detects similar entities or identities across multiple relational databases. This is a simplified explanation of the technology, although it demonstrates a key component of data analysis where currently unknown interrelationships in data ecosystems and data networking (comparison of differential data sources) make discarding data potentially riskier than retaining it.

The volume of raw data high-throughput genomics generates—on the order of terabytes to petabytes per day—can be overwhelming. With a 2025 target of between 100 million and 2 billion human genomes sequenced, according to a report published in the journal *PLoS Biology*, data storage demands for this alone will be expected to absorb 2 to 40 exabytes (1 exabyte is 10^{18} bytes) [5]. To illustrate: In comparison, YouTube projects annual storage needs of 1 to 2 exabytes of video by 2025, and Twitter projects 1 to 17 petabytes (PB) per year (1 PB is 10^{15} bytes). It even exceeds the 1 exabyte per year projected for what will be the world's largest astronomy project, the Square Kilometre Array, to be sited in South Africa and Australia. And even if we are able to meet the storage challenge, technology writer Antonio Regalado notes that "the unfolding calamity in genomics is that a great deal of life-saving information, though already collected, is inaccessible" [6]. This inaccessibility can be due to lack of compute resources and other limitations.

The raw storage, management, and infrastructure needs are only a small part of the challenge. The computing requirements for acquiring, distributing, and analyzing genomic data are far more demanding. The volume of data that must be stored for a single genome is 30 times larger than the size of the genome itself to account for errors incurred during sequencing and preliminary analysis. Only after the raw sequence data has been processed is it useful to the scientific community.

DATA TYPES

Data, of course, is not all the same. There are quite a few important differences, and data is often classified according to type. As with many typologies, data typologies are imperfect. Types of data overlap and blend into each other. Part of this is due to the fact that designations are often driven by vendors trying to lay claim to those terms (and to market share). Despite all this, it is very much worth our time to consider some of the major types of data and their most important differences.

Structured Data

The term "structured data" generally refers to any data type that resides in a fixed field, record, table, index, or file. In its most common sense, the term should be reserved for relational databases, spreadsheets, or query-based systems that utilize Structured Query Language (SQL). SQL has been a standard of the American National Standards Institute since 1986. Unlike many of the other data types, structured data has its own standards and a high degree of built-in organization, increasing its portability and adoption.

Unstructured Data

Unstructured data tends to serve as the big catchall for flat file types. The majority of genomics and biomedical research data is unstructured data. The term "flat file" typically refers to a file type that lacks descriptive details about its own identity, content, and provenance. A popular methodology for management of such data is object-based management, where thoughtful attributes are assigned to data/files and then made available for query in a structured or semistructured manner. Unstructured data tends to be the most populous as multiple copies tend to exist in storage silos where deduplication does not exist or where unstructured data types are stored both in native format and in an object-based repository. As discussed later, object storage is considered semistructured data because typically it is unstructured data along with structured metadata (data about data). Examples of some of the most common types of unstructured data are image data (JPEG, TIF, GIF, and PNG) or documents in PDF format. For a helpful complete listing of common image file formats, please visit the Cornell University Library (https://www.library.cornell.edu/preservation/tutorial/presentation/table7-1.html) or Wikipedia (https://en.wikipedia.org/wiki/Image_file_formats).

Semistructured Data

Semistructured data is commonly a database model where there is no schema, but which contains tags, markers, or metadata. Object storage in which unstructured data is stored along with metadata is the most common example of semistructured data in biomedicine. The creation of metadata is not only influenced by the data itself but by the purpose of the store. For example, a BAM, a binary file for sequence data storage, has known attributes based on the file; however, additional metadata could include parameters external to the file, such as "principal investigator" or "study used in." For a quick example consider this: a common medical record in PDF format is considered unstructured data, but it becomes semistructured data when you create metadata in the form of metadata tags for the unstructured file (often referred to as an object) where that metadata can be used to locate or organize the document. But remember, the document still lacks the high-level or complex organization to be considered structured data. Extensible Markup Language or XML, e-mail messages, JavaScript Object Notation or JSON, and Electronic Data Interchange or EDI are commonly used examples of semistructured data.

The primary advantage to this data management model is that data can be represented and compared and new relationships can be created and/or defined. It's best to consider this a database model where there is no separation between the data and the schema; therefore, information for data sources is not constrained by schema limitations requiring potentially costly schema redesign. Semistructured data also enables: flexibility for developers; support for nested and hierarchical data models; simplification of the representation of complex attributes/relationships between entities; and ease of serialization (typically), which in the Hadoop ecosystem plays a key role in reducing object-relational impedance mismatch (a set of technical difficulties that could occur when a relational database management system [RDBMS] is being used by an application written in an object-oriented programming language or style, particularly when objects or class definitions are mapped in a straightforward way to database tables or relational schemata). Hibernate.org explains:

> "Object-Relational Impedance Mismatch" (sometimes called the "paradigm mismatch") is just a fancy way of saying that object models and relational models do not work very well together. RDBMSs represent data in a tabular format (a spreadsheet is a good visualization for those not familiar with RDBMSs), whereas object-oriented languages, such as Java, represent it as an interconnected graph of objects [7].

When you move between the two, a number of mismatching problems can occur.

Most modern semistructured models have nonnative or SQL-like tool sets, although traditional RDBMS models are designed for SQL. However, semistructured data can be prone to inefficient data modeling by removing the typical restraints to a preorganized framework. The flexibility in design could lead to shortcuts in application design leading to "garbage in, garbage out" application design. MongoDB and Couchbase are databases/data stores that store data natively in JSON format, leveraging the advantages of semistructured data architecture.

Polystructured Data

Polystructured data, multistructured data, and semistructured data overlap, but all typically indicate a defined database management system. These new terms are lazy replacements for complex structured data types that contain both an organizational index and a "schema on demand" system where objects have both metadata and some metadata management framework. Complex structured data includes e-mail messages, text, voice, video, tagged images, spatial data, geographical information system (GIS) data, and others.

We often see polystructured data in computational archaeology, where we have objects with embedded images and metadata (i.e., a GIF with JSON reference). Usually complex structured data can be organized into simpler referential structures that can be easily located and retrieved. This organizational model is the closest match to data types within the biomedical informatics realm. Examples of polystructured data include data created by IoT devices, software components, social media, and high-performance analytics that create interdisciplinary data.

DATA SECURITY AND COMPLIANCE

Before diving into how to store and work with large quantities of genomics and biomedical data, we consider the current state and future directions of data security and compliance.

At the time of this writing, only a handful of federal granting agencies, most notably the National Science Foundation and the National Institutes of Health, require researchers to submit data management plans as part of their grant proposals. The research community is expecting the number of federal granting agencies requiring data management plans to increase as the agencies release how they will respond to the Office of Science and Technology Policy (OSTP) policy memorandum [8]. The memorandum, dated February 22, 2013, directs federal agencies with more than $100 million in research and development expenditures to develop plans to make the published results of federally funded research freely available to the public within one year of publication and requiring researchers to better account for and manage the digital data resulting from federally funded scientific research [9].

The U.S. Department of Energy Office of Science released the Statement on Digital Data Management on July 28, 2014. The NIH released the NIH Genomic data sharing policy on August 27, 2014. It is expected that human genome data and collected samples could soon fall under data classification as protected health information (PHI) and therefore also fall under the governance of Health Insurance Portability and Accountability Act controls.

As additional federal agencies require researchers to share their data as described in a data management plan, it will become more important for research institutions and universities to develop options for data repositories that meet compliance challenges.

Data repositories would provide:

- Centralized places for researchers to deposit their data.
- Ways to make data available, accessible, searchable, and durable.
- Increased confidence for universities and funding agencies regarding results, resources, and infrastructure.

The compliance models outlined next can provide guidance and some general considerations for your institution's data management. Many institutions are subject to one or more or none, depending on the types of research and institution.

Controls and Responsibility

Implementing Information Security Standards and Guidelines

For the research university the responsibilities, rights over research data (including research generated data), and stewardship of the scientific record for projects conducted fall under the auspices of the university and/or are based on both federal regulations and sound management principles. Some of the responsibility of research universities with respect to data management are listed below.

- Compliance with federal grant requirements with respect to the management, access, and retention of research data to support grant payments throughout the funding life cycle and at times beyond.
- Compliance with the terms of sponsored project agreements, including clinical trial agreements with partner institutions and external entities.
- Protection and security for the university's intellectual property rights; and facilitation for potential investigations in the event of allegations of research misconduct or conflict of interest.
- Protection of the rights of students, postdoctoral appointees, staff and other collaborators, including, but not limited to, their rights to access data from research in which they were a participant.
- Appropriate data management related to the use of human subjects, animals, recombinant DNA, biological agents or toxins, etiological agents, radioactive materials, and the like (partially defined in 45 Code of Federal Regulations 46) [10].
- Establishment of procedures for long-term research projects and protection of essential records in the event of a natural disaster or other emergency. Typically data retention and archive have not been clear elements outlined in funding opportunities.

National Institute of Standards and Technology, Federal Information Processing Standards, and Federal Information Security Management Act

For research labs and research institutions, controls and responsibilities are often less clear than they are for either enterprises or university information technology (IT). We hope that controls and responsibilities become more consistent for biomedicine, both in statute and in practice.

The first two controls we touch on are defined in Federal Information Processing Standards (FIPS) 200 and National Institute of Standards and Technology (NIST) Special Publication (SP) 800-53 [11, 12]. FIPS 200 and NIST SP 800-53, in combination, ensure that appropriate security requirements and security controls are applied to all federal information and information systems. What is provided within the documents are the tools for an organizational assessment of risk and validation for the initial security controls including determination if additional controls are applicable. The resulting set of security controls establishes a level of security and due diligence for the organization. The controls both stem from the Federal Information Security Management Act (FISMA) of 2002 [13]. FISMA is a significantly larger framework with defined levels and callouts. The key point here is to understand the hierarchical nature of the compliance frameworks and get comfortable with the acronyms and overall compliance family. For reference, FISMA has three levels: low, moderate, and high. FISMA accreditation is based on three primary security objectives: confidentiality, integrity, and availability of systems and data.

FISMA accreditation for a research university is not a one-size-fits-all proposition. Typically universities become interested in accreditation in direct response to a large-scale funding opportunity or emerging center. In those cases, the institution is seeking a public cloud partner that meets the desired FISMA level. Approximately 65% of accredited systems in the government today are moderate, another 15% are low, and the remaining 20% are high. It would be rare to find a research project requiring controls above moderate. Additional FISMA information can be found at: http://csrc.nist.gov/groups/SMA/fisma/.

As indicated, the policy frameworks at the federal level have continued to adapt to current and emerging threat levels and attack surfaces. As of this writing, NIST SP 800-53 (Version 4) represents the most comprehensive update to the security controls catalog since its inception in 2005. This revision of the document includes eight new families of privacy controls.

Key characteristics are the "Build It Right" strategy, which is the latest holistic strategy launched to address the increasingly widened attack surface for adversaries, foreign and domestic. Within the controls are security controls for "Continuous Monitoring" to give organizations near-real-time information essential for decision making. In Chapter 5, which focuses on big data, we briefly discuss how institutions have adopted tools like Splunk to collect enormous amounts of data to meet the goal of continuous monitoring. Continuous monitoring is not even on the horizon for most biomedical researchers, nor should it be; rather, it is the domain of IT and data managers.

NIST SP 800-53 aims to provide the following information:

- Assumptions related to security control baseline development
- Expanded, updated, and streamlined guidance tailored to particular situations

- Additional assignment and selection statement options for security and privacy controls
- Descriptive names for security and privacy control enhancements
- Consolidated tables for security controls and control enhancements by family with baseline allocations
- Tables for security controls that support development, evaluation, and operational assurance
- Mapping tables for international security standards of the International Organization for Standardization and the International Electrotechnical Commission (ISO/IEC) 15408 (Common Criteria)

The addition of these parameters makes the NIST SP 800-53 far more user friendly and readable than previous materials released by the Defense Information Systems Agency (DISA), which is the controlling body for the Security Technical Implementation Guides (STIGs) [14, 15]. The DISA STIGs supply technical implementation guides for Department of Defense– and National Security Agency–compliant infrastructure components from the perspective of configuration elements. The STIGs contain technical guidance to lock down information systems/software that might otherwise be vulnerable to malicious computer attacks. If you can achieve compliant lockdown status and still have a usable component, you have done enough to meet compliance with any and all of the other compliance requirements named in this chapter. The Centers for Medicare & Medicaid Services and other highly sensitive groups enforce DISA-STIG compliance for infrastructure components.

Figure 3.1 shows a small sampling of the technical implementation guides available on the Information Assurance Support Environment (IASE) web portal (IASE Information Assurance Support Environment).

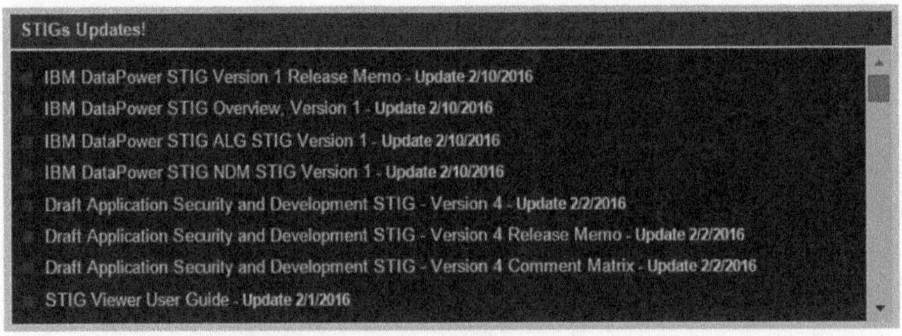

STIGs Updates!
IBM DataPower STIG Version 1 Release Memo - Update 2/10/2016
IBM DataPower STIG Overview, Version 1 - Update 2/10/2016
IBM DataPower STIG ALG STIG Version 1 - Update 2/10/2016
IBM DataPower STIG NDM STIG Version 1 - Update 2/10/2016
Draft Application Security and Development STIG - Version 4 - Update 2/2/2016
Draft Application Security and Development STIG - Version 4 Release Memo - Update 2/2/2016
Draft Application Security and Development STIG - Version 4 Comment Matrix - Update 2/2/2016
STIG Viewer User Guide - Update 2/1/2016

Figure 3.1 Security Technical Implementation Guides

Family Educational Rights and Privacy Act

The Family Educational Rights and Privacy Act (FERPA) (20 U.S.C. § 1232g; 34 CFR Part 99) is a federal law that protects the privacy of student education records [16]. The law applies to all schools that receive funds under an applicable program of the U.S. Department of Education. Generally FERPA controls apply only to central IT at the university, but they can lean into research depending on the nature of research and cohort involved.

Office of Science and Technology Policy

Congress established the Office of Science and Technology Policy (OSTP) in 1976 with a broad mandate to advise the president and others within the Executive Office of the President on the effects of science and technology on domestic and international affairs. The 1976 Act also authorizes OSTP to lead interagency efforts to develop and implement sound science and technology policies and budgets and to work with the private sector, state and local governments, the science and higher education communities, and other nations toward this end.

> The mission of the Office of Science and Technology Policy is threefold; first, to provide the President and his senior staff with accurate, relevant, and timely scientific and technical advice on all matters of consequence; second, to ensure that the policies of the Executive Branch are informed by sound science; and third, to ensure that the scientific and technical work of the Executive Branch is properly coordinated so as to provide the greatest benefit to society.
>
> **Strategic Goals and Objectives**
>
> - Ensure that Federal investments in science and technology are making the greatest possible contribution to economic prosperity, public health, environmental quality, and national security
> - Energize and nurture the processes by which government programs in science and technology are resourced, evaluated, and coordinated
> - Sustain the core professional and scientific relationships with government officials, academics, and industry representatives that are required to understand the depth and breadth of the Nation's scientific and technical enterprise, evaluate scientific advances, and identify potential policy proposals
> - Generate a core workforce of world-class expertise capable of providing policy-relevant advice, analysis, and judgment for the President and his senior staff regarding the scientific and

technical aspects of the major policies, plans, and programs of the Federal government [17]

In summary, NIST continues to be the prevalent provider of guidebooks for the greatest percentage of your research initiatives. FIPS 200 certification will be a key component of funding opportunities placed to federal agencies as the National Science Foundation (NSF), especially in programs directly related to information security. FISMA will serve as a control set for best practices for data center partners and external relationships where exposure of personally identification information (PII) or protected health information (PHI) are potential risk factors. OSTP will enact legislation and oversee funding critical to research and discovery of public value through thoughtful management of federal programs and initiatives. FERPA will have only limited application in the research domain but is a key compliance control for involvement in higher education where management of student data could be involved.

University Research Data Life Cycle

Now that we have reviewed security and compliance controls that would apply to research data management, we can start to look at the data life cycle within the research university. Figure 3.2 offers a conceptualized data life cycle for the research university. The life cycle for many research opportunities follows a common path from Proposal Creation, Project Launch (assuming successful funding), Data Collection, Data Analysis, Data Collaboration, and finally to Project Completion. The steps are described in somewhat greater detail next. Hopefully this schematic life cycle can help you and your organization think through data management needs and challenges over time.

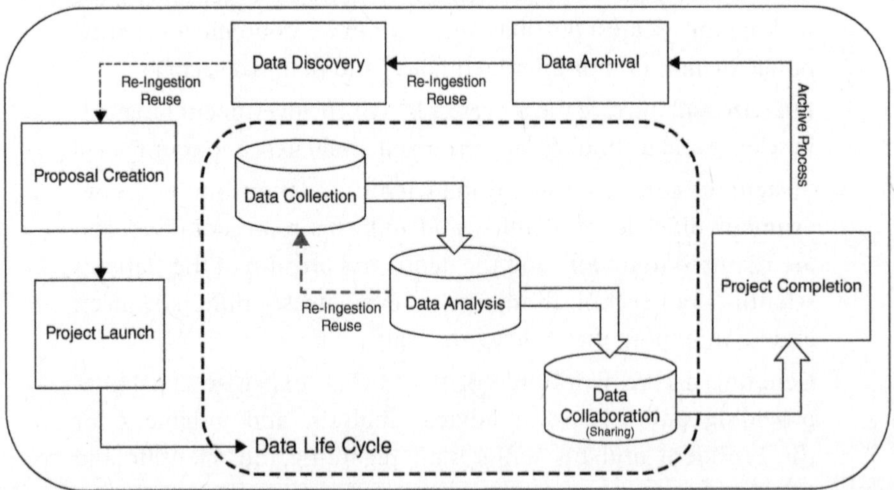

Figure 3.2 University Research Data Life Cycle

1. Proposal creation
   a. Audit of existing data sources assessment of applicability to current initiative.
   b. Determination of *de novo* data production in comparison to data reuse potential.
   c. Identification of stakeholders, data consumers, and applicable compliance regulations.
   d. Identification of data set performance requirements and storage performance tier.
   e. Map data life cycle to compliance regulations to create data management forecast.
2. Project launch
   a. Creation of data management plan.
   b. Creation of project-specific data life cycle policy.
   c. Identification of data sources for collection.
   d. Financial impact analysis.
3. Data collection
   a. Organization and execution of data collection/creation/download.
   b. Application and testing of access controls and security.
   c. Assignment of indexing parameters for metadata management.
   d. Staging and readiness.
4. Data analysis
   a. Data and document ingestion with analysis with metadata creation.
   b. File type(s) analysis including version control (normalization if applicable).
   c. Application and testing of access controls and security.
   d. Research testing with provenance assessment.
5. Data collaboration (publication/sharing)
   a. Reevaluation of desired collaborators with roles assignment.
   b. Publication methodologies and data sharing guidelines.
   c. Application and testing of access controls and security (internal audit).
   d. Documentation creation and publication of research-specific data sets.
6. Project completion
   a. Data relocation and migration strategy for retention and archive.
   b. Project completion audit with data validation/verification.
   c. Data search and access testing/index validation.

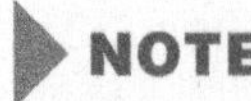

Additional concepts on managing data can be found at V. Van den Eynden, L. Corti, M. Woollard, and L. Bishop, *Managing and Sharing Data: A Best Practice Guide for Researchers* (Colchester, Essex: UK Data Archive University of Essex, 2009). http://www.data-archive.ac.uk/media/2894/managingsharing.pdf.

DATA STORAGE

As previously discussed and as you likely already know, biomedical data is growing extremely rapidly. Next-generation sequencing, precision medicine, electronic health records, and the IoT are all challenging our ability to store and manage data. Next we describe several promising approaches to biomedical data storage.

Object Storage

The majority of genomics data is unstructured data, and object storage is best suited to storing this sort of data. Two attributes of object storage make it particularly appealing to the biomedical community.

1. **Durable support for millions of files.** For example, Georgia Tech systems support 16 million JPG files in their remote-sensing GIS system. Typically, genomics produces millions of little files, not actually big data in the typical sense, but rather lots and lots of little data. The popular cloud storage provider Dropbox has a soft limit of 350,000 files and a hard limit of 1 million files, which makes it not ideal for this type of data.
2. **Editable metadata that is massively concurrent, highly durable, multitenant, and geographically distributed.** This is why Swift, the most popular object store, powers the largest cloud provider: Amazon S3 is a rolled version of Swift.

Object storage enables programmatic data management and the ability to create and maintain rich custom metadata within the object. Features such as data durability, access parameters, elasticity, and network accessibility are in-built features within most object storage offerings. The importance of individual components and features should be weighed on a case-by-case basis to determine which object storage will best fit your use case. The industry is moving quickly so it is worth doing your own research into the most current offerings.

Another major appeal of object storage is the ability to import external data from heterogeneous sources in disparate formats, publish through a common framework, and integrate with additional known relationship data. This allows data elements to be associated in a way that supports user-defined aggregated analyses. The metadata management components assist in the facilitation and extraction of knowledge from disparate data resources. This is of great value in biomedical research.

Object storage has been popular and widely used for more than 10 years. Originally produced at the Parallel Data Lab of Carnegie Mellon University in 1996, object storage became widely known as an EMC Centera product that debuted in 2002 and launched a multitude of software interfacing applications to interoperate with the technology. The original players all still have ongoing development in projects like the Google File System (GFS), Lustre, GlusterFS, and Amazon AWS S3. The OpenStack projects Ceph and Swift have also stimulated exponential growth in niche offerings, such as Caringo, Scality, Atmos, ViPR, DDN WOS, and Amplidata. There are many others, but we examine only ones that are open source and/or targeted toward bio-specific initiatives or use cases in biomedical informatics.

Below we offer an in-depth examination of SwiftStack (software built for Swift). Swift has become one of the most widely used object storage systems for the biological life sciences whether in its open source form or with SwiftStack. First, however, is a brief discussion of iRODS, a storage abstraction and federated service originally designed for use with block storage devices that is also relatively widely used in the biosciences.

Integrated Rule-Oriented Data System

The Integrated Rule-Oriented Data System (iRODS) is open source data management software that enables users to access, manage, and share data across any type or number of storage systems located anywhere while maintaining redundancy and security. At a high level, iRODS is a storage abstraction and federation service with support for a variety of backend storage products, including Amazon S3 and Swift (via Swift3 middleware). Although iRODS enables object storage features, it was originally designed to be used with block storage devices. iRODS lets users exercise precise control over their data with extensible rules that ensure the data is archived, described, and replicated in accordance with user needs and schedules. It also empowers users by supporting virtualization, which provides a one-stop shop for all data regardless of the heterogeneity of storage devices. Finally, iRODS supports data discovery through the use of descriptive metadata, workflow automation, and data sharing between collaborating or distributed teams.

iRODS is a second-generation data grid system that organizes distributed data into shared collections across large geographic areas and across administrative domains. iRODS was developed as open source data grid middleware based on experience gained with the development and deployment of the first-generation data grid system called the Storage Resource Broker (SRB). The first-generation SRB used data virtualization to hide the complexities and heterogeneity of storage systems from users and applications. The second-generation iRODS builds on data virtualization and extends it with policy virtualization to provide a transparent administrative and usage model for data grid services. One goal of iRODS is to enable object storage features on block storage systems.

Both iRODS and SRB were developed by the Data Intensive Cyber Environment Group (DICE) from 1995 to 2008 at the San Diego Supercomputer Center at the University of California, San Diego. The DICE group currently operates as a distributed virtual organization with team members located at the University of North Carolina at Chapel Hill (UNC), the Renaissance Computing Institute (RENCI), and the Institute for Neural Computation (INC) at the University of California, San Diego (UCSD). Development of the core iRODS data grid system is funded by grants to the DICE group from the Office of Cyber Infrastructure (OCI) at the NSF and from the National Archives and Records Administration (NARA). Discipline-centric and project-centric extensions to iRODS (and the earlier SRB) are provided by multiple grants from federal agencies including the NSF, NIH, Department of Energy (DOE), and National Aeronautics and Space Administration (NASA). An international collaboration participating in open source codevelopment of the iRODS technology is growing worldwide, with collaborators located in the United Kingdom, France, Taiwan, Australia, and the United States.

Storage Resource Broker (SRB) software was developed between 1995 and 2007. Currently major development of SRB has been suspended, and all the effort in the DICE group is focused on developing the iRODS software. But software support for SRB continues because of the rich and active user base that continues to rely on SRB for their data management needs. Bug fixes and minor features continue to be developed as per user requests and needs and releases of software versions are made periodically.

SRB has been used by over 200 projects all over the world. At University of California, San Diego, several domain-specific data grids are supported with collections containing a total of 200 million files and total size of over 1 PB. SRB is also used by the National Science Digital Library (NSDL), National Virtual Observatory (NVO), Biomedical Informatics Research Network (BIRN), and Southern California Earthquake Center (SCEC). Around the world, there are also large groups of users (Babar, UK eScience, Taiwan National Archives, French IN2P3, NOAO, NARA, etc.) that rely on the SRB system for distributed data management. Projects include local institutional data grids, regionally shared collections, and internationally shared collections. We believe the total size of collections in such usage to be over 2 PBs.

iRODS software development is funded by the National Science Foundation and National Archives and Records Administration. Multiple collaborative projects are under way, including an NSF DataNet Federation Consortium that is due to wrap up in August 2017. Under the current proposals, a rich development and deployment schedule is in process. Extensions to the core modules as well as new features are proposed.

Here are the main areas proposed for development:

- Extension to server architecture for additional drivers to access specific heterogeneous storage systems such as an object ring buffer
- Extension to the mounted collection feature for access to different kinds of bundled collections (zip files, AIP, SRB, gFarm, etc.)
- Extensions for structured resource access (OpenDAP, LDAP, etc.)
- Extensions for relational resource access (DB2, SQLserver, MySQL, etc.)
- Extensions to the iCAT catalog to support additional databases (DB2, SQLserver, MySQL, etc.)
- New version of the Rule Engine to support policies for federations of data grids
- Improvements to the Message Server to interact with enterprise bus architecture
- Improvements to batch and delayed execution servers for incorporating OOI control flow
- Extensions to iCAT to support an extensible schema and enhanced feature support in iCAT, including extended auditing and accounting
- Extensions for interactions with other third-party systems, such as SAML-based authorization, and extended authentication methods, such as LDAP and other user name services
- Deeper integration with digital library systems, such as Fedora Commons and Dspace, and indexing systems, such as Cheshire.
- Extensions to microservices for execution across multiple domains

These features have been proposed for design and development within the next five years by the DICE group and in collaboration with external partners.

The iRODS system is being used to support multiple, major projects, including:

NARA Transcontinental Persistent Archive Prototype (TPAP),

NSF Temporal Dynamics of Learning Center,

NSF Ocean Observatories Initiative, and the

French National Library.

Arizona State University is an iRODS consortium partner and is working to publish iRODS data management as a service.

While there is a lot of value to be drawn from the iRODS feature list, when considering whether it is a good fit for a particular solution, it is good to be aware of some risks.

Performance can suffer as iRODS adds an additional layer of systems that data has to pass through, and it adds additional database lookups to every data operation. iRODS is not easily scalable, in part because metadata is stored in multiple places that do not scale in the same way. Operations can be more complex because redundant metadata resides in multiple systems. Monitoring and alert diagnosis is also made more complicated by having to work through multiple systems to identify and repair the failure.

For these reasons, iRODS is best in situations where more than one storage system must be accessed via a common interface and unified namespace. Next we explore Swift, an object storage that redresses many of the shortcomings of iRODS. It is worth noting that many of the iRODS features just mentioned do not exist in a standard SwiftStack deployment. If some or all of those features are required, consider the following customization of SwiftStack that does not carry the same risks as iRODS. It is possible to add many additional capabilities and services to Swift. In summary, the best approach is to start with the set of requirements for a given project and then leverage all available options to develop the most robust, scalable, performant, and maintainable solution possible.

SWIFTSTACK*

SwiftStack is an object storage system that includes an unmodified, 100% open source release of OpenStack Swift at the core. In addition to Swift, SwiftStack provides extensive functionality for deploying, integrating, upgrading, and managing single- and multiregion Swift clusters coupled with enterprise support. SwiftStack object storage includes:

- OpenStack Swift Application Program Interface (API) and Amazon Web Services (AWS) S3 support
- Integrated filesystem access
- Erasure Codes and Replica storage policies
- Encryption
- Multiregion storage
- Storage policies
- Integrated load balancer
- Automated install process
- Capacity management
- No downtime, rolling upgrades

* Content contributed by Joe Arnold.

- LDAP and Active Directory integration
- Utilization API

A key characteristic of SwiftStack is that it decouples the control, management, and configuration of the Swift storage nodes from the physical hardware. Although the actual storage services run on the servers where Swift is installed, deployment, management, and monitoring are conducted out of band by a separate storage controller, which can manage one or more clusters. Figure 3.3 illustrates the main components of SwiftStack.

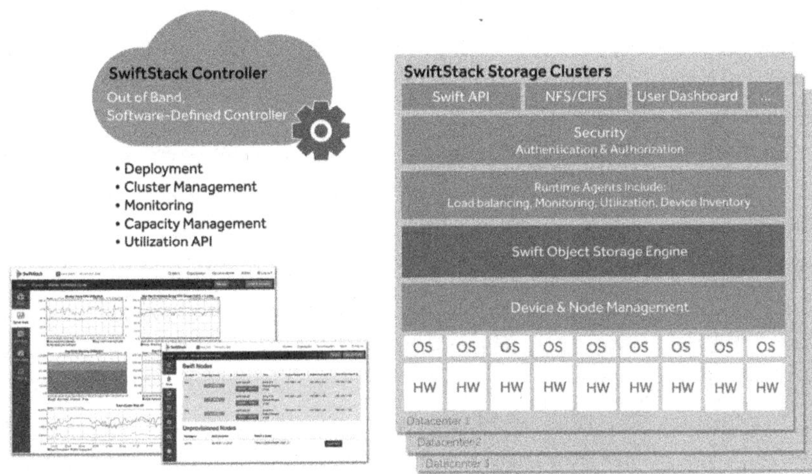

Figure 3.3 Components of SwiftStack

This approach has many benefits because operators can now: manage multiple, geographically distributed storage clusters from a single management system; dynamically tune clusters to optimize performance; respond to hardware failures; and upgrade clusters while they are still running. All of these capacities are driven programmatically for the entire storage tier, independent of where the storage resources are deployed.

Before exploring SwiftStack's capabilities in greater detail, we offer an overview of how genomic sequencing works with SwiftStack.

Genomic Sequencing with Object Storage

During the sequencing process, various storage and compute workflows are used in order to generate a genome sequence. In this section we cover the data that is generated during this process using Illumina sequencing instruments. Sequencing through a chemical and photographic process, Illumina sequencers analyze prepared genetic material on flow cells. Each lane is further subdivided and scanned multiple times.

The primary output of the sequencer is base call (BCL) files. While this data is initially stored on a workstation, it needs to be moved to a durable storage location that will be accessible for the next stage of the process.

This is where the first storage challenge comes in. With a fully running set of 10 Illumina HiSeq X sequencers, 4.6 million BCL files are generated in a three-day sequencing run. There are also millions of additional files and thumbnails, all of which are required for processing. The HiSeq X Ten System produces up to 13 terabytes (TB) across 20 million files over this three-day period.

This process requires the following storage characteristics:

Small-file ingest The storage system needs to be able to distribute files across a large number of individual storage devices (drives). This allows many drives to participate in the data ingest, increasing the throughput capability of the storage system. To accommodate this workload, OpenStack Swift/SwiftStack is architected to distribute data across many devices in a storage cluster, which provides high-throughput ingest of lots of small files over the course of multiple, back-to-back sequencing runs.

Highly durable writes As data is streaming from multiple sequencers, the storage system must be able to support a continuous ingest rate. Ideally, writes should be placed in a primary durable storage location. A write is fully durable to its primary locations with data placement algorithms in OpenStack Swift/SwiftStack. Either with multiple replicas or erasure codes, when a write is acknowledged, a durable write is complete.

Integration The workstation attached to a sequencer will either speak native object storage or will write to a filesystem Server Message Block (SMB) mount point. SwiftStack provides filesystem exports so that workstations can directly integrate with the object storage system with a filesystem mount point.

Raw data processing The next stage is consolidating the BCL data into a FASTQ format file. A compute cluster or large server is used for this processing. A typical FASTQ is a data file containing all sequence reads from a given instrument run. It summarizes the individual base calls and their associated quality scores for each read.

This consolidation process requires many high-throughput, small file reads. Each node in the compute cluster will be reading different sections of BCL files. This can place a lot of strain on a traditional file-based storage system. While some workloads can benefit from caching, this workload cannot. Each read into the storage system is for unique data. OpenStack Swift/SwiftStack scales horizontally for read requests. Read requests are distributed across the system, increasing performance.

Genome assembly/alignment The next operation is to map the reads in the FASTQ files to positions in the reference genome sequence. During the alignment processing DNA, schematically represented in Figure 3.4, sequences from the FASTQ files are aligned to the best-matching positions in the reference genome.

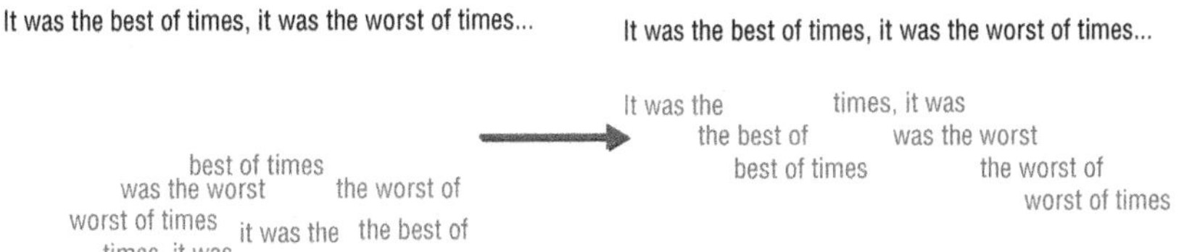

Figure 3.4 The Alignment Process Organizes Sequence Data

In the first step, software running in a compute cluster will generate an index of the FASTQ. This indexing process can be multithreaded. The second step is the alignment process itself, which is single-threaded but can be hardware accelerated.

The output of this process is a SAM file with aligned sequence data and metadata. SAM stands for Sequence Alignment Map and is a text file. This SAM file is compressed into binary format, BAM (Binary Alignment Map). This multigigabyte (GB) file is frequently stored, since it contains not just all sequence, quality, and position information but also is the product of significant computational steps that one might not want to repeat.

This alignment process outputs large files that require storage. If stored sequentially, large files can take a long time to write and read from a storage system. OpenStack Swift/SwiftStack supports large-file format that chunks up objects into smaller segments, making it possible to quickly load data in parallel.

Variant calling SAM files are around 400 GB for a whole human genome, and BAM files around 150 GB, depending on percentage of coverage and depth of coverage. The term "percentage of coverage" refers to how much of the reference genome was mapped. The "depth of coverage" is an average that describes how many times that given part of the genome was sequenced. The numbers just given represent 30-times coverage. Clinical sequencing of whole genomes may end up being two to three times deeper than research-grade genomes, which means two to three times more data. Sequencing of DNA from tissues made up of mixtures of cells (e.g., cancer and normal tissue, in a tumor) may be even deeper, to identify subpopulations with important variants.

In the variant calling step, the BAM file is analyzed to find differences (or variants) between the sample genome that was sequenced and the reference genome that the sample genome was aligned against. The most common kind of difference is a single nucleotide or base difference between the sample and reference, and these are called single nucleotide polymorphisms (SNPs). The entire set of variants is written to a file in a format called variant call format (VCF).

Variant calling requires high-throughput, large file uploads and downloads. These large input files benefit from parallel uploads and downloads for very fast transfer times. The files can be transferred into dedicated compute clusters for variant detection and visualization using BAM file viewers. OpenStack Swift/SwiftStack supports a standard method to upload a single file via multiple chunks. These chunks can also be used to do a multithreaded download of large objects so that they can be quickly transferred.

To review, the basic workflow of genomic sequencing with Swift is as follows:

1. **Genomic sequencing.** Cluster generates 13 TB of raw data across 20 million files in three days. Generates BCL files and images.
2. **Consolidation.** High-performance computing (HPC) cluster consolidates the BCL data into FASTQ format, which summarizes the individual base calls.
3. **Assembly/alignment.** Maps to a reference genome, generating a BAM file.
4. **Variant calling.** Analyzes BAM file to find differences between the sample and the reference genome.

Now that we are familiar with the genomics workflow with Swift, we move into a more detailed examination of how Swift and SwiftStack work.

Multiregion Management

SwiftStack provides a simple way to deploy, configure, and manage nodes across multiple regions and data centers. Swift organizes storage nodes by zones, regions, and possibly storage policies. Regions are a way to define parts of a cluster that are physically separate; most often this is geographic (regional). Within a region, the cluster can further be grouped into zones. Zones are generally created to help identify the failure points (e.g., all the nodes in one rack or all the nodes in one data center) so that the copies of the data can be placed in different zones and regions to isolate failures and ensure the durability and accessibility of the data in the cluster. We'll get into storage policies, which allow various data protection strategies, shortly, but the next example offers a look at how a two-region cluster with two zones per region might store four copies of one object as far from each other as possible in separate regions and zones. This shows how the object would still be available even if a zone (e.g., top of rack switch dies) or region (e.g., citywide power outage) was temporarily unavailable

In the life sciences, multiple regions would be useful for two reasons: data protection and data distribution. When a second region is used for data protection, fewer proxy nodes need to be deployed. When a second region is used for data distribution, storage requests can be routed to nearby data, improving latency and reducing network congestion.

SwiftStack makes configuration of regions and zones in a cluster simple by providing operators with a web interface, as shown in Figure 3.5, that easily allows the addition and removal of regions and zones.

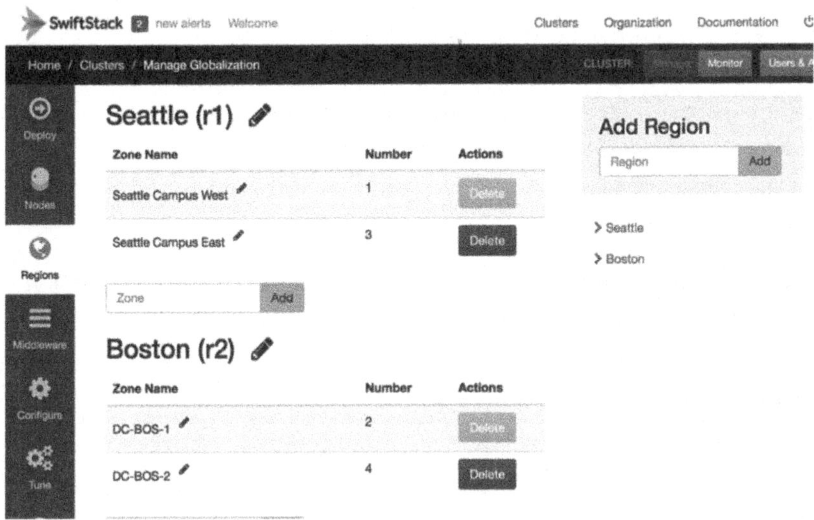

Figure 3.5 Multiregion and Zone Management with SwiftStack Controller

Storage Policy Management

While regions and zones serve as a way to organize nodes, storage policies are used in Swift as a way to organize and manage objects. This is done by applying storage policies to containers that hold objects. One policy is applied to one container, and then all objects placed in it will be handled according to that policy. The policies affect the objects, so they are object storage policies, but they are commonly referred to as storage policies.

The default configuration of a Swift cluster will have all nodes available for storage, and a default object storage policy is applied automatically to containers. This default policy says that objects should be copied so that a total of three copies will be saved across the cluster. In addition to replica storage policies, erasure codes can be used for single-region and multiregion storage policies. Custom storage policies are created when you want objects to be stored differently. For example, if the objects will be stored only on a subset of nodes (e.g., only the ones with solid-state drives (SSDs)) or if a different number of copies of the data should be stored.

Storage policies allow objects to be stored based on these criteria:

1. Data protection strategy—number of replicas or erasure code strategy
2. Performance of drives
3. Geographical location (region/zone)
4. Efficient data placement based on projected ring size

Example Use Cases

Swift's configuration options allow a great deal of flexibility in how data is stored in the cluster. Different options work better for different use cases. A benefit of using storage policies is that a single Swift deployment can offer multiple data storage options at the same time, allowing it to best serve multiple use cases. These use cases cover some common scenarios for life sciences data.

- Highly scalable flat storage (standard, 3-replica)
  - **Use case:** Large variety of files and access patterns. Availability and simplicity is most important.
  - **Number of replicas:** Three
- Highly available geodistributed
  - **Use case:** Data is created and accessed in multiple geodistributed regions. A failure at one site should not disrupt access to storage in another.
  - **Number of replicas:** Two per region
- Archive store
  - **Use case:** Data is stored and retrieved for archival purposes.
  - Use erasure coding storage policy with 27% overhead.

Storage policies are easy to manage through SwiftStack's web interface, as shown in Figure 3.6.

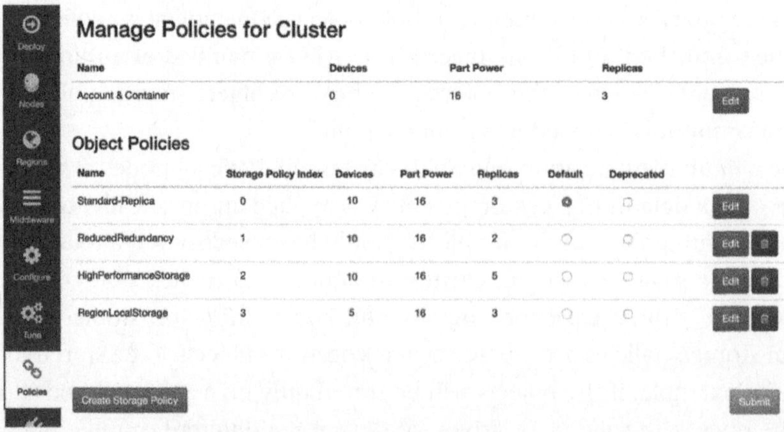

Manage Policies for Cluster

Name	Devices	Part Power	Replicas
Account & Container	0	16	3

Object Policies

Name	Storage Policy Index	Devices	Part Power	Replicas	Default	Deprecated
Standard-Replica	0	10	16	3		
ReducedRedundancy	1	10	16	2		
HighPerformanceStorage	2	10	16	5		
RegionLocalStorage	3	5	16	3		

Figure 3.6 Storage Policy Management with SwiftStack

Multigeneration Hardware Support

SwiftStack can incorporate multiple generations of storage hardware within the same storage cluster. This means there isn't a forklift upgrade. Instead, hardware can be replaced incrementally. This allows you to take advantage of the hardware upgrade cycle where performance/capacity to price ratios are continuously going up.

Data Placement

By default, SwiftStack places data in cluster locations that are as unique as possible. This lets Swift intelligently place data on any storage device in the cluster, preferring locations that are in different zones, nodes, and drives. All data stored in SwiftStack also has hand-off locations defined, which are alternative data placement locations in the cluster should one of the copies not be available due to a hardware failure.

Swift tries to evenly distribute data across all the devices (drives) and nodes in the system. Swift uses a consistent hashing ring to pseudorandomly distribute all copies of an object across the drives in the cluster according to the size of each.

Gradual Capacity Adjustment

When adding new capacity, you usually don't add just one hard drive. It is more typical to add a new server with many drives or a rack filled with servers. That's a pretty good chunk of data capacity. Swift has built-in capabilities that let administrators control the addition of capacity to a cluster, to prevent network bottlenecks and ensure that data is not left vulnerable during large capacity changes.

SwiftStack takes it a step further and automates the process so that administrators do not need to calculate and kick off round after round of gradual adjustments. Instead, the SwiftStack Controller automates the process of adding capacity (e.g., new drives or new nodes) to a Swift cluster.

Undelete and Delete Prevention

Certain sequence data may be precious due to limited availability of the sample, or particular sequence data may have to be retained for long periods of time due to regulatory concerns. SwiftStack provides a mechanism for data retention beyond the user deletion date. For example, if a user deletes an object, it can be configured to be recoverable for a certain number of days. Additionally, the system can also be configured to prevent user deletion of data.

OPENSTACK SWIFT ARCHITECTURE

We look at the key characteristics of Swift, explain the fundamental concepts (accounts, containers, and objects), examine Swift's architecture, and discuss how Swift places data. We finish by walking through a few scenarios to show how all these components work together. This chapter also introduces you to the basics of the Swift API.

Swift Characteristics

Here is an overview of Swift's characteristics:

- Swift is an object storage system that is part of the OpenStack project.
- Swift is open source and freely available.
- Swift can be used as a stand-alone storage system.
- Swift runs on standard Linux distributions and on standard x86 server hardware.
- Swift supports Amazon S3 API.
- Applications store and retrieve data in Swift via an industry-standard RESTful HTTP API.
- Objects can have extensive metadata, which can be indexed and searched.
- Failed nodes and drives can be swapped out while the cluster is running with no downtime. New nodes and drives can be added the same way.

Up to now, we have just been saying that Swift can store objects. To be more precise, Swift enables users to store, retrieve, and delete objects (with their associated metadata) in containers via a RESTful HTTP API.

Swift Requests and Responses

Communication with a Swift cluster is done via HTTP using a RESTful API, which results in every request having a response returned. This request and response pairing is a fundamental part of HTTP communication. All requests sent to Swift are made up of at least three and sometimes four parts:

1. HTTP verb (e.g., GET, PUT, DELETE)
2. Authentication information
3. Storage URL
4. Data or metadata to be written or read (optional depending on the request type)

The HTTP verb provides the action of the request. For example, "I want to PUT this object into the cluster" or "I want to GET this account information out of the cluster."

The authentication information confirms the identity of the sender and verifies that the request is allowed to be fulfilled. The storage URL has two purposes: it is the cluster address where the request should be sent, and it is the storage location in the cluster where the requested action should take place.

A storage URL in Swift for an object looks like this:

https://swift.example.com/v1/account/container/object

Using the example, we can break the storage URL into its two main parts:

1. Cluster location: swift.example.com/v1/
2. Storage location (for an object): /account/container/object

The storage location is given in one of three formats:

1. /account

   The account storage location is a uniquely named storage area that contains the metadata (descriptive information) about the account itself as well as the list of containers in the account.

   It is important to keep in mind that in Swift, an account is not a user identity. When you hear the word "account," think storage area.

2. /account/container

   The container storage location is the user-defined storage area within an account where metadata about the container itself and the list of objects in the container will be stored.

3. /account/container/object

   The object storage location is where the object itself and its metadata will be stored.

Figure 3.7 illustrates the relationship between accounts, containers, and objects.

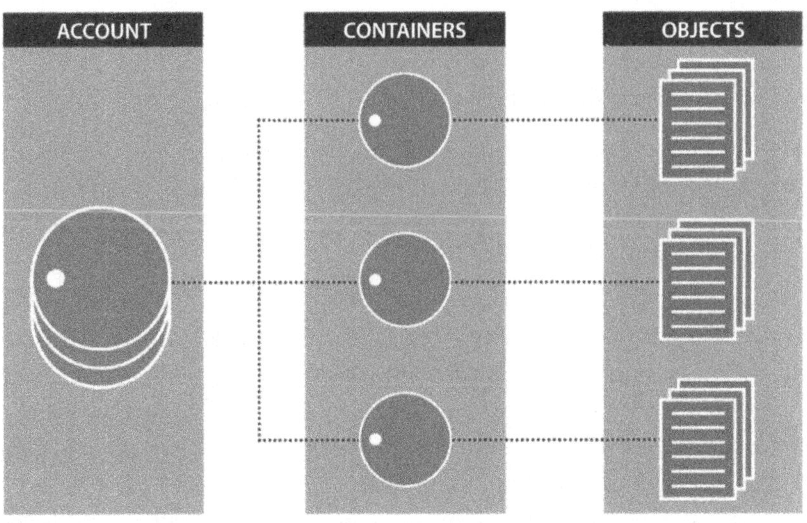

Figure 3.7 Account, Containers, and Objects

Swift HTTP API

A command-line client interface, such as curl, is all you need to perform simple operations on your Swift cluster. But many users require more sophisticated client applications. Behind the scenes, all Swift applications, including the command-line clients, use Swift's HTTP API to access the cluster.

Swift's HTTP API is RESTful, meaning that it exposes every container and object as a unique URL and maps HTTP methods (like PUT, GET, POST, and DELETE) to the common data management operations (Create, Read, Update, and Destroy—collectively known as CRUD).

Swift makes use of most HTTP verbs, including:

- **GET.** Downloads objects, lists the contents of containers or accounts
- **PUT.** Uploads objects, creates containers, overwrites metadata headers
- **POST.** Creates containers if they don't exist, updates metadata (accounts or containers), overwrites metadata (objects)
- **DELETE.** Deletes objects and containers that are empty
- **HEAD.** Retrieves header information for the account, container, or object

Client Libraries

Application developers can construct HTTP requests and parse HTTP responses using their programming language's HTTP client, or they may choose to use open source language bindings to abstract away the details of the HTTP interface. Open source client libraries are available for most modern programming languages, including Python, Ruby, PHP, C#/.NET, and Java.

What happens once a request is sent to the cluster? Before we take a look at how the cluster handles a request, first let's look at how a cluster is put together.

Swift Overview—Processes

A Swift cluster is the distributed storage system used for object storage. It is a collection of machines that are running Swift's server processes and consistency services. Each machine running one or more Swift processes and services is called a node.

The core Swift server processes are proxy, account, container, and object. When a node has only the proxy server process running, it is called a proxy node. Nodes running one or more of the other server processes (account, container, or object) often are called storage nodes. Storage nodes contain the data that incoming requests wish to affect (e.g., a PUT request for an object would go to the appropriate nodes running the object server processes). Storage nodes also have a number of other services running on them to maintain data consistency.

When talking about the same server processes running on the nodes in a cluster, we call it the server process layers (e.g., proxy layer, account layer, container layer, and object layer). Let's look a little more closely at the server process layers.

Server Process Layers

Proxy Services

The proxy server processes are the public face of Swift as they are the only ones that communicate with external clients. As a result, they are the first and last to handle an API request. All requests to and responses from the proxy use standard HTTP verbs and response codes.

Proxy servers use a shared-nothing architecture and can be scaled as needed based on projected workloads. A minimum of two proxy servers should be deployed for redundancy. Should one proxy server fail, the others will take over.

For example, if a valid request is sent to Swift, then the proxy server will verify the request, determine the correct storage nodes responsible for the data (based on a hash of the object name), and send the request to those servers concurrently. If the primary storage nodes are unavailable, the proxy will choose appropriate hand-off nodes to send the request to. The nodes will return a response and the proxy will, in turn, return the first response (and data if it was requested) to the requester.

Remember that the proxy server process is looking up multiple locations because Swift provides data durability by writing multiple complete copies or erasure coded fragments of the data and storing them in the system.

ProxyFS Services

The proxyFS server processes provide a filesystem using access using a native log-structured object format. These services include the proxy server processes and therefore include the logic of how individual objects are durably written into the object storage services.

Swift includes multiple object formats for defining how an object is represented. For example, large objects can be broken up into segments using a manifest file with static large objects (SLOs). To support the dynamic nature of filesystem access, a log-structured file format is used for both files and the directory tree.

With log-structured files in Swift, file or directory tree updates are written as new objects, and a corresponding filesystem log is updated. This permits file modifications without replacing an entire file. It also supports file renaming and moving files in the directory hierarchy. Log-structured files can also be serviced with object API requests. This enables data compatibility in workflows where applications use both filesystem and object APIs.

To facilitate coordination with other clients of the filesystem, proxyFS servers make use of a distributed key-value store to support filesystem clustering.

Account Services

The account server process handles requests regarding metadata for the individual accounts or the list of the containers within each account. This information is stored by the account server process.

Container Services

The container server process handles requests regarding container metadata or the list of objects within each container. It's important to note that the list of objects doesn't contain information about the location of the object, simply that it belongs to a specific container.

Object Services

The object server process is responsible for the actual storage of objects on the drives of its node. Objects are stored as binary files on the drive using a path that is made up in part of its associated partition (which we discuss shortly) and the operation's timestamp. The object's metadata (standard and custom) is stored in the file's extended attributes, which means that the data and metadata are stored together and copied as a single unit.

Consistency Services

A key aspect of Swift is that it was built with the knowledge that failures happen and works around them. When account, container, or object server processes are running on a node, it means that data is being stored there. This means that consistency services will also be running on those nodes to ensure the integrity and availability of the data.

The two main consistency services are auditors and replicators. There are also a number of specialized services that run in support of individual server processes (e.g., the account reaper that runs where account server processes are running).

Auditors

Auditors run in the background on every storage node in a Swift cluster and continually scan the disks to ensure that the data stored on disk has not suffered any bit rot or filesystem corruption. There are account auditors, container auditors, and object auditors that run to support their corresponding server process.

If an error is found, the auditor moves the corrupted object to a quarantine area.

Replicators

Account, container, and object replicator processes run in the background on all nodes that are running the corresponding services. A replicator will continuously examine its local node and compare the accounts, containers, and objects against the copies on other nodes in the cluster. If one of the other nodes has an old or missing copy, then the replicator will send a copy of its local data out to that node. Replicators only push their local data out to other nodes; they do not pull in remote copies if their local data is missing or out of date. For a schematic representation, see Figure 3.8.

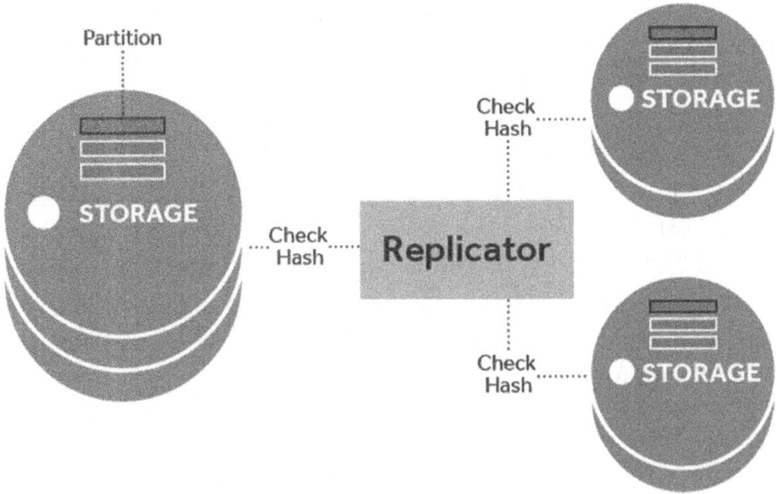

Figure 3.8 Replicators Examine the Checksums of Partitions

The replicator also handles object and container deletions. Object deletion starts by creating a zero-byte tombstone file that is the latest version of the object. This version is then replicated to the other nodes and the object is removed from the entire system.

Container deletion can happen only with an empty container. It will be marked as deleted and the replicators will push this version out.

Swift Overview—Cluster Architecture

Nodes

A node is a machine that is running one or more Swift processes. When multiple nodes are running that provide all the processes needed for Swift to act as a distributed storage system, they are considered a cluster.

Within a cluster, the nodes also belong to two logical groups: regions and nodes. Regions and nodes are user-defined and identify unique characteristics about a collection of nodes—usually geographical location and points of failure, such as all the power running to one rack of nodes. These ensure that Swift can place data across different parts of the cluster to reduce risk.

Regions

Regions are user-defined and usually indicate when parts of the cluster are physically separate—usually a geographical boundary. A cluster has a minimum of one region, and there are many single-region clusters as a result. A cluster that is using two or more regions is a multiregion cluster.

When a read request is made, the proxy layer favors nearby copies of the data as measured by latency. When a write request is made, the proxy layer, by default, writes to all the locations simultaneously. There is an option called write affinity that, when enabled, allows the cluster to write all copies locally and then transfer them asynchronously to the other regions.

Zones

Within regions, Swift allows availability zones to be configured to isolate failure boundaries. An availability zone should be defined by a distinct set of physical hardware whose failure would be isolated from other zones. In a large deployment, availability zones may be defined as unique facilities in a large data center campus. In a single data center deployment, the availability zones may be different racks. While there does need to be at least one zone in a cluster, it is far more common for a cluster to have many zones.

Swift Overview—Data Placement

We mentioned earlier that there are several locations for data because Swift makes copies and stores them across the cluster. This section covers this process in greater detail.

When the server processes or the consistency services need to locate data, they look at the storage location (/account, /account/container, /account/container/object) and consult one of the three rings: account ring, container ring, or object ring.

Each Swift ring is a modified consistent hashing ring that is distributed to every node in the cluster. The boiled-down version is that a modified consistent hashing ring contains a pair of lookup tables that the Swift processes and services use to determine data locations. One table has the information about the drives in the cluster; the other has the table used to look up where any piece of account, container, or object data should be placed. That second table—where to place things—is the more complicated one to populate. Before we further discuss the rings and how they are built, we should cover partitions and replicas as they are critical concepts to understanding the rings.

Partitions

Swift wants to store data uniformly across the cluster and have it be available quickly for requests. The developers of Swift tried various methods and designs before settling on the current variation of the modified consistent hashing ring.

Hashing is the key to the data locations. When a process, like a proxy server process, needs to find where data is stored for a request, it calls on the appropriate ring to get a value that it needs to correctly hash the storage location (the second part of the storage URL). The hash value of the storage location maps to a partition value.

This hash value is one of hundreds or thousands of hash values that could be calculated when hashing storage locations. The full range of possible hash values is the "hashing ring" part of a modified consistent hashing ring.

The "consistent" part of a modified consistent hashing ring is where partitions come into play. The full range of hash values in a hashing ring is chopped up into numerous smaller ranges. Each of these parts of the hashing ring, called partitions, can be mapped to a drive. As drives are added or removed storage would be mapped randomly around the ring and either take hash ranges from or release hash ranges to the mapped drives that were adjacent to it. Over time this would produce partitions with much larger and much smaller ranges than average, which increases the likelihood that objects will be unavailable during capacity changes.

To address the churn and availability issues, Swift uses a modified consistent hashing ring where the partitions are a set number and uniform in size. As a ring is built, the partitions are assigned to drives in the cluster. This implementation is conceptually simple—a partition is just a directory sitting on a disk with a corresponding hash table of what it contains.

Storage nodes have disks. Partitions are represented as directories on each disk. The relationship of a storage node, a disk, and a partition is represented in Figure 3.9.

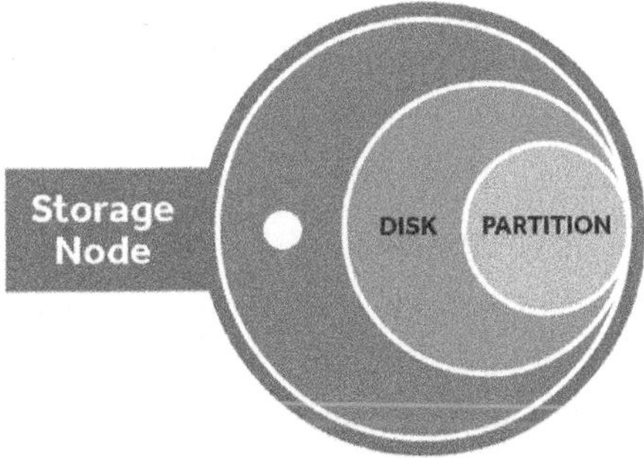

Figure 3.9 The Relationship of a Storage Node, a Disk, and a Partition

While the size and number of partitions does not change, the number of drives in the cluster does. The more drives in a cluster, the fewer partitions per drive. For a simple example, if there were 150 partitions and two drives, then each drive would have 75 partitions mapped to it. If a new drive is added, then each of the three drives would have 50 partitions.

Partitions are the smallest unit that Swift likes to work with—data is added to partitions, consistency processes check partitions, and partitions are moved to new drives. By having many of the actions happen at the partition level, Swift is able to keep processor and network traffic low. This also means that as the system scales up, behavior continues to be predictable because the number of partitions remains fixed.

Replicas

Swift's durability and resilience to failure depends in large part on its replicas. The more replicas used, the more protection against losing data when there is a failure. This is especially true in clusters that have separate data centers and geographic regions to spread the replicas across.

When we say "replicas," we mean partitions that are replicated. Most commonly a replica count of three is chosen. During the initial creation of the Swift rings, every partition is replicated, and each replica is placed as uniquely as possible across the cluster. Each subsequent rebuilding of the rings calculates which, if any, of the replicated partitions need to be moved to a different drive. Part of partition replication includes designating hand-off drives. When a drive fails, the replication/auditing processes notice and push the missing data to handoff locations. The probability that all replicated partitions across the system will become corrupt (or otherwise fail) before the cluster notices and is able to push the data to handoff locations is very small, which is why we say that Swift is durable.

Previously we talked about proxy server processes using a hash of the data's storage location to determine where in the cluster that data is located. We can now be more precise and say that the proxy server process is locating the three replicated partitions, each of which contains a copy of the data.

Erasure Codes

Erasure codes are like fractional replicas. The basic idea is to break up the original data into smaller pieces and compute a set of chunks of data so that you can re-create any missing pieces if you lose them, up to a certain number of chunks. With a Reed-Solomon–style encoding, data is broken into m data chunks, and then k parity chunks are computed (for a total of n chunks). So a 10+4 scheme has 14 total chunks and can withstand the loss of any four chunks.

In Swift, the ring stores a primary partition for each of the total number of chunks (e.g., 14 in a 10+4 scheme). As data comes into the cluster, it is encoded and the chunks are spread out throughout the cluster. This gives you very good durability without all the overhead of full replicas. In a 15+4 scheme, there is a 27% overhead in storage: 27 additional megabytes (MB) are stored for every 100 MB of content. In a triple-replicated scheme, there is a 200% overhead: 200 additional MB are stored for every 100 MB of content.

This method requires less disk usage and commensurate network utilization; however, erasure codes are not without cost. Erasure codes require more computation on the data every time it is read and written, but reduce total amount of data stored. Therefore, erasure-coded storage schemes are great for large objects that are less frequently accessed.

Rings

With partitions and replicas defined, we can now look at the data structure of the rings. Each of the Swift rings is a modified consistent hashing ring. This ring data structure includes the partition shift value, which processes and services use to determine the hash of a storage location. It also has two important internal data structures: the devices list and the devices lookup table.

The devices list is populated with all the devices that have been added to a special ring building file. Each entry for a drive includes its ID number, zone, weight, Internet Protocol (IP), port, and device name.

The devices lookup table has one row per replica and one column per partition in the cluster. This generates a table that is typically three rows by thousands of columns. During the building of a ring, Swift calculates the best drive to place each partition replica on using the drive weights and the unique-as-possible placement algorithm. It then records that drive in the table.

Recall the proxy server process that was looking up data. The proxy server process calculated the hash value of the storage location that maps to a partition value. The proxy server process then uses this partition value on the devices lookup table. The process checks the first replica row in the partition column to determine the device ID where the first replica is located. The process searches the next two rows to get the other two locations. In Figure 3.10 you can see that the partition value was 2 and the process found that the data was located on drives 1, 8, and 10.

	Partitions					
	0	1	2	3	4	...
Replicas 0	7	0	1	4	22	
Replicas 1	12	4	8	10	18	
Replicas 2	1	21	10	0	3	

Figure 3.10 Ring Component: Devices Lookup Table

For erasure codes, each partition is mapped to the total chunks for the erasure code scheme. For example, in a 10+4 scheme, the ring would have a partition mapped to 14 different devices.

The proxy server process can then make a second set of searches on the devices list to get the information about all three drives, including ID numbers, zones, weights, IPs, ports, and device names. With this information the process can call on the correct drives. In our example, Figure 3.11, the process determined the ID number, zone, weight, IP, port, and device name for device 1.

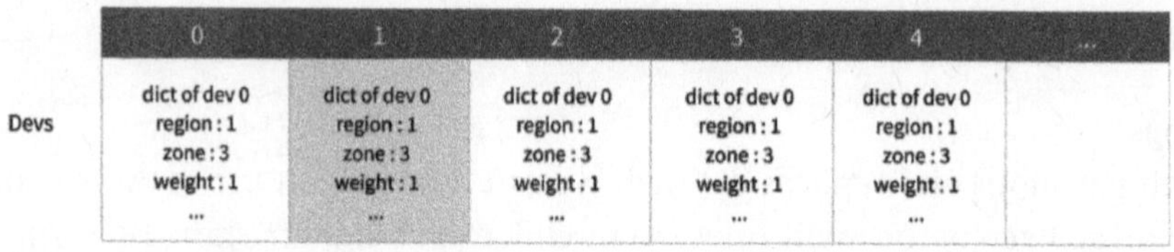

	0	1	2	3	4	...
Devs	dict of dev 0 region : 1 zone : 3 weight : 1 ...	dict of dev 0 region : 1 zone : 3 weight : 1 ...	dict of dev 0 region : 1 zone : 3 weight : 1 ...	dict of dev 0 region : 1 zone : 3 weight : 1 ...	dict of dev 0 region : 1 zone : 3 weight : 1 ...	

Figure 3.11 Ring Component: Devices List

Let's take a closer look at how partitions are calculated and how they are mapped to drives.

Building a Ring

When a ring is being built, the total number of partitions is calculated with a value called the partition power. Once the partition power is set during the initial creation of a cluster, it should not be changed. This means that the total number of partitions will remain the same in the cluster. The formula used is 2 raised to the partition power. For example, if a partition power of 13 is picked, then the total partitions in a cluster is 2^{13}, or 8,192.

During the very first building of the rings, all partitions will need to be assigned to the available drives. When the rings are rebuilt, called rebalancing, only partitions that need to be moved to different drives, usually because drives were added or removed, will be affected.

The placement of the partitions is determined by a combination of replica count, replica lock, and data distribution mechanisms such as drive weight and unique-as-possible placement.

Replica Count

Remember that it is not just partitions but also the replicated copies that must be placed on the drives. For a cluster with a partition power of 13 and a replica count of 3, a total of 8,192 partitions and 24,576 (which is 3 × 8,192) total replicated partitions will be placed on the drives. For erasure codes, the replica count is the total number of nodes for the algorithm used (e.g., 19 in a 15+4 scheme).

Replica Lock

While a partition is being moved, Swift locks that partition's replicas so that they are not eligible to be moved for a period of time to ensure data availability. This locking is used both when rings are being updated and operationally when data is moved. It is not used with the very first building of the rings. The exact length of time to lock a partition is set by the min_part_hours configuration option, which is often set to a default of 24 hours.

Weight

Swift uses a value called weight for each drive in the cluster. This user-defined value, set when the drive is added, is the drive's relative weight compared to the other drives in the ring. The weight helps the cluster calculate how many partitions should be assigned to the drive. The higher the weight, the greater number of partitions Swift should assign to the drive.

Unique-as-Possible Placement

To ensure that the cluster is storing data evenly across its defined spaces (regions, zones, nodes, and disks), Swift assigns partitions using a unique-as-possible placement algorithm. This algorithm identifies the least-used place in the cluster to place a partition. First it looks for the least used region; if all the regions contain a partition, it then looks for the least-used zone, then server (IP:port), and finally the least-used disk, and places the partition there. The least-used formula also attempts to place the partitions as far from each other as possible.

If a cluster cannot be balanced (e.g., if it has different-size zones), then Swift attempts to balance it such that every drive is evenly filled until the smallest zone is full. Then any remaining partitions to be placed are put into the larger zones, overweighting them but enabling cluster capacity to be effectively utilized. This allows for clusters to easily expand with new zones and regions without immediately causing a huge amount of data movement in the cluster.

Once Swift calculates and records the placement of all the partitions, then the ring can be created. One account ring is generated for a cluster and is used to determine where the account data is located. One container ring is generated for a cluster and is used to determine where the container data is located. One object ring is generated for a cluster and is used to determine where the object data is located.

There is a great deal to say about how Swift works internally. We encourage those who are interested in learning more to read the OpenStack Swift documentation (http://docs.openstack.org/developer/swift/).

Swift HTTP Requests: A Closer Look

Now that we have covered the basics of Swift, we can look at how this all works together. Let's see how a cluster handles an incoming request.

As mentioned earlier, all requests sent to Swift are made up of at least three parts*:

1. HTTP verb (e.g., GET, PUT, DELETE)
2. Authentication information

3. Storage URL (swift.example.com/v1/account)
   - Cluster location: swift.example.com/v1/
   - Storage location (for an object): /account/container/object
4. *Optional data or metadata (depending on the request)

The request is sent to the cluster location, which is a hook into the proxy layer. The proxy layer first handles the request verifying auth. Once the request passes auth, the proxy layer routes the incoming request to the appropriate storage nodes.

For our next examples, we assume that the client has valid credentials and permission for the actions being taken and that the cluster uses three replicas.

Example: PUT

A client uses the Swift API to make an HTTP request to PUT an object into an existing container. Swift receives the request and one of the proxy server processes will handle it. First the proxy server process verifies auth and then it takes the hash of the storage location and looks up all three partition locations (the drives) where the data should be stored using the object ring. The process then uses the object ring to look up the IP and other information for those three devices.

Having determined the location of all three partitions, the proxy server process sends the object to each storage node, where it is placed in the appropriate partition. When a quorum is reached—in this case when at least two of the three writes are returned as successful—then the proxy server process notifies the client that the upload was successful.

Next, the container database is updated asynchronously to reflect the new object in it.

Example: GET

A client uses the Swift API to make an HTTP request to GET an object from the cluster. Swift receives the request and one of the proxy server processes will handle it. First the proxy server process verifies auth, and then it takes the hash of the storage location and looks up all three partition locations (the drives) where the data should be stored using the object ring. The process then uses the object ring to look up the IP and other information for those three devices.

Having determined the location of all three partitions, the proxy server process requests the object from each storage node and returns the object to the client.

Additional Swift Capabilities

Swift is very flexible and can be extended with middleware that plugs into a python Web Server Gateway Interface (WSGI) pipeline. By adding middleware in Swift's proxy layer, Swift can be extended with additional features not possible in other storage systems. Some of these features and integrations include:

- **Encryption.** Swift can be configured for object data and user metadata to be encrypted at rest. Each object is encrypted with a unique encryption key.
- **Active checksum checking.** Swift stores an MD5 checksum with each object. The checksum is not only checked by internal auditing processes but is also returned in the header with each request. If the checksum doesn't match, both the storage system and the client can toss away the result and fetch one of the other protected replicas.
- **Static website hosting.** You can host and serve files, such as BAM/VCF files, directly from the storage system. Rather than building a custom application, these files can be directly served from the cluster using HTTP. Static websites can be built to host and serve the data.
- **Automatically expiring objects.** During some stages of a genomics workflow, data needs to be stored only temporarily. Objects can be given an expiry time after which they are no longer available and will be deleted.
- **Time-limited URLs.** Some applications create data that needs to be temporarily public. URLs can be generated that are valid for only a limited period of time. These URLs can be used to build a drop box for large files that enable temporary write permissions without needing to hand out full credentials to an unauthenticated party.
- **Direct-from-HTML-form uploads.** Working with time-limited URLs, web forms can be built that upload data directly into Swift so that the data does not have to be proxied through another server.
- **Quotas.** Storage limits can be set on containers and accounts.
- **Versioned writes.** When a new version of an object is uploaded, a container can be configured so that older versions of the object will be retained.
- **Support for chunked transfer encoding.** Users can upload data to Swift without knowing ahead of time how large the object is.
- **Multirange reads.** Users can read one or more sections of an object with only one read request.
- **Access control lists.** Users can configure access to their data to enable or prevent others' ability to read or write the data.
- **Programmatic access to data locality.** Deployers can integrate Swift with HPC systems and take advantage of locality information to lower network requirements when processing data.

Applications: How to Access Object Storage

Several applications provide an integration directly with Swift.

Command-Line Tool: Swift CLI

The Swift command line is a great way to use a Swift cluster. The Swift CLI is part of the python-swiftclient package and can be installed on any computer running Python. Detailed installation instructions can be found at: https://swiftstack.com/docs/integration/python-swiftclient.html.

The Swift command simplifies things for users by saving some typing and making several common types of requests easier.

```
$ swift stat
   Account: AUTH_account
Containers: 2
   Objects: 2
     Bytes: 2048
```

You can get a listing of all the containers in the account with the list command:

```
$ swift list
animals
vegetables
```

Here you see that you have two containers. You can create new containers with the post command:

```
$ swift post minerals
$ swift list
animals
minerals
vegetables
```

To get a listing of objects within a container, you can again use the list command, this time passing the container as a parameter:

```
$ swift list animals
lions.txt
tigers.txt
```

To upload objects to the cluster, you use the upload command, passing both the container and the object file name as parameters:

```
$ swift upload animals bears.txt
```

You can specify multiple files to upload in one command by passing additional parameters. If you specify a directory (folder) to upload instead of a file, all the files and directories within that directory will be uploaded too.

Similarly, to download objects, use the download command, passing the container and object names as parameters:

```
$ swift download animals lions.txt
```

Finally, to remove an object from a container, use the delete command:

```
$ swift delete animals bears.txt
```

To remove a container and all the objects within it, pass only the container name:

```
$ swift delete animals
$ swift list
minerals
vegetables
```

Command-Line Tool for HPC: Swift Commander

Swift Commander was developed by the Fred Hutchinson Cancer Research Center to be optimized for small-file workloads to archive and restore data sets in HPC environments. Swift Commander was written by the author of the postmark file system benchmark who is experienced in building tools to handle small files.

Swift Commander is actively maintained and available at: https://github.com/FredHutch/swift-commander/. It is a simple shell wrapper for the Swift client, curl, and some other tools and makes working with Swift very easy:

```
$ swc upload /my/posix/folder /my/swift/folder
$ swc compare /my/posix/folder /my/swift/folder
$ swc download /my/swift/folder /my/scratch/fs
```

Subcommands, such as swc ls, swc cd, swc rm, and swc more, give you a feel that is similar to a Unix file system.

Swift Commander for HPC Archive

Lots of small files are problematic regardless of the storage system used. A common strategy is to create an archive of the entire directory structure via tar. However, in genomics research, a single tar file can grow quite large.

The solution with Swift Commander is to create a tarball for each level:

```
/folder1.tar.gz
/folder1/folder2.tar.gz
/folder1/folder2/folder3.tar.gz
```

Restoring folder2 and below, we just need folder2.tar.gz + folder3.tar.gz.

Swift Commander also contains an archiving module:

```
$ archive:  swc arch /my/posix/folder /my/swift/folder
$ restore:  swc unarch /my/swift/folder /my/scratch/fs
```

With Swift Commander, the archiving module uses multiple processes. It has a measured performance of up to 400 MB from one Linux box. Each process uses pigz multithreaded gzip compression. (Example: compressing 1 GB DNA string down to 272 MB: 111 sec using gzip, 5 seconds using pigz.) Restore can use standard gzip.

Filesystem Access

OpenStack Swift supports native filesystem access with proxyFS services. This permits both filesystem access and object API access in the same workflow for the same set of data. Additionally, desktop clients and various filesystem gateways provide additional methods to provide filesystem access.

Object storage enables large, distributed storage systems to be built with standard x86 storage servers. This has dramatically reduced the costs of deploying data-intensive applications, particularly for life sciences organizations. Swift (in either its OpenStack Swift or SwiftStack versions) is helping to improve processing time and realize the promise of personal genomics. Speed is critical for clinical genomics applications, and Swift clusters make both compute and storage more efficient. By lowering costs, Swift can help accelerate innovations in personal genomics, which depend on cheap storage and compute. One main appeal of Swift is that you can use standard x86 server components and buy only the storage equipment needed, when it is needed.

CONCLUSION

In this chapter you learned about challenges and potential solutions for managing biomedical data. After surveying some prevalent data types, we offered a high-level review of security and compliance and a discussion of the research data life cycle. We covered iRODS and presented how to use SwiftStack object storage. Three case studies follow this chapter. The first considers the data demands of genomic sequencing. The second offers specifications for HudsonAlpha's SwiftStack storage cluster. The third focuses on the use of Nimble Storage's predictive flash storage at ASU.

NOTES

1. Francis Collins. 2015. "Keynote Address." Lecture, Health Data Palooza, Washington, DC, May 31.
2. Atul Butte. 2012. "E Pluribus Genome." TEDxSF (7 Billion Well), TEDx Talks, November 17. https://www.youtube.com/watch?v=TYcE-HJHST8.
3. Chris Anderson. 2008. "The End of Theory: The Data Deluge Makes the Scientific Method Obsolete." *WIRED*, June 23. http://www.wired.com/2008/06/pb-theory/.

4. "Jeff Jonas—IBM Fellow and Chief Scientist, Entity Analytics." IBM News Room. January 2013. https://www-03.ibm.com/press/us/en/biography/40087.wss.
5. Albert Geskin, Elizabeth Legowski, Anish Chakka, et al. 2015. "Needs Assessment for Research Use of High-Throughput Sequencing at a Large Academic Medical Center." *PLoS ONE* 10, no. 6. doi: 10.1371/journal.pone.0131166.
6. Antonio Regalado. 2015. "Internet of DNA." MIT Technology Review. https://www.technologyreview.com/s/535016/internet-of-dna/.
7. "What Is Object/Relational Mapping?" Hibernate ORM. http://hibernate.org/orm/what-is-an-orm/#the-object-relational-impedance-mismatch.
8. Office of Science and Technology Policy. 2013 Memorandum. "Increasing Access to the Results of Federally Funded Scientific Research." February 22. Office of Science and Technology Policy. https://www.whitehouse.gov/sites/default/files/microsites/ostp/ostp_public_access_memo_2013.pdf.
9. National Academies of Science, Engineering, and Medicine, Division of Behavioral and Social Sciences and Education. "Public Access to Federally-Supported Research and Development." http://sites.nationalacademies.org/DBASSE/CurrentProjects/DBASSE_082378.
10. Office for Human Research Protections. 2016. "45 CFR 46." HHS.gov. http://www.hhs.gov/ohrp/regulations-and-policy/regulations/45-cfr-46/index.html.
11. Federal Information Processing Standards Publication. 2016. "FIPS 200: Minimum Security Requirements for Federal Information and Information Systems." http://csrc.nist.gov/publications/fips/fips200/FIPS-200-final-march.pdf.
12. Joint Task Force Transformation Initiative. April 2013. "Security and Privacy Controls for Federal Information Systems and Organizations," NIST Special Publication 800-53 Revision 4. http://nvlpubs.nist.gov/nistpubs/SpecialPublications/NIST.SP.800-53r4.pdf.
13. NIST Computer Security Division. Federal Information Security Management Act (FISMA) Implementation Project. http://csrc.nist.gov/groups/SMA/fisma/.
14. Defense Information Systems Agency. Home page. http://www.disa.mil/.
15. Security Technical Implementation Guides (STIGs). Home page. http://iase.disa.mil/stigs/Pages/ind.ex.aspx.
16. U.S. Department of Education. "Family Educational Rights and Privacy Act (FERPA)." http://www2.ed.gov/policy/gen/guid/fpco/ferpa/index.html.
17. "About OSTP." https://www.whitehouse.gov/administration/eop/ostp/about.

CASE STUDY

CASE STUDY 2: IS SEQUENCING A BIG DATA PROBLEM?

Christopher Mueller

At this point I am sure we agree that sequencing is a big data problem, with our focus on the scale of data generated by sequencing instruments. Here we look at the problem from the context of biology to help understand the fundamental reasons why sequencing will always be a big data problem.

We derive two main conclusions, one for DNA applications and one for RNA applications:

1. For DNA applications, noise and bias drive how much data must be collected.

(*Continued*)

(*Continued*)

2. For RNA applications, the distribution of transcripts drives the sampling depth.

Let's look into the basic (and admittedly simplified) math behind these two important conclusions.

DNA

The goal of most DNA sequencing experiments is to identify locations where a sample differs from a reference genome. These can be single-point mutations (e.g., SNPs, indels), translocations, copy number variations, or differences in the way the bases have been modified by external factors (e.g., methylation). In all cases, each location on the genome must be measured repeatedly, as shown in Figure CS3.1,

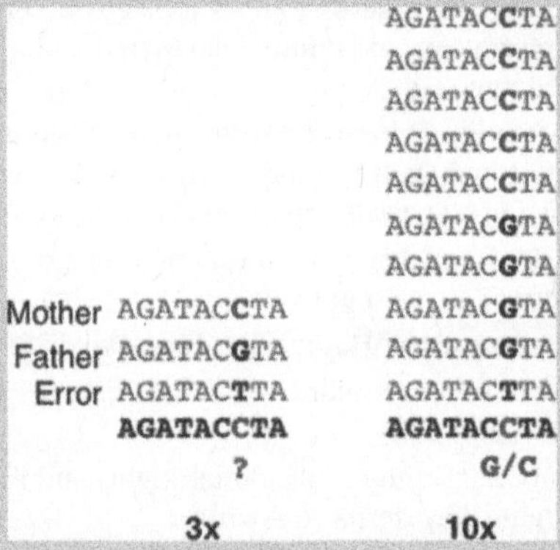

Figure CS3.1 Repeated Measurement of DNA Ensures Accuracy

until the actual base present at the location can be called with confidence.

DNA sequencing depth is driven by the types of variations and the number of times a base value must be seen to call it with confidence.

A number of factors can lead to different measurements at the same location, including:

- In polyploidal organisms, two or more distinct bases are possible at each location.
- Basic mutation rates ensure that over time individual bases will diverge as cells evolve.
- Instruments and prep methods can induce read errors or biases.

Each of these factors requires oversampling at a particular location to call the base (or bases, for polyploidal genomes) correctly. Most variant calling methods require 10 to 30 times coverage at a given location to correctly call a base.

For a small genome, such as *E. coli*, with 5 million bases, 10 to 30 times coverage corresponds to 125 to 375 megabytes of sequence data (quality scores and metadata increase the amount of data by about 2.5 times compared to number of bases measured). For larger genomes, such as human with 3 billion bases, 75 to 225 gigabytes of sequence data must be collected.

RNA

Expression levels are one of the primary measurements made in RNA experiments. Expression levels measure (1) if a transcript is expressed at all and (2) what the relative proportion of that transcript is to the other actively expressed transcripts in the sample. Expression measurements are made by counting the number of reads that map to a given transcript. Highly expressed transcripts have more reads than rarely expressed transcripts.

Each cell contains a number of active transcripts that represent the current genomic activity in the cell. Active transcripts vary by cell type and the cell's stage in its life cycle. Copy numbers for transcripts within a cell vary greatly—a few highly expressed genes account for the bulk of the active transcripts in a cell.

Consider an RNA preparation from a collection of cells containing 10,000 active genes in which ribosomal RNA has been removed and only transcripts with poly(A) tails are included. The top 20 expressors likely account for the bulk of the copies of active transcripts, and the top 10 expressors account for 95% percent of the active transcripts.

Given 1 million reads, 950,000 reads will map to the top 10 expressors, leaving 50,000 reads for the remaining transcripts. Of these, 95% will likely represent the next 10 top expressors, leaving 2,500 reads for the next 9,980 transcripts. Assuming the remaining transcripts are present in similar copy numbers, there is only a one in four chance of seeing a single read from one of them.

Increasing the number of reads to 5 million starts to ensure that most transcripts may be counted at least once. However, more than one read is required to ensure detection and provide enough counts for differential expression analysis.

For RNA experiments, this sets a lower bound on the amount of data that must be collected. If the transcripts of interest are highly expressed, then only a few million reads are necessary. But, for rare transcripts, tens of millions of reads are needed, as shown in Figure CS3.2.

RNA sequencing depth is driven by the relative abundance of the target gene. Highly expressed genes require less depth for accurate expression measurements.

RNA-Seq is based on read-counting instead of coverage. The goal is to assign read counts to a region of the genome instead of ensuring even coverage across the whole genome. For counting experiments, shorter reads can be used, reducing the amount of data and instrument run time. For counting applications, 35-base-pair

(*Continued*)

(*Continued*)

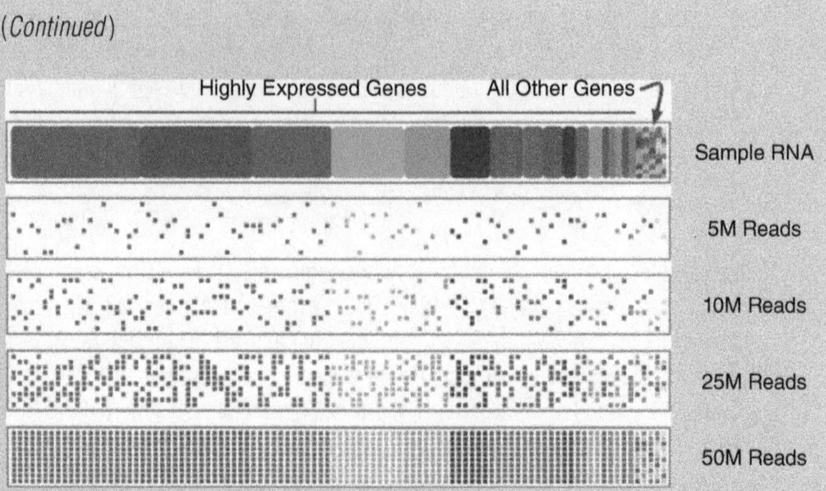

Figure CS3.2 Rare Transcripts Require More Reads

(bp) reads are generally considered sufficient. (As an aside: Longer reads and full coverage of transcripts are helpful for identifying transcripts and splice events, but for straight counting, they are not necessary.)

Back to our discussion of data scale: For studies that target highly expressed genes where 5 million 35-bp reads are sufficient, 450 MB of actual data will be collected per replicate. For studies that target transcripts with fewer copies in any given sample, up to 50 million 35-bp reads may be required, or around 4.5 GB of data per replicate. RNA experiments compare multiple samples with multiple replicates, quickly pushing the data scale for a single experiment into the hundreds of GBs.

BIOLOGY DRIVES DATA SCALE

As these two examples show, basic tenets of biology and measurement systems determine the amount of data needed to answer specific questions using sequencing. Without NGS instruments, these types of measurements would not be practical.

As a stopgap to reduce data scales, different prep methods have been developed to target specific regions of the genome. Exome sequencing sequences only DNA in known coding regions. Gene panels have probes for transcripts of interest along with a few reference transcripts to allow for targeted differential expression studies.

In the early days of NGS, I was approached by a local research and development group about designing a cluster for their two new SOLiD instruments. The budget was modest—tens of thousands of dollars—and the expectations were high—a run every 10 days for each instrument or one run a week for the lab. Some quick back-of-the-envelope calculations yielded some disappointing results: With the proposed budget, the best solution would be a nice workstation that would take at least 10 days to process a single run. Even if everything worked perfectly, it simply would not be possible to keep up with the instrument output.

To reset expectations and develop a more appropriate solution, we took a step back and looked at the problem from a systems perspective: How does data move from the instrument through analysis? What are the main bottlenecks? What else will the cluster be used for? What solutions exist that will allow us to meet our development and production goals?

Next, we go through the basic analysis we performed. Along the way, we identify the main components of a sequencing informatics system, discuss the parameters that matter the most when planning a system, and set guidelines for designing a sequencing informatics system to meet your specific requirements.

MODEL NGS PIPELINE

To start, consider the basic steps in a bioinformatics workflow:

1. Translate raw data into short reads.
2. Map reads to the reference genome.
3. Perform protocol-specific analysis (e.g., expression analysis for RNA-Seq, variant calling for resequencing).
4. Report results.

At each step, data is transformed and prepared for the next stage. In between stages, data may be moved between different compute resources. These steps are common enough across sequencing protocols that steps 1 to 3 are often simply referred to as primary, secondary, and tertiary analysis.

We use this basic model to help think about our sequencing informatics system.

SEQUENCING AS A BIG DATA PROBLEM

What sets NGS apart from many other data collection methods is the sheer amount of data generated by each run. In fact, aside from a couple of physics instruments, such as the Hubble Space Telescope and the Large Hadron Collider, few other scientific instruments generate as much data as NGS instruments.

Figure CS3.3 shows the workflow for sequencing informatics. From a pure operations perspective, the amount of data at each analysis stage is driven by the output of primary analysis, which generally occurs on the instrument. A HiSeq run can generate anywhere from a few hundred GB to a few TB of read data. Our SOLiD instruments originally generated around 40 GB per run but quickly grew, through improvements in chemistry, to generate over 300 GB.

Secondary analysis maps all the reads against a genome reference and generates a file with one or more entries per read, identifying all the locations the read mapped against the reference. The type of data stored for each mapped read takes roughly the same amount of storage as the read itself, essentially doubling the data size for

(*Continued*)

(*Continued*)

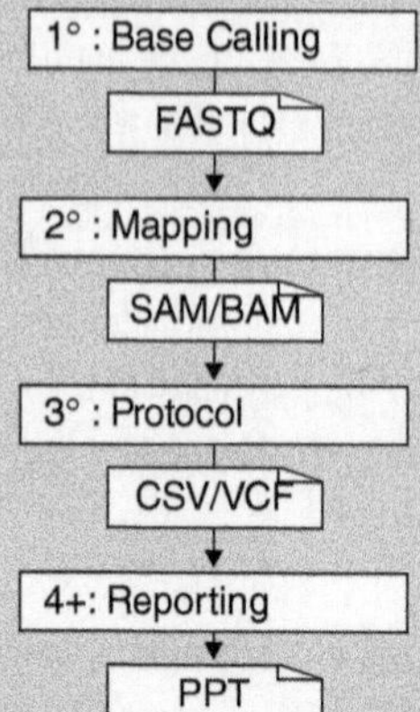

Figure CS3.3 Common Sequencing Informatics Workflow Steps

the run. Binary compressed formats are often used for mapped data, reducing the storage requirements.

Tertiary analysis further processes the mapped reads based on the specific protocol. Results for tertiary analysis are often reported from the perspective of the reference rather than the reads and are much smaller. For example, RNA-Seq results report how many reads mapped to each gene or transcript. Even with 80,000 to 100,000 transcripts, basic read count reports are small in comparison to the actual read data.

While it is tempting to focus on the results of tertiary analysis and disregard the data from the other stages, any sequencing informatics system must take into account all working data and the actual, not just ideal, usage patterns. Secondary analysis is often repeated using different aligners and parameters to help validate results. Pipelines fail and need to be restarted. Bioinformaticians replicate past results to develop new methods. Data retention polices may require reads and other intermediate results to be stored for a period. As a rule of thumb, any sequencing run will require around 2.5 times the size of the FASTQ file in online storage, and the data will need to remain available for at least the duration of the project.

Table CS3.1 summarizes the basic data scales for different types of instruments. FASTQ file sizes are computed as (Read Length × 2 + 50) × (Reads) where the factor of 2 accounts for the read and quality values and 50 bytes are added for the identifier (paired end runs have an additional 2x multiplier). Total data uses the 2.5x multiplier on the FASTQ size. Read length and number of reads are from the product websites, except for Proton 2, which is just a guess for a future proton.

Given these results, it might seem prudent to simply use ION Torrent PGMs or MiSeqs and sidestep the big data problem entirely. Of course, that ignores another

Table CS3.1 Basic Data Scales for Different Types of Instruments

Instrument	Read LENGTH	Paired End	Reads (millions)	FASTQ (GB)	Total Data (GB)
HiSeq 2500	36	No	3,000	366	915
	100	Yes	6,000	600	1,500
MiSeq	36	No	15	1.5	3.75
	100	Yes	30	3	7.5
	250	Yes	30	33	82.5
SOLiD 4	110	75+35	1,400	378	945
ION PGM 318	35	No	8	0.96	2.4
	200	No	8	3.6	9
	400	No	8	6.8	17
ION Proton 1	200	No	80	36	90
ION Proton 2	200	No	160	72	180

important factor in sequencing: basic biology drives how much data must be collected for a given experiment.

Perhaps biology itself is the big data problem?

CASE STUDY

CASE STUDY 3: HUDSONALPHA INSTITUTE FOR BIOTECHNOLOGY AND SWIFTSTACK

Joe Arnold

HudsonAlpha Institute for Biotechnology is a nonprofit institute that provides genomic sequencing services for research and clinical use. Its Genomic Services Laboratory deals with petabyte-scale data and operates more than 12 high-performance sequencing instruments including Illumina HiSeq X Ten systems. See: https://gsl.hudsonalpha.org/.

Additionally, the Clinical Services Laboratory at HudsonAlpha provides physicians with clinical-grade whole-genome sequencing for patients to enable clinical personalized medicine. See: https://csl.hudsonalpha.org/.

Throughout the process of bringing NGS online, the infrastructure team faced these challenges:

- Maintain current staffing levels and expertise.
- Maintain geographic redundancy and distribution.
- Ensure high durability and availability for the valuable data being generated.

(*Continued*)

(*Continued*)

- Make use of commodity hardware.
- Avoid vendor lock-in.

HUDSONALPHA SOLUTION

HudsonAlpha stores FASTQ, BAM, and VCF data generated by Illumina HiSeq X Ten sequencers and the data generated by related applications that process, align, and analyze that data. A rack-level architecture was designed to simplify operations and provide a standard unit of incremental scaling.

In this configuration, approximately 3 PB of raw capacity is available in a single rack. A rack is provisioned on-site near the genomic sequencers. Additional racks are also available in two remote locations for distribution of BAM and VCF files to scientists who perform additional analysis in outside facilities. All three sites participate in the same multiregion Swift cluster, and storage policies allow control over what data is distributed to which remote locations.

RACK CONFIGURATION

The standard rack contains the following hardware:

- PAC—Proxy/Account/Container Node (x2)
    - 1u Standard x86 server
    - 64 GB DRAM
- 2x 8-core CPUs
- 2x 200 GB HDDs (RAID-1 for operating system)
- 2x 200 GB SSD (for Account/Container data)
- 2x 10GbE dual-port NIC
- O—Object Storage Node (x6)
- 60–90 drive storage enclosure
- 60–90 6 TB HDDs
- 1U Standard x86 server
- 128 GB DRAM
- 2x Intel E5–2630 CPUs
- 2x HDDs (RAID-1 for operating system)
    - 1x 10 GbEdual-port NIC
    - 4x 1 GbE onboard NIC ports
    - 1x SAS HBA

CASE STUDY

CASE STUDY 4: NIMBLESTORAGE DEPLOYMENT AT ARIZONA STATE UNIVERSITY

NimbleStorage

NimbleStorage, founded in 2008 in San Jose, California, was started with the core belief that flash, cloud, and big data analytics would disrupt the storage market and that these catalysts created an opportunity to deliver unprecedented application performance and infrastructure with nonstop availability. NimbleStorage is headquartered in San Jose, California, with over 8,000 customers in 50 countries.

NimbleStorage offers predictive flash storage solutions, through a platform that combines flash performance with predictive analytics to predict and prevent barriers to real-time performance caused by complex IT infrastructure. The Nimble platform is comprised of two core technologies: a Unified Flash Fabric and InfoSight Predictive Analytics.

The Unified Flash Fabric is a single consolidation architecture, powered by the Nimble flash optimized file system, which combines All Flash and Adaptive Flash arrays into a single managed entity. InfoSight is the Nimble cloud-connected management system that monitors Nimble customers' infrastructure in real time to predict and prevent downtime and radically simplify planning.

NIMBLE/ASU OVERVIEW

Summary: NimbleStorage donated IT infrastructure to enable research scientists and entrepreneurs from Arizona State University's venture-capital firm, The Mill, to bring their ideas from genesis to production. The Mill supports businesses globally, providing financial backing for researchers developing ideas and patents within the university in exchange for shares in the company and in the patents developed.

Background: NimbleStorage's engagement with ASU began with the Translational Genomics Research Institute (TGen), a nonprofit organization focused on developing earlier diagnostics and smarter treatments. Following the initial trials, Varun Mehta, cofounder and vice president of Product Operations for NimbleStorage, and Jay Etchings, director of Operations, research computing at the high-performance computing (HPC) group at ASU, further collaborated on a vision to support the small businesses coming out of The Mill.

Results and benefits: A NimbleStorage CS700 Adaptive Flash array currently supports four small businesses, one of which focuses on genomics and discovering a cure to cancer. The processing of raw sequence data can be demanding on compute resources as well as storage, and requires rapid speed of data from a highly available source.

(*Continued*)

(*Continued*)

Through this donation, Mehta aims to support the small businesses as they grow to their full potential, both in size and in customers attained. With the CS700 array, NimbleStorage has created an on-premise cloud so other research scientists can also be granted access to this private cloud held by ASU, at a lower cost.

Technology: NimbleStorage donated a CS700 array with an 8 TB cache in the head and an all-flash shelf partially populated, equating to about 600 raw TB.

The Nimble Adaptive Flash array is based on two groundbreaking storage innovations: the Nimble patented Cache-Accelerated Sequential Layout (CASL) architecture and InfoSight, the company's automated cloud-based management and support system. The arrays leverage CASL to accelerate read and write performance, optimize capacity, protect data, and seamlessly scale to meet the changing demands of diverse enterprise workloads.

The CS700 array is a part of the NimbleStorage CS-Series, designed for consolidating multiple large-scale critical applications within aggressive performance demands. Organizations have struggled to build out storage infrastructure quickly and cost-effectively to handle unpredictable data growth and to meet changing requirements. As such, they have been forced to create storage silos to meet a single functional benefit: high performance or high capacity. The NimbleStorage Adaptive Flash platform enables institutions to eliminate the trade-off between flash performance and capacity, delivering the performance of all-flash arrays and the cost-efficient capacity of hybrid and legacy storage solutions, within a small data center footprint.

CHAPTER 4

Designing a Data-Ready Network Infrastructure

Computer networking can productively be thought about through an analogy with human anatomy. Networks are, after all, startlingly complex systems for the circulation of data and the allocation of resources. Imagine if you would the human circulatory system with its communication system where blood cells are transmission control packets. Plasma as the fluid content supports blood cells that circulate throughout the vasculature, picks up oxygen molecules, and transports them to remote systems that need them to operate. If an oxygen molecule is lost or if low oxygenation were to occur, the body has a fault-tolerant system whereby the next molecule is delivered and acknowledged. We can imagine computer networks in similar terms, if we replace oxygen molecules with data packets and vasculature with physical network media, such as optical cable, coaxial, twisted pair, or Category 6 (CAT6). This can prove a useful thought experiment, especially for those in the biosciences.

Computer networking began with systems that now seem startlingly simple. On November 11, 1973, a 2.94 Mbps Carrier Sense Multiple Access with Collision Detection (CSMA/CD) system connected about 100 workstations on a 1-kilometer cable in the Xerox Palo Research Center [1]. From there Xerox filed the patent, and Robert Metcalfe founded 3Com and over the next handful of years launched collaborative efforts with Digital Equipment Corporation, Intel, and Xerox to cooperatively promote Ethernet as an Institute of Electrical and Electronics Engineers (IEEE) Standard [2]. Ethernet evolved rapidly and, as they say, the rest is history.

To return to our analogy of the human body, we can ask whether the circulatory system is the only component. The answer, of course, is no. Our bodies contain multiple interconnected systems that depend on each other. For instance, the lymphatic system is critical for waste removal, the central nervous system is a low-voltage messaging network, and the digestive system is an intricate processing plant for energy. These systems closely parallel modern-day enterprise network infrastructure. A fully functioning circulatory system is of little use without the continual movement of waste through the lymphatic system or the interconnectivity of the central nervous system.

Now let us consider a simple networking task. We would like to transport some genetic data from one facility to another. As is the case with the human body, this task involves multiple interconnected and interdependent systems. For example, the Transmission Control Protocol (TCP) stack is reliant on the physical media, much as blood cells rely on the vasculature. And this simple data transfer depends on source and destination negotiations, methods of authentication, acknowledgment of delivery, and much more. To make matters more complicated, networks depend on other networks. Communication networks are of little use without wide area or Internet connectivity (which support a wide variation of external protocols, discussed later). Storage networks also support application-centric protocols. Security and management networks include private networks and security-specific networks like virtual private networks (VPNs); differentiated media and/or alternate network types, such as Fibre Channel, InfiniBand, wireless, and software-defined networking (SDN); and application-specific or content networks. Networks also use a seemingly endless and ever-growing assortment of protocols (agreed rules for connections), media types (physical componentry [vasculature]), topologies, and proprietary implementations for provision of service assurance and securing all of the above from threats.

To understand complexity in network protocols above the physical media, please refer to Figure 4.1, which shows the Open Systems Interconnection (OSI) model. Medical professionals with only cursory knowledge of networks might assume that information systems are nowhere near as complex as human anatomy and physiology. However, Figure 4.1 calls that assumption into question.

OSI (Open Systems Interconnection) 7 Layer Model

Layer	Application/Example		Central Device/ Protocols			DOD4 Model
Application (7) Serves as the window for users and application processes to access the network services.	**End User layer Program that opens what was sent or creates what is to be sent** Resource sharing • Remote file access • Remote Printer access • Directory services • Network management		**User Applications** SMTP		GATEWAY	Process
Presentation (6) Formats the data to be presented to the Application layer. It can be viewed as the "Translator" for the network.	**Syntex layer encrypt & decrypt (if needed)** Character code translation • Data conversion • Data compression • Data encryption • **Character Set Translation**		JPEG/ASCII EBDIC/TIFF/GIF PICT			
Session (5) Allows session establishment between processes running on different stations.	**Synch & send to ports (logical ports)** Session establishment, maintenance and termination • Session support - perform security, name recognition, logging, etc.		**Logical Ports** RPC/SQL/NFS NetBIOS names			
Transport (4) Ensures that messages are delivered error-free, in sequence, and with no losses or duplications.	**TCP Host to Host, Flow Control** Message segmentation • Message acknowledgement • Message traffic control • Session multiplexing	PACKET FILTERING	TCP/SPX/UDP			Host to Host
Network (3) Controls the operations of the subnet, deciding which physical path the data takes.	**Packets ("letter", contains IP address)** Routing • Subnet traffic control • Frame fragmentation • Logical-physical address mapping • Subnet usage accounting		**Routers** IP/IPX/ICMP		Can be used on all layers	Internet
Data Link (2) Provides error-free transfer of data frames from one node to another over the Physical layer.	**Frames ("envelopes", contains MAC address)** [NIC card — Switch — NIC card] (end to end) Establishes & terminates the logical link between nodes • Frame traffic control • Frame sequencing • Frame acknowledgment • Frame delimiting • Frame error checking • Media access control		**Switch Bridge WAP** PPP/SLIP	Land Based Layers		Network
Physical (1) Concerned with the transmission and reception of the unstructured raw bit stream over the physical medium.	**Physical structure Cables, hubs, etc.** Data Encoding • Physical medium attachment • Transmission technique - Baseband or Broadband • Physical medium transmission Bits & Volts		**Hub**			

Figure 4.1 Basic OSI Model
Phil Zito, "What Is the OSI Model," Building Automation Monthly, *May 3, 2013, http://buildingautomationmonthly.com/what-is-the-osi-model/.*

We hope that this quick thought experiment and consideration of networks has shown that networks are complex and should be regarded as complex adaptive systems. In the rest of this chapter, we offer a brief history of computer networking and then examine research networks. After presenting some current challenges in networking, we examine several areas in which networking advances are being made. These include: InfiniBand, a communications standard used in high-performance computing (HPC) that features very high throughput and very low latency; high-performance fabrics; network function virtualization (NFV); and SDN. Both NFV and SDN allow for greater network flexibility and much lower cost due to their ability to run on commodity hardware. The bulk of the chapter is devoted to OpenDaylight, an open source SDN platform.

RESEARCH NETWORKS: A PRIMER

Much of the key research conducted at universities today depends on the ability to process, store, and share massive volumes of data. For instance, the Data Center at CERN—the European laboratory that houses the Large Hadron Collider—processes approximately 1 petabyte of data each day. CERN distributes its data to research institutions throughout the world. Across the biosciences large-scale data transfers are also becoming commonplace and elongated wait times are no longer acceptable. Few research programs understand the need for shared data across infrastructure but most are still maxed out at 10 gigabit (Gb) per second Ethernet speeds, and some are even bottlenecked at 1 gigabit Ethernet (GbE). While 10 GbE was once considered state of the art, institutions today are straining the capacity of those networks especially where 10 GbE was deployed as an aggregate link. The IEEE introduced a standard for transmitting Ethernet frames at 100 Gb per second in 2010; operating 10 times faster than the previous generation, this technology offers a clear advantage to universities that adopt it. Many institutions have started to consider an upgrade to 100 GbE. Some have already deployed this technology and, as a result, are beginning to observe significant practical benefits. Universities are upgrading by connecting to the Research Education Network and adopting Internet2 (100 GbE). Before discussing Internet2 in more detail, we examine the Energy Sciences Network (ESnet), which has been an important driver of networking innovation. ESnet is the mission network of the U.S. Department of Energy (DOE).

Next we reprint an excellent overview of ESnet. More secure data on ESnet utilizes the Science DMZ (demilitarized zone), a portion of the network, built at or near the campus or laboratory's local network perimeter, that is designed such that the equipment, configuration, and security policies are optimized for high-performance scientific applications rather than for general-purpose business systems or "enterprise" computing. ESnet recommends that its members create a Science DMZ with 100 GbE capabilities, plus SDN using OpenFlow technology. Non-blocking switch fabrics in the routers ensure unimpeded data flow and are another key configuration element suggested by ESnet.

ESNET AT 30: EVOLVING TOWARD EXASCALE AND RAISING EXPECTATIONS*

In tandem with high-performance computing, high-speed nationwide and global infrastructure networks provide the essential backbone for today's collaborative science workflows. In the United States, the Energy Sciences Network (ESnet) is the mission network of the U.S. Department of Energy. This high-performance, unclassified network that is managed by Lawrence Berkeley National Laboratory is moving into the newly constructed Wang Hall on the Berkeley Lab campus.

ESnet links 40 DOE sites across the country and scientists at universities and other research institutions via a 100 gigabits per second backbone network. One of these sites, the National Energy Research Scientific Computing Center (NERSC), has made the move to the Berkeley campus from its previous 15-year home in Oakland, California. ESnet has built a 400 gigabit per second (Gbps) super-channel between the Berkeley and Oakland sites to support this transition over the next year. This is the first-ever 400G production link to be deployed by a national research and education network, and will also be part of a research testbed for assessing new tools and technologies that are necessary to support massive data growth as supercomputers approach the exascale era.

"We are often the first organization to adopt new networking technologies because our scientists are really pushing the envelope when it comes to data transfer and access of large data sets," commented ESnet Director Greg Bell in an interview with *HPCwire*. Along with Internet2, ESnet also built the first nationwide continental-scale 100 Gbps network in 2012. "If you think of ESnet as being the national labs network, you can think of Internet2 as being the university network in the US," Bell clarified.

In his role as ESnet director, Bell oversees all of the operational activities of one of the largest and fastest networks in the world—there are network engineers on call 24/7, a cybersecurity team, storage experts, data collection and data analysts, and others engaged in building out the network. Bell also oversees teams that help make the network useful to scientists. There is a team of people who build software tools to help the network be less of a black box. Then there is another team focused just on science engagement, helping scientists make the best possible use of the network and raising expectations about the network's capabilities.

"This team directly engages with scientific collaborations large and small, but mostly large to medium-sized," noted Bell, "and it also teaches scientists and networkers around the country and around the world best practices for

---

*This section is reproduced from an article of the same title by Tiffany Trader in *HPCwire*, December 10, 2015. https://www.hpcwire.com/2015/12/10/esnet-evolving-toward-exascale/. Used with permission.

networking so we can all build networks that are better and make it easier to move data and make it easier to accelerate scientific outcomes."

Over the last 10 years, the ESnet team has seen a move away from the sneakernet model, in which data is moved using a storage medium that is carried on a person or sent via a postal service.

"We aren't ideologically opposed to sneakernet," said Bell. "If you just need to move data once and you know you never need to access it again, it can sometimes be the most efficient solution, but in general, people need to move data over and over again, and they need to combine it with other data sets and they need to share it and they need to access it later and for that, networks are just great.

"We are trying to raise everyone's expectations and let them know that networks can do much more than they could just a few years ago. In fact, the great vision that we have for networks is not only as a scientific instrument in their own right, but that they can glue together big scientific instruments like a particle accelerator or a light source and a computational facility, for example, a DOE supercomputer center. This enables a scenario where we can take data in real-time from the source and move it at high-speed over the network and process it in real-time at the supercomputer center so the scientists can get immediate feedback about the experimental parameters that they have chosen and then adjust them in real-time.

"Doing this requires that the network glue together two or three other instruments," Bell added. "If we can do that, we can make the DOE science complex and the US science complex more than the sum of its parts. We can enable discovery workflows that wouldn't have been possible without excellent high-speed networks."

Esnet Then and Now

ESnet will be 30 years old in 2016, which makes it one of the oldest networks in the world. "It actually predates the creation of the commercial network," Bell shared. The DOE network was created at a time when two DOE science activities, one in high-energy physics and one in fusion energy—each had their own network before the Internet had really settled down into one technical architecture. In 1986, it was decided to create a single unified mission network and to choose a single architecture, which was TCP/IP, which is the way that the Internet evolved.

"ESnet was created out of the merger of these two domain specific science networks and since then, fusion and most especially high-energy physics has pushed us to be at the bleeding edge of networking for those 30 years," Bell added.

The Department of Energy's Office of Science funds nearly half of the physical science research in the US and provides about a billion dollars a year to university campuses. ESnet provides the high-bandwidth, reliable connections that link scientists at national laboratories, universities and other research institutions, enabling them to collaborate on some of the world's most important scientific challenges within energy, climate science, and the origins of the universe.

The fundamental challenge for ESnet is keeping up with data growth, which has increased at a fairly steady exponential rate since its inception. Since 1990, ESnet's average traffic has grown by a factor of 10 every 47 months, roughly along a Moore's law growth curve. Recently, the network moved 36 petabytes of traffic.

What's interesting, though, is that there has been a change in the source of this data, as Bell explained. "It used to come from very large experiments like Large Hadron Collider (LHC), ATLAS and CMS detectors," he said. "Now, it's still coming from those large experiments but increasingly it's coming from a lot more sources that are smaller and cheaper, for instance, the detectors at the DOE Advanced Light Source beamline. Those are conceptually like the cameras in a mobile phone and they are getting much more high-resolution and the refresh rate is getting faster and faster. That compounded effect of high-resolution and faster refresh rates means that individual detectors are capable of sending out 10 Gbps or much more and soon this will be 80–100 Gbps.

"So it actually is a tremendous challenge to engineer the network so it can grow cost-effectively," said Bell. "We don't have exponential budgets, we actually have at best linear budgets and sometimes flat budgets, so the question is how can we keep up with the demand.

"The light sources are just one example," Bell added. "Tiny inexpensive genomic sequencers are producing a lot of data, as are environmental sensors, telescopes, and cosmology experiments, so for us it adds up to this exponential growth curve that is the fundamental challenge of ESnet, which is to evolve its architecture to accommodate and stay ahead of this growth curve."

Over the years, ESnet has continued to rise to the challenge of supporting this exponential growth. ESnet5, the moniker for the current ESnet instantiation, is the 100 Gbps transcontinental and transatlantic network that was constructed a few years ago. They are now planning for the next network, ESnet6, which will probably need to use a different technology, according to Bell. To that end, he and his staff are keeping a close eye on developments in software-defined networking to produce more efficient use of the network as well as a consolidation of networking layers.

INTERNET2 INNOVATION PLATFORM

To be competitive as a university, you have to give your faculty the ability to collaborate on projects involving big data.

—Dr. Erik Deumens, Director of Research Computing, University of Florida

Internet2 is another major U.S. advanced networking community, founded by a consortium of higher-education institutions in 1996. The Internet2 Innovation Platform is an orchestration of new technologies and services that provide a leading-edge, end-to-end architecture and a unique set of unified capabilities at the national, regional, and campus level to create an environment for innovation in research and education. Internet2 provides network services to 247 universities, plus corporations and government agencies, and supports and provisions a deployed 100 GbE in its backbone network. The Innovation Platform architecture creates an end-to-end networking environment that will enable new and unique applications in addition to supporting current science requirements. Included in the Innovation Platform are key components, such as massive amounts of bandwidth through 100 GbE Layer 2 connections. SDN capabilities support the development and deployment of new applications, including a host of NFV opportunities that create pluggable, programmable research networks. The traditional bottlenecks challenging hybrid campus cloud models for "X as a Service" are met with aggregation points to pass high-bandwidth traffic providing performance monitoring/verification through implementation and support of the Science DMZ, a model developed by the DOE's ESnet.

Participants commit to implementation of the three key components of the innovation platform architecture: 100 GbE Layer 2 connection, SDN, and the Science DMZ model. The Next Generation Cyber Capability (NGCC) team at Arizona State University, in collaboration with advanced networking and systems experts, has targeted the development of applications and application programming interfaces (APIs) for end-to-end optimization of research collaboration. (The NGCC is discussed in much greater detail in Chapter 8.) In brief, the overarching initiative includes network management modules facilitating point-to-point dynamic communications with application path optimization, integration, and interface to Internet2's Open Exchange Software Suite; collaboration with international research partners via the International Consortium for Technology in Biomedicine (ICTBioMed) network; participation in larger collaborative commons models for conformant clouds with the National Institutes of Health, National Cancer Institute Cancer Cloud Genomics pilots, Big Data to Knowledge (BD2K) initiative, as well as a full spectrum of programs, such as Genomics Data Commons and the National Institute of Allergy and Infectious Diseases/National Human Genome Research Institute (NIAID/NHGRI) Human Microbiome Cloud. ASU's immediate development plans include security enhancements identifying and addressing essential challenges to building a robust firewall within the SDN/NFV layer that is stateful, distributed, and portable (virtual). In addition to protocol enhancements, robust security measures will be applied to SDN controllers to create secure enforcement kernels.

Figure 4.2 outlines the logical connections that are part of the Innovation Platform. As with any Innovation Platform, a diverse range of connections and applications are expected, but at minimum it includes: 100 GbE Advanced Layer 2 ports, SDN, and a Science DMZ connecting campuses.

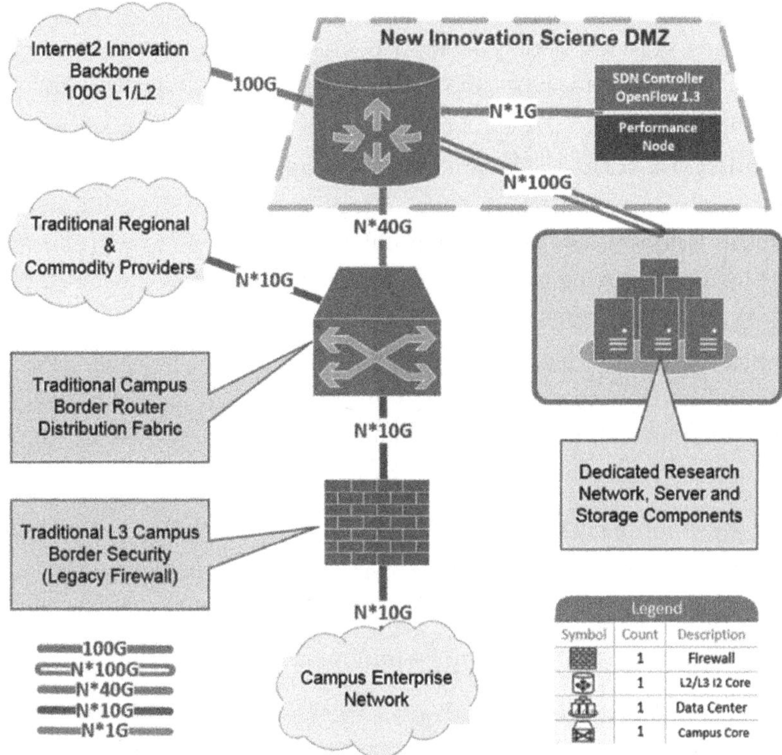

Figure 4.2 Innovation Platform Components
Jay Etchings, Research Computing Senior Architect, Arizona State University, presented at the Internet2 Innovation Platform, March 2, 2015.

ADVANCES IN NETWORKING

A number of computing trends are particularly important factors driving the need for a new network paradigm. These factors are discussed next.

Changing traffic patterns. Applications that commonly access geographically distributed databases and servers through public and private clouds require extremely flexible traffic management and access to bandwidth on demand.

"Consumerization of IT". The bring your own device (BYOD) trend requires networks that are both flexible and secure.

Rise of cloud services. Users expect on-demand access to applications, infrastructure, and other IT resources.

"Big data" means more bandwidth. Handling today's mega-datasets requires massive parallel processing that is fueling a constant demand for additional capacity and any-to-any connectivity.

In trying to meet the networking requirements posed by evolving computing trends, network designers find themselves constrained by the limitations of current networks. Some limitations are described next.

Complexity that leads to stasis. Adding or moving devices and implementing network-wide policies are complex, time-consuming, and primarily manual endeavors that risk service disruption. This discourages network changes.

Inability to scale. The time-honored approach of link oversubscription to provision scalability is not effective with the dynamic traffic patterns in virtualized networks—a problem that is even more pronounced in SPNs with large-scale parallel processing algorithms and associated datasets across an entire computing pool.

Vendor dependence. Lengthy vendor equipment product cycles and a lack of standard, open interfaces limit the ability of network operators to tailor the network to their individual environments. Drawbacks of vendor dependence include:

- Need for logical centralization
- Discrete, vertically integrated stacks—no end-to-end policy
- Performance or features—must choose
- Multivendor infrastructure—multiplying points of management

A core tenet of network design over the past 20 years has been segmentation at Layer 2 in the form of virtual local area networks (VLANs). The main challenge to VLANs is the lack of flexibility and adaptation to modern "microsegmented" areas of the network.

A number of promising developments in networking are redressing many of these challenges. We discuss them in the sections that follow. InfiniBand is a communications standard used in HPC that features very high throughput and very low latency. InfiniBand relies on traditional HPC and can be complex and costly so its future, particular in the research sciences, might be limited. The future of networking is certainly in the direction of NFV and SDN, both of which make networking more flexible and less costly. You can, of course, combine SDN and NFV. The bulk of this chapter focuses on SDN and more specifically OpenDaylight. SDN, which is still in its youth, offers mechanisms to not only add modularity in the form of dynamic segmentation but to inject additional capabilities of path selection and on-the-fly rerouting of traffic. The OpenDaylight Project, a collaborative open source project hosted by the Linux Foundation with the goal of accelerating the adoption of SDN, launched in 2013. We explore OpenDaylight in detail as it is an excellent way to implement SDN and NFV.

INFINIBAND AND MICROSECOND LATENCY

Microsecond or even submillisecond latency will be expected in the near future. Currently Ethernet fails to deliver this type of quick turnaround without layers of complexity or layered protocol approaches, such as RoCE,

RDMA over Converged Ethernet, or simply Remote Direct Memory Access (RDMA), leaving InfiniBand as the best selection when this type of speed is required for transactions.

InfiniBand is a network communications protocol that offers a switch-based fabric of point-to-point bidirectional serial links between processor nodes as well as between processor nodes and input/output nodes, such as disks or storage. Every link has exactly one device connected to each end of the link, such that the characteristics controlling the transmission (sending and receiving) at each end are well defined and controlled.

InfiniBand creates a private, protected channel directly between the nodes via switches, and facilitates data and message movement without CPU involvement with RDMA and send/receive offloads that are managed and performed by InfiniBand adapters. The adapters are connected on one end to the CPU over a PCI Express interface and to the InfiniBand subnet through InfiniBand network ports. This provides distinct advantages over other network communications protocols, including higher bandwidth, lower latency, and enhanced scalability.

The InfiniBand Trade Association (IBTA), established in 1999, chartered, maintains, and furthers the InfiniBand specification and is responsible for compliance and interoperability testing of commercial InfiniBand products. Through its roadmap, the IBTA has pushed the development of higher performance more aggressively than any other interconnect solution, ensuring an architecture that is designed for the 21st century. InfiniBand network products are, however, expensive. Table 4.1 provides the existing data rates and specifications.

Table 4.1 InfiniBand Data Rates

Name	Abbreviation	Raw Signaling Rate	Applied Encoding (b = bits)	Effective Data Rate	Aggregated (4x) Throughput
Single Data Rate	SDR	2.5 Gbps	8b/10b	2 Gbps	8 Gbps
Double Data Rate	DDR	5 Gbps	8b/10b	4 Gbps	16 Gbps
Quad Data Rate	QDR	10 Gbps	8b/10b	8 Gbps	32 Gbps
Fourteen Data Rate	FDR	14.1 Gbps	64b/66b	13.64 Gbps	54.5 Gbps
Enhanced Data Rate	EDR	25.8 Gbps	64b/66b	25 Gbps	100 Gbps
High Data Rate	HDR	51.6 Gbps	64b/66b	50 Gbps	200 Gbps
Next Data Rate	NDR	Tbd	Tbd	Tbd	Tbd

Tbd = to be determined.
Adapted from "InfiniBand FAQ, Rev 1.3," white paper, last updated December 22, 2014, Mellanox, http://www.mellanox.com/related-docs/whitepapers/InfiniBandFAQ_FQ_100.pdf.

For more information on InfiniBand, please see: https://cw.infinibandta.org/document/dl/7268.

What Is RDMA, and What Are Its Benefits?

InfiniBand uses RDMA as its method of transferring the data from one end of the channel to the other. RDMA is the ability to transfer data directly between the applications over the network with no operating system involvement and while consuming negligible CPU resources on both sides (zero-copy transfers). The application on the other side simply reads the message directly from the memory, and the message has been transmitted successfully.

This reduced CPU overhead increases the network's ability to move data quickly and allows applications to receive data faster. The time interval for a given quantity of data to be transmitted from source to destination is known as latency, and the lower the latency, the faster the application job completion.

How Is InfiniBand Different from Traditional Network Protocols?

InfiniBand is designed to enable the most efficient data center implementation. It natively supports server virtualization, overlay networks, and SDN.

InfiniBand takes an application-centric approach to messaging, finding the path of least resistance to deliver data from one point to another. This differs from traditional network protocols (such as TCP/IP and Fibre Channel), which use a more network-centric method for communicating.

Direct access means that an application does not rely on the operating system to deliver a message. In traditional interconnect, the operating system is the sole owner of shared network resources, meaning that applications cannot have direct access to the network. Instead, applications must rely on the operating system to transfer data from the application's virtual buffer to the network stack and onto the wire, and the operating system at the receiving end must have similar involvement, only in reverse.

InfiniBand's primary advantages over other interconnect technologies are listed next.

Higher throughput. 56 Gbps per server and storage connection, and soon 100 Gbps, compared to up to 40 Gb Ethernet and Fibre Channel (FC supports 16-32-64 GB connections and most higher bandwidth levels are over Ethernet in the form of FCoE, Fibre Channel over Ethernet at 100-200-400 GB; 256 GB is projected to be available by 2020) [3].

Lower latency. RDMA zero-copy networking reduces operating system overhead so data can move through the network quickly.

Enhanced scalability. InfiniBand can accommodate theoretically unlimited-sized flat networks based on the same switch components simply by adding additional switches.

Higher CPU efficiency. With data movement offloads the CPU can spend more compute cycles on its applications, which will reduce run time and increase the number of jobs per day.

Better return on investment. Higher throughput and CPU efficiency.

THE FUTURE OF HIGH-PERFORMANCE FABRICS*

Current standards-based high-performance fabrics, such as InfiniBand, were not originally designed for HPC, resulting in performance and scaling weaknesses that currently impede the path to exascale computing. Intel Omni-Path Architecture (OPA) is being designed specifically to address these issues and scale cost-effectively from entry-level HPC clusters to larger clusters with 10,000 nodes or more. While both Intel OPA and InfiniBand Enhanced Data Rate (EDR) will run at 100 Gbps, there are many differences. The enhancements of Intel OPA will help enable progress toward exascale while cost-effectively supporting clusters of all sizes with optimization for HPC applications at both the host and fabric levels for benefits that are not possible with the standard InfiniBand-based designs.

Intel OPA is designed to provide the:

- Features and functionality at both the host and fabric levels to greatly raise levels of scaling.
- CPU and fabric integration necessary for the increased computing density, improved reliability, reduced power, and lower costs required by significantly larger HPC deployments.
- Fabric tools to readily install, verify, and manage fabrics at this level of complexity.

Intel Omni-Path Key Fabric Features and Innovations

Adaptive Routing

Adaptive routing monitors the performance of the possible paths between fabric end points and selects the least congested path to rebalance the packet load. While other technologies also support routing, the implementation is vital. Intel's implementation is based on cooperation between the Fabric Manager and the switch application-specific integrated circuits (ASICs). The Fabric Manager—with a global view of the topology—initializes the switch ASICs with several egress options per destination, updating these options as

*This section is taken from "Intel® Omni-Path Architecture: The Next-Generation Fabric," http://www.intel.com/content/www/xr/en/high-performance-computing-fabrics/omni-path-architecture-fabric-overview.html. Used with permission.

the fundamental fabric changes when links are added or removed. Once the switch egress options are set, the Fabric Manager monitors the fabric state, and the switch ASICs dynamically monitor and react to the congestion sensed on individual links. This approach enables adaptive routing to scale as fabrics grow larger and more complex.

Dispersive Routing

One of the critical roles of fabric management is the initialization and configuration of routes through the fabric between pairs of nodes. Intel Omni-Path Fabric supports a variety of routing methods, including defining alternate routes that disperse traffic flows for redundancy, performance, and load balancing. Instead of sending all packets from a source to a destination via a single path, dispersive routing distributes traffic across multiple paths. Once received, packets are reassembled in their proper order for rapid, efficient processing. By leveraging more of the fabric to deliver maximum communications performance for all jobs, dispersive routing promotes optimal fabric efficiency.

Traffic Flow Optimization

Traffic flow optimization optimizes the quality of service beyond selecting the priority—based on virtual lane or service level—of messages to be sent on an egress port. At the Intel OPA link level, variable length packets are broken up into fixed-size containers that are in turn packaged into fixed-size link transfer packets for transmitting over the link. Since packets are broken up into smaller containers, a higher-priority container can request a pause and be inserted into the Inter-Switch Link (ISL) data stream before completing the previous data.

The key benefit is that traffic flow optimization reduces the variation in latency seen through the network by high-priority traffic in the presence of lower-priority traffic. It addresses a traditional weakness of both Ethernet and InfiniBand in which a packet must be transmitted to completion once the link starts even if higher-priority packets become available.

Packet Integrity Protection

Packet integrity protection allows for rapid and transparent recovery of transmission errors between a sender and a receiver on an Intel OPA link. Given the very high Intel OPA signaling rate (25.78125 G per lane) and the goal of supporting large-scale systems of 100,000 or more links, transient bit errors must be tolerated while ensuring that the performance impact is insignificant. Packet integrity protection enables recovery of transient errors, whether it is between a host and switch or between switches. This eliminates the need for transport-level timeouts and end-to-end retries. This is done without the heavy latency penalty associated with alternate error recovery approaches.

Dynamic Lane Scaling

Dynamic lane scaling allows an operation to continue even if one or more lanes of a 4x link fail, saving the need to restart or go to a previous checkpoint to keep the application running. The job can then run to completion before taking action to resolve the issue. Currently, InfiniBand typically drops the whole 4x link if any of its lanes drops, costing time and productivity.

NETWORK FUNCTION VIRTUALIZATION

Research institutions are beginning to embrace NFV and partner to develop new and interesting applications and use cases. The concepts within the NFV stack continue to evolve and augment software-defined networking. For simplicity it may be better to think of SDN as the holistic whole and network function virtualization as the individual parts of the whole. For example, consider a standard firewall. What happens in a firewall, and what are the specific steps in packet processing? You have some switched interface that performs packet switching either through software or an ASIC (application-specific independent circuitry), then there is some type of a basic routing mechanism that forwards to an inspection engine of sorts, which then, based on a wide array of conditions, makes yet another routing decision to send the packet on to its destination or send it to the bit bucket. Each individual operation is a "network function," and the traversal of the network flow can be mapped with ease back to the OSI model of operations as the packet travels through the layer 1 interface (physical) to the layer 2 switching (datalink) to the layer 3 routing (network) and so on. Think of NFV as the decoupling of those elements and the optimization of each within hardware/software design and development. Expect the requisite amount of vendor-driven confusion as NFV moves into production offerings.

If NFV is a subcomponent of SDN, then virtualized network function (VNF) is yet another step toward granularity within the same network stack. Therefore, if the same analogy as above is utilized, we can further decouple and look at this added operation within the firewall after the initial layer 1-2-3 operations have succeeded and the inspection engine attempts to look at the traffic to determine its validity. At this point it may need to perform yet another step. Say the packet is encrypted, as so many are these days (and rightfully should be). Furthermore, say the packet is on port 443 and HTTPS traffic. The inspection engine then needs to perform two additional operations, decryption and reencryption. Those introduce latency. Years ago the firewall manufacturer

Palo Alto Networks was most notable for separating those functions. That granular operation, albeit small, is critical, and it could be regarded as a VNF. That is where vendors will focus as SDN and NFV proliferate, as will research and development institutions. Multiple funding and patent opportunities will arise as a result.

As a quick example, here are some functions that can and will benefit the most from this granular approach to network optimization:

- Data and network security—inspection, identification of security threats
- Network optimizations—quality of service and traffic prioritization (QOS)
- SSL/private key encryption (PKE) and Internet Protocol Security (IPSec) encryption optimization, including authentication and decryption
- Inspection optimization, pattern matching, and next-generation cryptography
- Identification of OpenFlow topology changes and path optimizations
- Separation of "compute-intensive" network operations from "bandwidth-intensive" operations
- End-to-end (E2E) network service chaining (the connecting of functions to each other creating a larger operation)
- Acceleration of packet flows and thoughtful noise control or packet reduction
- Data compression and deduplication (network level within the hardware)

These solutions will increase in availability and mature in interoperability using software-based network functions completely decoupled from hardware through granular virtualization. NFV, networks, and networking will be redefined to be more open, flexible, and economical and run on commodity hardware or general-purpose computing platforms instead of traditional proprietary, purpose-built appliances. However, this transition is highly reliant on the development efforts to increase performance, reduce latency, and control costs. Latency or performance impact associated with virtualization on general-purpose platforms is well known and has been an area for improvement. The wider range of network-dependent cloud applications, which are highly susceptible and intolerant of adverse network events, will slow adoption as improvements in the area of interrupt-intensive, packet processing move forward.

To recap, the principal advantages of NFV are:

- Reduced equipment costs. Dynamic placement can reduce resource demands.
- Reduced operational costs. Reduced power, reduced space, and improved network monitoring.

- Flexibility to easily, rapidly, and dynamically provide and instantiate new services in various locations.
- Dynamic scaling. Should be able to change size and quantity easily.

SOFTWARE-DEFINED NETWORKING*

SDN is the physical separation of the network control plane from the forwarding plane, and where a control plane controls several devices. It is an emerging architecture that is dynamic, manageable, cost-effective, and adaptable, making it ideal for the high-bandwidth, dynamic nature of today's applications. This architecture decouples the network control and forwarding functions, enabling the network control to become directly programmable and the underlying infrastructure to be abstracted for applications and network services. The OpenFlow Standard is an SDN standard and a foundational element for building SDN solutions.

The OpenFlow Standard created by the Open Networking Foundation is a communications protocol that gives access to the forwarding plane of a network switch or router over the network. OpenFlow is the first standard communications interface defined between the control and forwarding layers of an SDN architecture.

The Open Networking Foundation lists the following as central characteristics of SDN architecture:

> **Directly programmable** Network control is directly programmable because it is decoupled from forwarding functions.
>
> **Agile** Abstracting control from forwarding lets administrators dynamically adjust network-wide traffic flow to meet changing needs.
>
> **Centrally managed** Network intelligence is (logically) centralized in software-based SDN controllers that maintain a global view of the network, which appears to applications and policy engines as a single, logical switch.
>
> **Programmatically configured** SDN lets network managers configure, manage, secure, and optimize network resources very quickly via dynamic, automated SDN programs, which they can write themselves because the programs do not depend on proprietary software.
>
> **Open standards–based and vendor-neutral** When implemented through open standards, SDN simplifies network design and operation because instructions are provided by SDN controllers instead of multiple, vendor-specific devices and protocols [4].

Figure 4.3 shows the separation of network layers in SDN.

---

*This section is taken from "OpenFlow." Open Networking Foundation, https://www.opennetworking.org/sdn-resources/openflow. Used with permission.

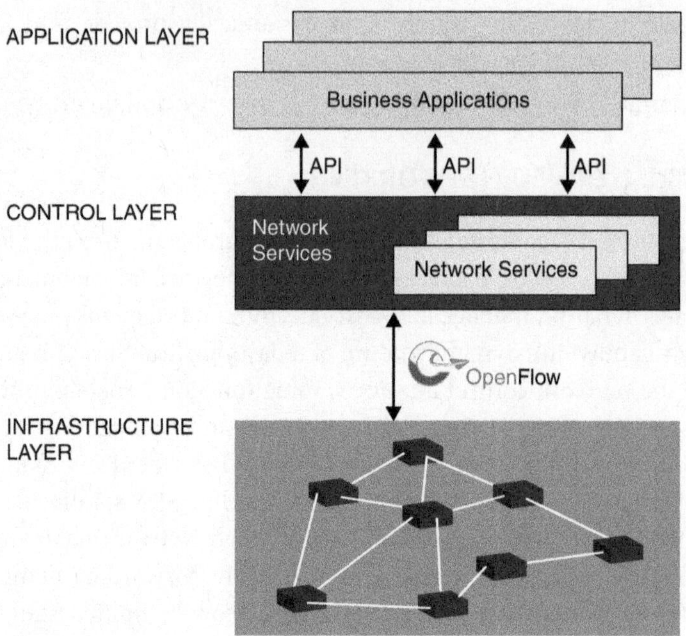

Figure 4.3 Separation of Network Layers with OpenFlow (SDN)

OPENDAYLIGHT*

OpenDaylight (ODL) is the open source SDN solution and is an excellent fit for academia. National Science Foundation panel reviews are one sign of a shift toward open source development. A recent announcement even informed panel reviewers that proposals with closed source or proprietary solutions in their proposals would need to include an addendum to validate the usage of proprietary software or the creation of software for profit (on public funding).

ODL and Open SDN ecosystem are projects of the OpenDaylight Foundation. ODL collaborates "with developers, end users and our members to produce the most relevant programs, events, and resources. We strongly believe in working together to solve our industry's shared challenges, and fostering a community where we all 'leave our company badges at the door'" [5]. I should note that I am a member of the ODL user advisory group. To learn more about this project and its governance, the staff and board of directors, and how your institution can support and advance ODL and the open SDN ecosystem, please visit: https://www.opendaylight.org/.

* This section is taken from "OpenDaylight Performance: A Practical, Empirical Guide." The OpenDaylight Platform. https://www.opendaylight.org/resources/odl-performance. Used with permission.

Because ODL is becoming widely adopted and is open source, our deep dive into SDN will focus on ODL. We present a number of common end-to-end scenarios for ODL.

End-to-End Scenarios for Common Usage in Large Carrier, Enterprise, and Research Networks

OpenDaylight is designed to serve a broad set of use cases and end user types. It does so by supporting a wide variety of southbound protocols to control network devices, providing a wide variety of network services, and allowing for the easy addition of new functionality in the form of southbound plugins, network services, and applications.

In order to deploy OpenDaylight, it is critical to understand not only the functionality it provides (and what subset a deployment might use) but also the performance characteristics of that functionality to evaluate whether it will meet the deployment's needs.

The goals of our tests were to measure end-to-end performance in the underlying protocols and technologies that support the body of OpenDaylight deployments in the world's largest networks for our major use case categories:

- Automated service delivery
- Network resource optimization
- Cloud and NFV

Most important, the performance we are measuring includes the complete end-to-end loop from application on top of the controller all the way to the network device and back, utilizing both northbound (application to controller) and southbound (controller to device) interfaces. Only by emulating this end-to-end scenario can test results be deemed representative of actual real-world deployments.

As closely as possible, we are simulating real-world scenarios that utilize:

- Emulating an application that programs a set of OpenFlow switches through the controller's northbound REST API.
- Emulating a network restart, where the controller needs to program a set of OpenFlow switches when the network restarts and the switches are brought online. We measured the rate of flow installation in the switches and the rate at which the controller was able to collect data about a large number of flows.
- BGP/BGP-Flow-Spec for flow redirection (selecting the egress point for the BGP next hop for a targeted flow); we measured both the route ingestion rate (i.e., the rate at which ODL is able to receive routes from a

peer) as well as route the advertisement rate (i.e., the rate at which ODL is able to advertise routes to a peer).

- PCEP for the optimal routing of MPLS LSPs.
- Emulating an application that programs a set of NETCONF devices through the controller's northbound REST API. In the NETCONF devices, we chose a YANG model roughly equivalent to flow programming through OpenFlow to determine the relative performance achievable by the two protocols (NETCONF and OpenFlow).
- Emulating the network scaling of a set of NETCONF devices (i.e., how many NETCONF devices can be connected to the controller).
- Emulating OpenFlow with Open vSwitch Database (OVSDB).

Provided in this report is data for other SDN controllers for general comparative reference only. They should not be considered as definitive maximum performance values for those platforms.

This report is the first in a series. As the team went through this exercise, we discovered several variables within the test environments that had a significant effect on performance of OpenDaylight and the other controllers we tested as comparative benchmarks. In addition, there are many other real-world scenarios that should be explored. We hope to collaborate with other open source communities focused on SDN and continue to provide interesting performance data to our communities.

OpenDaylight Architecture

The following sections provide a brief architectural overview of ODL.

Microservices Architecture

ODL employs a model-driven approach to describe the network, the functions to be performed on it, and the resulting state or status achieved. By sharing YANG data structures in a common data store and messaging infrastructure, OpenDaylight allows for fine-grained services to be created and then combined to solve more complex problems. In the ODL Model Driven Service Abstraction Layer (MD-SAL), any app or function can be bundled into a service that is then loaded into the controller. Services can be configured and chained together in any number of ways to match fluctuating needs within the network.

- Only install the protocols and services you need
- Ability to combine multiple services and protocols to solve more complex problems as needs arise
- Modular design allows anyone in the ODL ecosystem to leverage services created by others

Multiprotocol Support

ODL includes support for the broadest set of protocols in any SDN platform—both traditional and emerging—that improve programmability of modern networks and solve a range of user needs.

For example, the platform supports OpenFlow and OpenFlow extensions such as Table Type Patterns (TTP) as well as traditional protocols, including NETCONF, BGP/PCEP, and CAPWAP. Additionally, ODL interfaces with OpenStack and Open vSwitch through the OVSDB Integration Project. The ODL community will continue to evaluate and integrate protocols to provide the best level of support for its user base:

- Deploying into existing or greenfield networks
- Broadest set of protocol support available—from NETCONF to OpenFlow
- Open source development model allows for continuous innovation

Policy and Intent

With SDN we can achieve network programmability and abstraction, but then comes the question of how we manage it. By publishing common API frameworks, app developers can create abstractions north or south of the controller without having to look under the hood. There are several approaches to intent and policy that allow users to do this within ODL. In fact, as the industry's emerging de facto open SDN platform, ODL is the primary place for the development and testing of different approaches to policy and intent, such as ALTO, Group Based Policy, and Network Intent Composition. We are working closely with a number of industry groups, such as Open Networking Foundation and IETF, to vet and test the different approaches.

- ODL is the epicenter for development and testing of policy and intent approaches.
- App developers can write abstractions without having to dive under the hood.
- A growing list of APIs is included in the platform.

S3P: Security, Scalability, Stability, and Performance

The ODL community provides continual improvements across all its projects in the areas of security, scalability, stability, and performance, or "S3P" as we call it. Our Testing and Integration groups, along with people from each individual project, work together to run ongoing tests that give developers real-time results to see how changes affect S3P. We continue to evolve our development process to ensure that we can understand and monitor improvements in each of these four areas.

ODL is also working with OPNFV in support of a Controller Performance Testing project (CPerf) that would create industry-wide performance tests for SDN controllers in realistic, large, automated deployments. Those involved intend to foster collaboration between benchmarking experts from academic/standards backgrounds and the upstream engineers who implement actual performance benchmarks in modern Continuous Integration environments.

Security is another key area of focus for ODL, with each new release including better, tighter security features. The platform provides a framework for Authentication, Authorization, and Accounting (AAA) as well as automatic discovery and securing of network devices and controllers. Additionally, we have a strong security team and process to respond to any vulnerabilities immediately. In general, open source software has major advantages when it comes to security: Anyone can find and report vulnerabilities; we can draw on a wide array of experts and developers across companies to discuss and fix them; and the community at large can see how such issues are addressed transparently and understand whether the issue really has been fixed.

- Strong focus on security, scalability, stability, and performance of ODL
- Continuous integration and testing of all projects
- Documented and transparent security process to identify and enable immediate fixes

Test Environment

For this report, the ODL community ran all tests on a common set of hardware to achieve uniform performance results. To get a broader view of OpenDaylight's performance characteristics and to determine the impact of the environment on performance, the tests were run in two different test environments. In the following sections, for each set of results, we describe which environment was used. The complete details on the two test environments are provided below.

Environment #1

This is the base environment setup #1 for all the test cases unless stated otherwise:

- Hardware:
  - CPU: Intel® Xeon® CPU E5-2690 v2 @ 3.00GHz, 40 cores
  - Total RAM: 128GB

- Operating System: Ubuntu Linux 4.2.0-30-generic x86_64
- Network:
  - Every test component is run directly on the machine.
  - All communication happens over the 127.0.0.1/8 loopback network.
- Java Virtual Machine (JVM):
  - Oracle 1.8.0_73
  - 8G of Java Heap
  - Default garbage collector
- ODL: Beryllium

Environment #2

This is the base environment setup #2 for all the test cases unless stated otherwise:

- Hardware:
  - CPU: 2 Intel Xeon E5-2699 v3sz @ 2.30 GHz, 72 cores
  - Total RAM: 64GB
- Operating System: Fedora release 23 Linux 4.2.3-300.fc23.x86_64 x86_64
- Network:
  - Test component is run directly on the machine
  - All communication happens over 127.0.0.1/8 loopback network
  - Exception: OVSDB Scale Tests that use multiple other identical systems to scale test tools
- JVM:
  - OpenJDK 64-Bit 1.8.0_72
  - 8G of Java Heap
  - Default garbage collector
- ODL: Beryllium

Performance Results

OpenFlow

This section provides performance measurements related to the OpenFlow protocol in OpenDaylight. All tests have been performed in Environment #1. We have also added other SDN controller results for reference. Figure 4.4 shows the test setup.

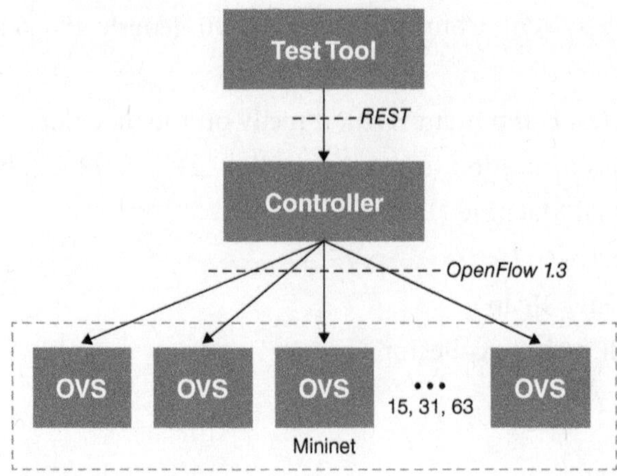

Figure 4.4 Test Setup

Northbound REST API Benchmark

The purpose is to perform an *end-to-end performance* test from a REST API all the way down to the network to simulate real-world scenarios. With OpenFlow, most applications use the controller's northbound APIs. This test uses Flow Programming APIs that are typically available on all controllers.

The test is performed as follows: We configure 100,000 (100k) flows through the REST APIs and wait until the flows are "read back" (collected) from the network by the controller. We measure the flow programming time at the controller and in the network and the flow confirmation time. After a short delay the flows are deleted from the controller, and again we measure the flow deletion time at the controller and in the network and flow confirmation time.

Controllers use different flow programming confirmation:

- OpenDaylight: "Confirmation" means flows are added or removed from the operational datastore.
- ONOS: "Confirmation" means flows change their states from 'PENDING_ADD' to 'ADDED' or from 'PENDING_ REMOVE' to be effectively removed.

Detailed information about the test scenario, test setup, and a step-by-step guide can be found at https://wiki.opendaylight.org/view/Openflow:Testing.

The columns in the tables are defined as follows:

- **Add controller time.** Time for all add REST requests to be sent and their response to be received.
- **Add switch time.** Time from the first REST request until all flows are present in the network.
- **Add confirm time.** Time period started after the last flow was configured until we receive "confirmation" (see above paragraph) all flows are added.

- **Remove controller time.** Time for all delete REST requests to be sent and their response to be received.
- **Remove switch time.** Time from the first delete REST request until all flows are removed from the network.
- **Remove confirm time.** Time period started after the last flow was unconfigured until we receive "confirmation" all flows are removed.

OpenDaylight Beryllium "Old Plugin" Results

OpenDaylight RESTconf REST API supports any flow programming granularity, from one flow per REST call to programming all desired flows in a single REST call. So we run two tests: 1 flow request per REST API call and 200 flow requests per REST API call. This way we can evaluate the effects of batching on performance. See Tables 4.2 through 4.5.

Table 4.2 Environment #1: Beryllium Release
1 Flow Add/Remove per REST Call

Switches	Add Controller Time (s)	Add Controller Rate (Flows/s)	Add Switch Time (s)	Add Confirm Time (s)	Remove Controller Time (s)	Remove Switch Time (s)	Remove Confirm Time (s)
15	81.13	1,232.58		143	67.08		2
15	76.88	1,300.72		151	68.16		2
15	80.47	1,242.69		152	66.37		2
31	78.46	1,274.53	81	49	66.98	63	5
31	76.16	1,313.02	78	50	67.33	64	2
31	76.28	1,310.96	80	56	69.39	65	2
63	77.69	1,287.16	83	23	70.06	65	3
63	76,96	1,299.37	79	22	70.10	68	5
63	78.25	1,277.95	82	23	67.11	64	6

Table 4.3 Environment #2 (using SSD drive, persistence disabled and tuned): Beryllium Release
1 Flow Add/Remove per REST Call

Switches	Add Controller Time (s)	Add Controller Rate (Flows/s)	Add Switch Time (s)	Add Confirm Time (s)	Remove Controller Time (s)	Remove Switch Time (s)	Remove Confirm Time (s)
15	52.02	1,922.37	53		37.45	37	2
15	51.86	1,934.13	53		38.89	37	2
15	53.15	1,881.64	54		37.59	37	2
31	52.53	1,903.55	53		40.62	40	2
31	53.81	1,858.39	54		40.48	40	2

(*Continued*)

Table 4.3 *(Continued)*

Switches	Add Controller Time (s)	Add Controller Rate (Flows/s)	Add Switch Time (s)	Add Confirm Time (s)	Remove Controller Time (s)	Remove Switch Time (s)	Remove Confirm Time (s)
31	53.04	1,885.49	55	26s	43.36	44	3
63	54.19	1,845.49	58		44.47	46	4
63	53.85	1,856.90	57	31	43.66	47	2
63	53.20	18,79.72	56	31	45.88	46	4

Table 4.4 Environment #1: Beryllium Release
200 Flows Add per REST Call/Remove All Flows in One REST Call

Switches	Add Controller Time (s)	Add Controller Rate (Flows/s)	Add Switch Time (s)	Add Confirm Time (s)	Remove Controller Time (s)	Remove Switch Time (s)	Remove Confirm Time (s)
31	10.60	9,434.84	12	158	1	4	6
31	13.57	7,370.40	15	149	1	5	6
31	11.89	8,409.69	13	152	1	6	6
63	12.59	7,944.23	14	81	1	5	6
63	11.44	8,741.29	13	87	1	5	7
63	11.26	8,880.94	14	86	1	5	6

Table 4.5 Environment #2 (using SSD drive, persistence disabled and tuned): Beryllium Release
200 Flows Add per REST call/Remove All Flows in One REST Call

Switches	Add Controller Time (s)	Add Controller Rate (Flows/s)	Add Switch Time (s)	Add Confirm Time (s)	Remove Controller Time (s)	Remove Switch Time (s)	Remove Confirm Time (s)
31	9.70	10,309.12	11		1	2	2
31	9.31	10,741.95	11		1	3	2
31	9.84	10,157.47	12	26	1	2	3
63	9.70	10,306.85	12	26	1	2	4
63	10.45	9,567.79	12	26	1	3	4
63	10.21	9,796.16	12	26	1	2	5

OpenDaylight Boron "New Plugin" Results

Again we run two tests: 1 flow request per REST API call and 200 flow requests per REST API call. Here we are using OpenDaylight Boron (which is the next ODL release). See Tables 4.6 through 4.9.

Table 4.6 Environment #1: Beryllium Release
200 Flows Add per REST Call/Remove All Flows in One REST Call

Switches	Add Controller Time (s)	Add Controller Rate (Flows/s)	Add Switch Time (s)	Add Confirm Time (s)	Remove Controller Time (s)	Remove Switch Time (s)	Remove Confirm Time (s)
15	70.85s	1,411.43	73	10	56.74	53	4
15	69.12s	1,446.75	71	9	57.28	55	4
15	68.77s	1,454.12	70	9	59.21	57	4
31	72.07s	1,387.54	77	15	58.43	56	4
31	69.26s	1,443.83	70	9	59.30	58	4
31	70.16s	1,425.31	73	9	58,75	56	4
63	69.49s	1,439.05	70	15	59.45	58	5
63	68.18s	1,446.70	70	15	58.75	59	4
63	69.04s	1,448.43	71	15	60.26	60	5

Table 4.7 Environment #2 (using SSD drive, persistence disabled and tuned): Beryllium Release
200 Flows Add per REST Call/Remove All Flows in One REST Call

Switches	Add Controller Time (s)	Add Controller Rate (Flows/s)	Add Switch Time (s)	Add Confirm Time (s)	Remove Controller Time (s)	Remove Switch Time (s)	Remove Confirm Time (s)
15	51.32	1,948.44	53	8	38.86	37	4
15	52.10	1,919.54	53	9	41.27	39	4
15	51.16	1,954.76	52	7	40.12	38	4
31	53.85	1,857.13	56	8	41.86	39	4
31	56.04	1,784.52	58	8	39.50	36	4
31	53.44	1,871.21	56	8	41.44	39	4
63	52.78	1,894.51	54	8	40.01	37	4
63	52.98	1,887.66	54	9	39.99	40	4
63	54.04	1,850.57	56	8	40.41	40	4

Table 4.8 Environment #1: Beryllium Release
200 Flows Add per REST Call/Remove All Flows in One REST Call

Switches	Add Controller Time (s)	Add Controller Rate (Flows/s)	Add Switch Time (s)	Add Confirm Time (s)	Remove Controller Time (s)	Remove Switch Time (s)	Remove Confirm Time (s)
31	12.45	8,029.84	12	8	1	10	12
31	11.04	9,057.56	14	14	1	9	12
31	11.54	8,661.92	13	13	1	9	11
63	11.07	9,034.00	15	13	1	11	13
63	11.03	9,064.82	15	14	1	12	13
63	11.21	8,923.72	15	14	1	11	11

Table 4.9 Environment #2 (using SSD drive, persistence disabled and tuned): Beryllium Release 1 Flow Add/Remove per REST Call

Switches	Add Controller Time (s)	Add Controller Rate (Flows/s)	Add Switch Time (s)	Add Confirm Time (s)	Remove Controller Time (s)	Remove Switch Time (s)	Remove Confirm Time (s)
31	11.58	8,634.79	14	10	1	5	10
31	11.01	9,079.21	14	8	1	6	9
31	10.19	9,810.51	12	7	1	7	11
63	10.07	9,932.58	11	7	1	8	12
63	10.72	9,330.09	12	7	1	8	9
63	11.69	8,552.72	13	7	1	7	11

ONOS Results

We used 1 flow request per REST API call, because that's what the REST API supports in ONOS Falcon 1.5.0. See Tables 4.10 and 4.11.

Table 4.10 Environment #1: ONOS Falcon 1.5.0-rc2

Switches	Add Controller Time (s)	Add Controller Rate (Flows/s)	Add Switch Time (s)	Add Confirm Time (s)	Remove Controller Time (s)	Remove Switch Time (s)	Remove Confirm Time (s)
15	41.65	2,400.96	43	404	95.54	80	NA **
31	41.83	2,390.62	53	100	41.84	43	181
31	42.15	2,372.48	61	400	48.83	50	387
31	40.68	2,548.21	45	NA *	55.93	57	300
63	40.63	2,561.23	53	55	40,63	31	3s
63	40.53	2,467.31	43	32	33.41	33	49
63	41.07	2,434.87	57	98	35.50	37	115

NA * After 500+s all 100k flows in PENDING_ADD state

NA ** After 500+s all 100k flows still in PENDING_REMOVE state

Table 4.11 Environment #2 (using SSD drive and tuned): ONOS Falcon 1.5.0

Switches	Add Controller Time (s)	Add Controller Rate (Flows/s)	Add Switch Time (s)	Add Confirm Time (s)	Remove Controller Time (s)	Remove Switch Time (s)	Remove Confirm Time (s)
15	65.34	1,530.46	99	477	382.9	391	NA*
31	66.01	1,514.92	72	98	207.14	170	283
31	65.36	1,529.99	79	125	213.56	206	299
31	63.31	1,579.52	65	230	246.28	238	531
63	65.01	1,538.22	75	221	171.07	160	321
63	66.05	1,514.00	69	346	202.92	196	374
63	54.04	1,850.57	56	8	40.41	40	4

NA * After 500+s all 100k flows in PENDING_REMOVE state

We had difficulty collecting statistics with ONOS on smaller networks (15 and 31 nodes) with 100k flows. We had no difficulty with statistics collection in larger networks (63 nodes). We also observed that the time to push all the flows to the switches could be up to 25 percent longer than the time to program all of the flows into the controller.

Floodlight Results

We used 1 flow request per REST API call, as that is what the REST API supports. See Table 4.12.

Table 4.12 Environment #1: Floodlight
1 Flow Add/Remove per REST Call

Switches	Add Controller Time (s)	Add Controller Rate (Flows/s)	Add Switch Time (s)	Add Confirm Time (s)	Remove Controller Time (s)	Remove Switch Time (s)	Remove Confirm Time (s)	Note (Dangling Flows)
15	52.99	1,887.31	54	NA	35.45	48	NA	453
15	52.98	1,887.43	55	NA	35.04	45	NA	533
15	53.54	1,867.69	56	NA	35.14	46	NA	3173
31	51.84	1,927.28	55	NA	35.75	57	NA	6,175
31	51.75	1,932.51	54	NA	35.34	46	NA	280
31	52.02	1,922.50	54	NA	35.92	48	NA	8,111
63	52.65	1,899.19	59	NA	35.54	64	NA	4,371
63	54.66	1,829.45	60	NA	35.92	58	NA	843
63	51.64	1,936.59	56	NA	35.73	57	NA	5,449

Floodlight does not have an API to verify added flows on the switch and that is the reason why confirmation time remains not available (NA). We also observed that Floodlight does not support secure HTTP (i.e., calls to Floodlight's REST API are neither encrypted nor authenticated).

For every test run we observed that dangling flows remained configured on switches after the flows had been removed from the controller. The number of dangling flows for each run is shown in the last column.

Conclusion

For single flow request per REST call programming, both the OpenDaylight Beryllium plugin and the Boron plugin support up to 1,900 flows per second. Flow Add Switch times are also similar in both plugins: 100k flows programmed in 53 seconds with almost no delay (1–3 seconds) between the last flow was configured in the controller and the last flow was programmed in the switch. Flow Confirmation is faster and more stable in the Boron plugin, spending less than 10 seconds to confirm 100k flows after the last flow was configured in the controller regardless of the topology used.

OpenDaylight northbound REST "batch" OpenFlow operation enables fast network flow programming. When using 200 flow requests per REST call, OpenDaylight supports up to 9,000 flows per second. This is five times faster than with a single request. Flow Add Switch times are also shorter with "batch" programming: 100k flows programmed in 11 seconds with almost no delay (1–3 seconds) between the time the last flow was configured in the controller and the last flow was programmed in the switch. Flow Confirmation is still faster and more stable in the Boron plugin, spending less than 10 seconds for 100k flows regardless of the topology used.

Southbound (OpenFlow) Benchmark

The purpose of this test is to benchmark a real stress scenario wherein several switches reboot and reconnect to the controller.

We use same setup as the northbound test (see Figure 4.6).

The test is performed as follows: We configure 100,000 (100k) flows through the REST APIs, and wait until the flows are programmed in the network by the controller. We then restart the network (mininet) and measure the flow programming time in the network and the flow confirmation time. Controllers tested use different flow programming confirmations:

- OpenDaylight: "confirmation" means flows are added to operational datastore.
- ONOS: "confirmation" means flows change their states from 'PENDING_ADD' to 'ADDED'.

Detailed information about the test scenario, test setup, and a step-by-step guide can be found at https://wiki.opendaylight.org/view/Openflow:Testing.

The columns in Tables 4.13 through 4.16 are defined as follows:

- **Add switch time.** Time since mininet is reconnected until all flows are present in the network.
- **Add confirm time.** Time period started after the last flow was programmed until we receive "confirmation" (see above paragraph) all flows are added.

Table 4.13 OpenDaylight Beryllium "Old Plugin" Results

Switches	Add Switch Time (s)	Add Switch Rate (flows/s)	Add Confirm Time (s)
31	4	25,000	171
31	5	20,000	160
31	5	20,000	160
63	9	11,111	202
63	9	11,111	198
63	9	11,111	204

Table 4.14 OpenDaylight Boron "New Plugin" Results

Switches	Add Switch Time (s)	Add Switch Rate (flows/s)	Add Confirm Time (s)
31	9	11,111	9
31	9	11,111	10
31	9	11,111	7
63	9	11,111	9
63	10	10,000	8
63	10	10,000	9

Table 4.15 ONOS Results

Switches	Add Switch Time (s)	Add Switch Rate (flows/s)	Add Confirm Time (s)	Note
31	104	932*	NA*	100,093 flows expected, but after 500+ sec only 97,007 flows were on the switches and verification showed {u'ADDED': 100086, u'PENDING_REMOVE': 1}
31	208	468*	NA*	100,093 flows expected, but after 500+ sec only 97,382 flows were on the switches and verification showed {u'ADDED': 100088, u'PENDING_REMOVE': 1}
31	96	988*	NA*	100,093 flows expected, but after 500+ sec only 94,855 flows were on the switches and verification showed {u'ADDED': 100087, u'PENDING_REMOVE': 2}
63	8	12,500	64**	100,189 flows expected, but only 100,182 got
63	7	14,285	61**	100,189 flows expected, but only 100,179 got
63	40	2,500	1**	100,189 flows expected, but only 100,175 got

*The rate is counted as "number of flows on the switches"/"Add Switch Time," but performance didn't look like slow adding flows. Just after switches were connected 93 flows (3 on each) were programmed. There was a long pause, and then in a few seconds (3–6) all other flows were programmed (but some flows remained missing).

**Some flow loss was noticed for every mininet restart. See the last column ("Note") in the table.

Table 4.16 Floodlight Results

Switches	Add Switch Time (s)	Add Switch Rate (flows/s)	Add Confirm Time (s)
31	5	20,000	NA
31	5	20,000	NA
31	4	25,000	NA
63	10	10,000	NA
63	9	11,111	NA
63	10	10,000	NA

Floodlight does not have API to get confirmation time.

Conclusion

With a reduced number of switches, OpenDaylight Beryllium plugin programs flow at about 20,000 flows/s. This is faster than the Boron plugin at 11,111 flows/s; however, this difference decreases and even disappears when we increase the number of switches. When it comes to collecting flow operational information from the network, the OpenDaylight Boron plugin is clearly superior (to the Beryllium plugin), confirming 100,000 flows in less than 10 seconds for any topology.

NETCONF

This section presents scale and performance measurements tied to the NETCONF protocol in OpenDaylight.

Southbound Scale

NETCONF southbound in ODL relies on asynchronous IO to establish and retain the sessions. This allows ODL to keep a relatively high number of active NETCONF sessions with limited resources.

The goal of this test is to measure the number of NETCONF devices the ODL NETCONF southbound plugin can mount with a certain amount of RAM. All of the devices are simulated with the same set of YANG models:

- ietf-netconf-monitoring
- ietf-netconf-monitoring-extension. ODL extensions to ietf-netconf-monitoring
- ietf-yang-types
- ietf-inet-types

To configure the connections in ODL, config pusher and config subsystem are utilized. NETCONF devices are simulated by ODL's netconf testtool, and no complex operations are performed once they are mounted.

The complete scenario is shown in Figure 4.5.

Detailed information about the test scenario, test setup, and a step-by-step guide can be found at ODL wiki: http://wiki.opendaylight.org/.

Results

All test runs were performed in Environment #1. Each simulated device starts its own NETCONF server bound to a dedicated port on the loopback IP address.

The following attributes were configured and observed in the test runs:

- **Heap size.** Max memory used by ODL.
- **Connection batch size.** Number of connections configured in a single config transaction. Batching is used to minimize the overhead in config subsystem.

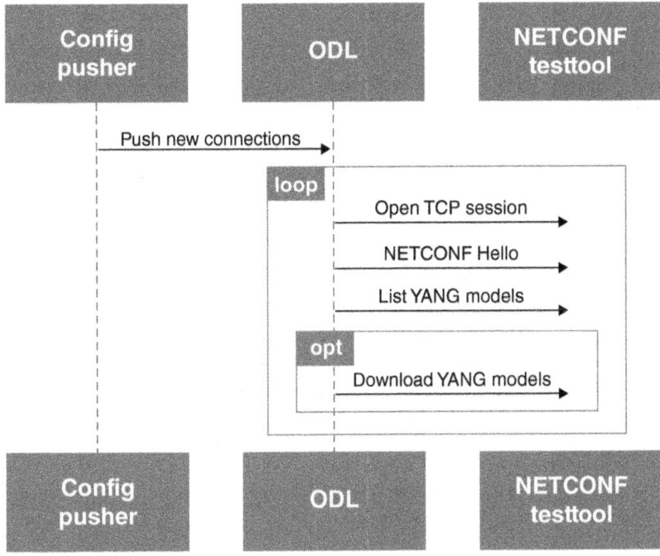

Figure 4.5 ODL Network Configuration

Measured numbers:

- **TCP max devices.** Number of mounted NETCONF devices by ODL before it runs out of resources, with an upper limit of 30,000 devices.
- **TCP execution time.** Total time between ODL start and last device successfully mounted, with timeout after 20 minutes. List of fully mounted devices is periodically queried from NETCONF topology via RESTCONF, and the time when last update occurred is read as the execution time.
- **SSH max devices.** Same as TCP max devices, but using SSH protocol between ODL and devices instead of TCP.
- **SSH execution time.** Same as TCP execution time, but using SSH protocol between ODL and devices instead of TCP. See Table 4.17.

Table 4.17 NETCONF Southbound Scale Results

Heap Size	Connection Batch Size	TCP Max Devices	TCP Execution Time	SSH Max Devices	SSH Execution Time
2GB	4k	20 000	6m 03s	8 000	3m 40s
2GB	1k	21 000	18m 54s	9 000	12m 16s
4GB	2k	28 000	17m 27s	14 000	9m 28s
4GB	1k	24 000	18m 31s	15 000	17m 20s

Conclusion

For minimalistic NETCONF devices (small set of YANG models), it is possible to mount 21k (9k with SSH) of them using just 2 GB of RAM in ODL. With 4 GB of RAM, the numbers are even higher: 28k (15k for SSH). For devices with bigger model sets, it is expected that the number of maximum mounted devices will be lower. However, thanks to the fully model-driven, pass-through nature of NETCONF southbound, the difference should not be dramatic. To confirm, additional tests of NETCONF scale are required for comparison.

It is important to note that the size of batched connections affects the maximum number of mounted devices as well as the execution time. Config-pusher and config subsystem of ODL were utilized to spawn NETCONF connectors, with each new connector having a dedicated config module instance. This presents considerable overhead, but it is the traditional way of connecting to NETCONF devices. With the Beryllium release of ODL, there is an alternative of using the NETCONF topology directly, bypassing the config subsystem altogether. We believe that using the NETCONF topology instead of the config subsystem would produce better results when trying to mount as many devices as possible. This should be the subject of additional NETCONF scale tests.

The difference between TCP and SSH is significant, with SSH being able to mount approximately 50% of what's possible with TCP.

Northbound Performance

NETCONF northbound in ODL provides an interface to the MD-SAL. Much like RESTCONF, it allows external users and applications to interact with ODL applications and services in terms of data, RPCs, and notifications. It fully leverages the model-driven approach, making the interface available to any MD-SAL based ODL application.

The goal of this test is to measure the performance of pushing data into ODL's global datastore via the NETCONF northbound interface. The data is a list of l2-fib entries. Each entry consists of a physical address and an assigned action. A small l2-fib YANG model has been developed to represent the l2-fib entries:

```
module ncmount-l2fib {
...
   container bridge-domains {
      list bridge-domain {
         key "name";
         leaf name { type string; }
         list l2-fib {
            key "phys-address";
               leaf phys-address {
                  type yang:phys-address;
                }
                  leaf action {
                     type enumeration {
                        enum "forward";
```

```
                enum "filter";
            }
        }
    }
...
```

XML rendered data according to this model used in the test:

```
<bridge-domain>
   <name>a</name>
   <l2-fib>
      <phys-address>08:00:27:08:5d:f2</phys-address>
      <action>forward</action>
   </l2-fib>
   <l2-fib>
      <phys- address>08:00:27:08:5d:f3</phys-address>
      <action>forward</action>
   </l2-fib>
...
```

The complete scenario is shown in Figure 4.6.

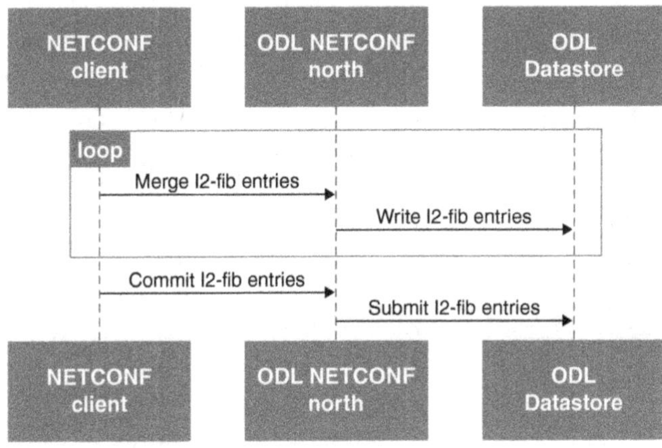

Figure 4.6 NETCONF Northbound Performance Test Results

Detailed information about the test scenario, test setup, and a step-by-step guide can be found at ODL wiki: http://wiki.opendaylight.org/.

Results

All test runs were performed in Environment #1 (some of them replicated in Environment #2) with two deviations:

- **ODL.** Stable/Beryllium build of ncmount sample ODL application using custom l2-fib model
- **ODL Heap.** 8GB

The following attributes were configured and observed in the test runs:

- **Clients**. Number of concurrent NETCONF clients used to push the data in. Each client handles *1/Clients* of total l2-fibs.
- **Client type.**
  - **Sync.** Client thread waits for response (OK) to every request (edit-config, commit) it sends out before sending the next one.
  - **Async.** Not waiting for the results in the thread responsible for sending out requests. Instead receiving requests in a dedicated thread without having to block any of the threads.
- **L2-fib per request.** How many l2-fib entries were sent per batch (1 edit-config RPC).
- **Total l2-fibs.** Total number of l2-fib entries pushed into ODL.

Measured numbers:

- **TCP performance.** Rate of l2-fib processing and storing in ODL. Measured as: Total l2-fibs / Duration between first request sent and last response received.
  - **edits/s.** Rate of edit-config rpcs processing in ODL.
  - **L2-fibs/s.** edits/s multiplied by number of l2-fibs per edit-config.
- **SSH performance.** Same as TCP but using SSH protocol for NETCONF instead of plain TCP.

Tables 4.18 – 4.20 show NETCONF performance test results.

Table 4.18 Single External NETCONF Client Results In Environment #1: Netconf Northbound Single Client Performance

Client Type	L2-Fib per Request	TCP Performance	SSH Performance	Total L2-Fibs
Sync	1	1,730 edits/s 1 730 l2-fibs/s	1,474 edits/s 1,474 l2-fibs/s	100k
Async	1	7,063 edits/s 7,063 l2-fibs/s	6,600 edits/s 6,600 l2-fibs/s	100k
Sync	100	233 edits/s 23,372 l2-fibs/s	148 edits/s 14,850 l2-fibs/s	500k
Async	100	421 edits/s 42,179 l2-fibs/s	386 edits/s 38,600 l2-fibs/s	500k
Sync	500	61 edits/s 30,935 l2-fibs/s	13 edits/s 6,590 l2-fibs/s	1M
Async	500	81 edits/s 40,894 l2-fibs/s	69 edits/s 34,500 l2-fibs/s	1M
Sync	1,000	35 edits/s 35,365 l2-fibs/s	13 edits/s 13,248 l2-fibs/s	1M
Async	1,000	38 edits/s 38,099 l2-fibs/s	19 edits/s 19,898 l2-fibs/s	1M

Table 4.19 Single External NETCONF Client Results In Environment #2: NETCONF Northbound Single Client Performance

Client Type	L2-Fib per Request	TCP Performance	SSH Performance	Total L2-Fibs
Syncl	1	1,178 edits/s 1,178 l2-fibs/s	655 edits/s 655 l2-fibs/s	100k
Async	1	5,107 edits/s 5,107 l2-fibs/s	4,791 edits/s 4,791 l2-fibs/s	100k
Sync	100	227 edits/s 22,700 l2-fibs/s	137 edits/s 13,700 l2-fibs/s	500k
Async	100	449 edits/s 44,900 l2-fibs/s	416 edits/s 41,600 l2-fibs/s	500k

Table 4.20 Concurrent External NETCONF Client Results: NETCONF Northbound Concurrent Clients Performance

Clients	Client Type	L2-Fib per Request	TCP Performance	SSH Performance	Total L2-Fibs
8	Sync	1	23,010 edits/s 23,010 l2fibs/s	13,847 edits/s 13,847 l2fibs/s	400k
8	Async	1	41,114 edits/s 41,114 l2fibs/s	12,527 edits/s 12,527 l2fibs/s	400k
16	Sync	1	31,743 edits/s 31,743 l2fibs/s	15,879 edits/s 15,879 l2fibs/s	400k
16	Async	1	43,252 edits/s 43,252 l2fibs/s	12,496 edits/s 12,496 l2fibs/s	400k
8	Sync	100	852 edits/s 85,215 l2fibs/s	769 edits/s 76,989 l2fibs/s	1,6M
8	Async	100	984 edits/s 98,419 l2fibs/s	869 edits/s 86,923 l2fibs/s	1,6M
16	Sync	100	808 edits/s 80,885 l2fibs/s	723 edits/s 72,345 l2fibs/s	1,6M
16	Async	100	852 edits/s 85,224 l2fibs/s	749 edits/s 74,962 l2fibs/s	1,6M

Conclusion

For a single NETCONF client, it is possible to achieve a maximal rate of 42,179 (38,600 with SSH) l2-fib entries pushed into ODL via NETCONF northbound interface per second. However, the key to this rate is batching and utilization of an asynchronous client. Without batching (single l2-fib per edit) the performance is much lower due to the overhead of NETCONF RPC processing in the NETCONF ODL pipeline. Asynchronous client utilization is actually a performance optimization on the client side to fully load the ODL threads in NETCONF northbound. Tests run in Environment #2 provided comparable results, being able to top the maximal rate.

For a multiclient setup, a maximal rate of 98,419 (86,923 for SSH) l2-fib entries per second was achieved with 8 concurrent asynchronous clients.

Again, batching and using asynchronous clients is important when trying to achieve the best performance.

Comparing performance using SSH to TCP shows an overall decrease of performance, from an approximately 10% decrease with small batches and up to 80% decrease with very big batches per message using synchronous clients.

Southbound Performance

NETCONF southbound in ODL provides a way for both internal and external applications to access remote, NETCONF-capable devices in a unified way. Exposing mountpoints into MD-SAL allows any application, internal or external, to manage and monitor NETCONF devices in terms of data, RPCs, and notifications. A model-driven approach is again utilized, allowing connections to any NETCONF-capable devices with existing YANG models.

The goal of this test is to measure the performance of pushing data into a BA (Binding Aware) ODL application via NETCONF southbound interface (NETCONF notifications flowing in from a mounted device). The data is a list of IPv4 prefixes sent from a fast, simulated NETCONF device. Each entry consists of a prefix and a single next hop. In this test, Cisco IOS XR models for router static configuration are utilized:

```
module Example-notifications {
...
   notification vrf-route-notification {
      uses ip-static-cfg:VRF-PREFIX-TABLE;
      description
      "Artificial notification based on Cisco-IOS-XR-ip-static-cfg model";
   }
...
module Cisco-IOS-XR-ip-static-cfg {
...
   grouping VRF-PREFIX-TABLE {
      description "Common node of vrf-unicast, vrf-multicast";
      container vrf-prefixes {
         description "The set of all Static Topologies for this AFI.";
         list vrf-prefix {
            key "prefix prefix-length";
            description "A static route";
            leaf prefix {
               type inet:ip-address;
               description "Destination prefix";
            }
         leaf prefix-length {
            type uint32 { range "0..128"; }
            description "Destination prefix length";
            }
         uses VRF-ROUTE;
```

```
        }
    }
...
```

XML rendered data according to this model used in the test:

```
<vrf-route-notification>
   <vrf-prefixes>
     <vrf-prefix>
       <prefix>127.0.0.1</prefix>
       <prefix-length>32</prefix-length>
     <vrf-route>
    <vrf-next-hops>
      <next-hop-address>
      <next-hop-address>10.0.0.1</next-hop-
address>
...
```

The complete scenario is shown in Figure 4.7.

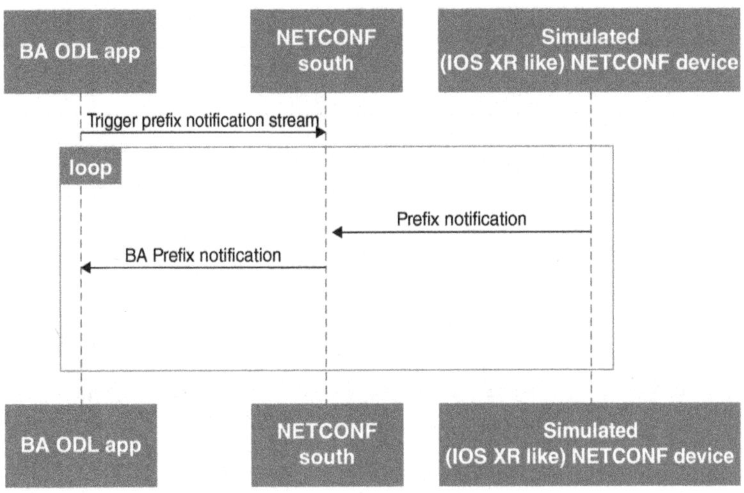

Figure 4.7 NETCONF Southbound Performance Test Results

Results

All test runs were performed in both environments with two deviations:

- **ODL.** Stable/Beryllium build of ncmount sample ODL application
- **ODL Heap.** 8 GB

The following attributes were configured and observed in the test runs:

- **Prefix per notification.** How many prefix entries were sent per batch (i.e., notification).
- **Total prefixes.** Total number of prefixes sent into ODL.

Measured numbers:

- **TCP performance.** Rate of prefix processing in ODL. Measured as: Total prefixes / Duration between first notification received and last notification processed in ODL.
    - **Notifications/s,** Rate of notification processing in ODL.
    - **Prefixes/s.** Notifications/s multiplied by number of prefixes per notification.
- **SSH performance.** Same as TCP but using SSH protocol for NETCONF instead of plain TCP.

Detailed information about the test scenario, test setup, and a step-by-step guide can be found at the ODL wiki: http://wiki.opendaylight.org/. See Tables 4.21 and 4.22.

Table 4.21 Single Device NETCONF Notification Results Environment #1: NETCONF Southbound Single Device Performance

Prefix per Notification	TCP Performance	SSH Performance	Total Prefixes
1	10,716 notifications/s 10,716 prefixes/s	9,828 notifications/s 9,828 prefixes/s	100k
2	7,112 notifications/s 14,224 prefixes/s	5,496 notifications/s 10,992 prefixes/s	200k
10	1996 notifications/s 19, 965 prefixes/s	1,635 notifications/s 16,356 prefixes/s	1M

Table 4.22 Single Device NETCONF Notification Results Environment #2: NETCONF Southbound Single Device Performance

Prefix per Notification	TCP Performance	SSH Performance	Total Prefixes
1	11,967 notifications/s 11,967 prefixes/s	10,576 notifications/s 10,576 prefixes/s	100k
2	8,468 notifications/s 16,936 prefixes/s	8,118 notifications/s 16,237 prefixes/s	200k
10	2,579 notifications/s 25,796 prefixes/s	2,429 notifications/s 24,296 prefixes/s	1M

Conclusion

With a single mounted NETCONF device using just a single NETCONF session in Environment #1, it is possible to achieve the rate of 19,965 (16,356 for SSH) prefixes per second being uploaded (using notifications) into a BA, ODL application. As with other NETCONF performance tests, the results show the importance of batching. Environment #2 produced even better results for every test run.

Comparing performance using SSH to TCP shows an average decrease in performance of approximately 20%. The decrease is more significant with bigger batches per notification. However, repeating the runs using SSH indicates a memory leak in ODL Beryllium, since the performance decreased with every next run and the JVM process was using more and more RAM without freeing it. This issue has been reported to the ODL community for further analysis.

End-to-End Performance

The goal of this test is to measure the end-to-end performance of pushing data into one or more mounted NETCONF devices from an external client utilizing ODL's RESTCONF northbound interface. The data is a list of IPv4 prefixes, identical to the ones in the southbound performance test. However, in this test the prefixes are flowing from ODL into the NETCONF device. And the way they get into ODL is an invocation of a custom RPC handler developed in a Binding Aware (BA) sample application via a RESTCONF northbound interface. The responsibility of that handler is to receive prefixes rendered in a generic model, transform them using device-specific models, and send to the device. This is a sample generic prefix model for a custom RPC handler:

```
rpc write-routes {
  input {
    leaf mount-name {
      type string;
      description "Id of mounted note to write the l2-fibs to";
    }
    leaf vrf-id {
      type string;
      description "Id of Vrf which should be modified (add new routes)";
    }
    list route {
     key "ipv4-prefix";
      leaf ipv4-prefix { type inet:ipv4-address; }
      leaf ipv4-prefix-length { type uint16; }
      leaf ipv4-next-hop { type inet:ipv4-address; }
    }
  }
}
```

JSON rendered data according to this model used in the test:

```
"input": {
  "mount-name": "17830-sim-device",
    "vrf-id" : "1",
    "route": [
    {
    "ipv4-prefix" : "1.2.1.4",
    "ipv4-prefix-length" : "24",
    "ipv4-next-hop" : "4.3.2.1"
```

```
    },
    {
    "ipv4-prefix" : "1.2.2.4",
    "ipv4-prefix-length" : "24",
    "ipv4-next-hop" : "4.3.2.1"
    },
...
```

The complete scenario is shown in Figure 4.8.

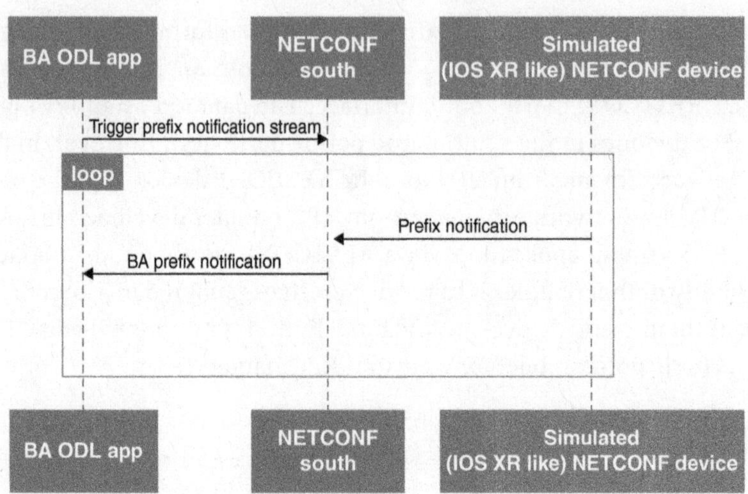

Figure 4.8 NETCONF End-to-end Performance Test Results

Detailed information about the test scenario, test setup, and a step-by-step guide can be found at the ODL wiki: http://wiki.opendaylight.org/.

Results

All test runs were performed in Environment #1 with two deviations:

- **ODL.** Stable/Beryllium build of ncmount sample ODL application
- **ODL Heap.** 8 GB

The following attributes were configured and observed in the test runs:

- **Prefix per request.** How many prefix entries were sent per batch (i.e., RESTCONF) request.
- **Total prefixes.** Total number of prefixes sent into ODL.
- **Clients.** How many clients were sending requests into ODL.

Measured numbers:

- **TCP performance.** Rate of prefix processing in ODL. Measured as: Total prefixes / Duration between first request sent and last request processed in ODL.

- **requests/s.** Rate of request processing in ODL.
- **prefixes/s.** Requests/s multiplied by number of prefixes per request.

- **SSH performance.** Same as TCP but using SSH protocol for NETCONF instead of plain TCP.

See Tables 4.23 through 4.26.

Table 4.23 NETCONF End-to-End Single Client Performance

Client Type	Prefixes per Request	TCP Performance	SSH Performance	Prefixes Total
Sync	1	254.4 requests/s 254.4 prefixes/s	165.6 requests/s 165.6 prefixes/s	20k
Async	1	3,187.3 requests/s 3,187.3 prefixes/s	2,288.6 requests/s 2,288.6 prefixes/s	20k
Sync	10	198.9 requests/s 1,989 prefixes/s	143.2 requests/s 1,432 prefixes/s	200k
Async	10	2,816.4 requests/s 28,164 prefixes/s	1,941.4 requests/s 19,414 prefixes/s	200k
Sync	50	123.7 requests/s 6,185 prefixes/s	83.3 requests/s 4,165 prefixes/s	1M
Async	50	1,706.5 requests/s 85,325 prefixes/s	1,220.8 requests/s 61,040 prefixes/s	1M

Table 4.24 NETCONF End-to-End Performance, 16 Clients

Client Type	Prefixes per request	TCP Performance	SSH Performance	Prefixes Total
Sync	1	8,940 requests/s 8,940 prefixes/s	5,904.9 requests/s 5,904.9 prefixes/s	20k
Async	1	13,362.2 requests/s 13,362.2 prefixes/s	8,510.6 requests/s 8,510.6 prefixes/s	20k
Sync	10	6,957.4 requests/s 69,574 prefixes/s	4,809.2 requests/s 48,092 prefixes/s	200k
Async	10	9,632.7 requests/s 96,327 prefixes/s	6,956.2 requests/s 69,562 prefixes/s	200k
Sync	50	3,400.5 requests/s 170,025 prefixes/s	2,600.6 requests/s 130,030 prefixes/s	1M
Async	50	3,999.6 requests/s 199,980 prefixes/s	3,455.8 requests/s 172,790 prefixes/s	1M

Table 4.25 NETCONF End-to-End Performance, 32 Clients

Client type	Prefixes per Request	TCP Performance	SSH Performance	Prefixes Total
Sync	1	12,043.6 requests/s 12,043.6 prefixes/s	6,976.5 requests/s 6,976.5 prefixes/s	320k
Async	1	13,531.2 requests/s 13,531.2 prefixes/s	8,329.8 requests/s 8,329.8 prefixes/s	320k

(Continued)

Table 4.25 *(Continued)*

Client type	Prefixes per Request	TCP Performance	SSH Performance	Prefixes Total
Sync	10	8,986.9 requests/s 89,869 prefixes/s	5,760 requests/s 57,600 prefixes/s	3.2M
Async	10	9,834.3 requests/s 98,343 prefixes/s	6,722.2 requests/s 67,222 prefixes/s	3.2M
Sync	50	3,998.1 requests/s 199,905 prefixes/s	2,974 requests/s 148,700 prefixes/s	16M
Async	50	4,094.7 requests/s 204, 735 prefixes/s	3,417.2 requests/s 170,860 prefixes/s	16M

Table 4.26 NETCONF End-to-End Performance, 64 Clients

Client Type	Prefixes per Request	TCP Performance	SSH Performance	Prefixes Total
Sync	1	11,809.8 requests/s 11,809.8 prefixes/s	7,570.9 requests/s 7,570.9 prefixes/s	320k
Async	1	11,187.2 requests/s 11,187.2 prefixes/s	7,056.6 requests/s 7,056.6 prefixes/s	320k
Sync	10	8,756.3 requests/s 87,563 prefixes/s	6,225.1 requests/s 62,251 prefixes/s	3.2M
Async	10	8,897.5 requests/s 88,975 prefixes/s	6,291.2 requests/s 62,912 prefixes/s	3.2M
Sync	50	3,848.9 requests/s 192,445 prefixes/s	3,142.6 requests/s 157,130 prefixes/s	16M
Async	50	3,811.2 requests/s 190,560 prefixes/s	3,143.2 requests/s 157,160 prefixes/s	16M

Conclusion

The important thing to note regarding the end-to-end test is that the simulated devices don't do anything with the data past XML parsing. So it would be unfair to expect the same performance with real NETCONF devices, pushing so much data into them. However, we are focusing on the performance of ODL here, not on the remote devices.

With a single mounted NETCONF device using just a single external REST client in Environment #1, it is possible to achieve the rate of 85,325 (61,040 for SSH) prefixes per second being pushed into a BA, ODL application, then translated and pushed into a mounted NETCONF device. As with other NETCONF performance tests, the results show the importance of batching and utilization of asynchronous clients.

With multiple (16, 32, 64) NETCONF devices mounted in ODL and multiple (one for each mounted device) external REST clients, it is possible to achieve rates of around 200k prefixes flowing through ODL toward the devices.

Comparing performance using SSH to TCP shows an overall decrease comparable to all the other performance tests.

OVSDB

Overview

ODL's OVSDB southbound plugin provides internal and external applications access to remote Open vSwitch instances via the OVSDB management protocol (RFC7047). The OVSDB management protocol uses JSON as its wire format and provides remote procedure calls (RPC) based on JSON-RPC. This allows the OVSDB client to call methods that exist on the OVSDB server, allowing the provisioning of bridges, ports, interfaces, tunnels, and more in the database. An RPC request is formatted as follows:

```
{
 "method":<string>,
 "params":[<object>],
 "id":<string> or <integer>
}
```

This will invoke the value given in "method" on the server, passing in the parameters specified in order. Parameters can be simple strings or complicated JSON objects. RPC response messages also have a standard formatting:

```
{
 "result":[<object>],
 "error":<error>,
 "id":<string> or <integer>
}
```

The goal of this test is to measure the number of OVSDB host devices the ODL OVSDB southbound plugin can support with a certain amount of RAM. All of the OVS host devices are simulated with mininet.

JSON rendered data according to the model used by OVSDB southbound plugin in the test:

```
"topology-id": "ovsdb:1",
   "node": [
   {
      "node-id": "ovsdb://uuid/a2f4efb4-
bffc-4fc7-b16b-3dbff8249a59/bridge/s546",
      "ovsdb:datapath-id": "00:00:00:00:00:00:02:22",
      "ovsdb:datapath-type": "ovsdb:datapath-type-system",
      "ovsdb:fail-mode": "ovsdb:ovsdb-fail-mode-secure",
      "ovsdb:bridge-other-configs": [
         {
            "bridge-other-config-key": "disable-in-band",
            "bridge-other-config-value": "true"
         },
         {
            "bridge-other-config-key": "datapath-id",
```

```
            "bridge-other-config-value": "0000000000000222"
            }
        ],
        "ovsdb:protocol-entry": [
            {
                "protocol": "ovsdb:ovsdb-bridge-protocol-openflow-13"
            }
        ],
        "ovsdb:bridge-name": "s546",
        "ovsdb:bridge-uuid": "c4cb317e-3567-4dc8-b418-1c789b837834",
        "ovsdb:managed-by": "/
network-topology:network-topology/
network-topology:topology[network-
topology:topology-id='ovsdb:1']/
network-topology:node[network-
topology:node-id='ovsdb://uuid/a2f4efb4-
bffc-4fc7-b16b-3dbff8249a59']",
        "ovsdb:controller-entry": [
            {
                "target": "ptcp:7179", "is-connected": false,
                "controller-uuid": "5a44519d-3f90-484a-afab-39820ecfabc5"
            },
            {
                "target": "tcp:10.11.23.30:6653",
                "is-connected": false,
                "controller-uuid": "c114419a-1656-4273-84d4-917aba52fa67"
            }
        ],
        "termination-point": [
            {
                "tp-id": "s546-eth2",
                "ovsdb:interface-uuid":
"1401c95d-8341-47bf-9345-5b19d311276e",
                "ovsdb:ofport": 2,
                "ovsdb:port-uuid": "ce399220-72e6-4b4b-b311-b207ef162bd3",
                "ovsdb:name": "s546-eth2",
                "ovsdb:ofport_request": 2
            }
        ]
    }
```


In the following test, multiple systems running mininet connect to the OVSDB southbound plugin. Each OVS host emulated by mininet is configured to connect and use the OVSDB southbound plugin as its OVSDB manager. Once the connection is established, the OVSDB southbound plugin requests, with JSON-RPC, the OVSDB database schema. This request is quickly followed by another JSON-RPC request to monitor OVSDB update notifications for specific tables of the OVSDB. When the OVS host sends update notifications to the OVSDB southbound plugin, the plugin creates, and subsequently updates, an OVSDB topology node in the operational MD-SAL for that OVS host.

The test verifies via RESTCONF that every node is present in the operational MD-SAL topology. When the mininet topologies are torn down and disconnected from the OVSDB southbound plugin, the test verifies via RESTCONF that each node has been removed from the operational MD-SAL. Detailed information about the test scenario, test setup, and a step-by-step guide can be found at the ODL wiki: http://wiki.opendaylight.org/.

Results

All test runs were performed in Environment #2. Though the max nodes tested was 1,800, this appears to be a limitation of the testing environment and not of the OVSDB southbound plugin.

Measured numbers, OVSDB southbound plugin nodes:

- OVSDB Nodes: 1,800

BGP

Overview

The OpenDaylight Border Gateway Protocol (BGP) plugin can serve as a BGP speaker capable of peering with multiple neighbors with different roles (iBGP, eBGP, RR-Client). The BGP speaker is able to learn and readvertise routing information; in addition, a programmable RIB (Application RIB/Peer) is provided to allow route injection and deletion.

The BGP plugin supports several BGP Multi-Protocol extensions—IPv4/IPv6 Unicast, IPv4/IPv6 Flowspec, IPv4 Labeled Unicast, and Linkstate, with each carrying different routing information.

The routing information is stored in RIBs (Adj-Rib-In, Effective-Rib-In, and Adj-Rib-Out on a per-peer basis) and a global Loc-Rib where only best paths are held. Moreover, the BGP plugin provides IPv4/IPv6 reachability and link state topology information.

The following tests use (with small changes due to environment specifics) the Robot Framework tests suites, which are also run as part of ODL's Continuous System Integration tests. Instead of a real device, the "play.py" Python utility is used to simulate a BGP peer. It is not part of ODL, but it is available from the integration/test repository: https://git.opendaylight.org/gerrit/gitweb?p=integration/test.git;a=blob_plain;f=tools/fastbgp/play.py;hb=2b171413a8168bb7d147c3c6d5cf3eced42fb8ec.

Raw information about test implementation, steps to reproduce, and performance numbers are located at: https://wiki.opendaylight.org/view/BGP_LS_PCEP:Specific_Performance_Testing#Tests.

BGP Data Ingestion

Upon start, the play.py tool connects to ODL and starts sending BGP simple Update messages (with one prefix/one next hop per message). After sending 1 million Updates, it goes quiet, sending only Keepalive messages.

In order to determine whether ODL has finished processing all the Updates, two monitoring methods were used. In the "Prefix Counting" method, the complete ipv4-topology data was repeatedly downloaded once per second via RESTCONF and the number of prefixes was counted. In the "Data Change Counting" method, only the value of the data change counter was periodically retrieved (once per second); after the counter stabilized, the final prefix count was validated. Note that the value of the data change counter differs from the number of Update messages, due to Updates batching in the ODL code.

When a BGP peer disconnects, ODL is supposed to remove route information advertised by the peer. With one million routes, it takes ODL some time to process. Once again this time was determined by either prefix counting or by data change counting.

The "routes per second" value is computed as 1,000,000 divided by time between when play.py is started (or stopped) and when ODL processing is finished.

The route ingest and removal rates measured on Environment #1 are shown in Table 4.27.

Table 4.27 Environment 1: Ingest and Removal Rates

Test Run	Prefix Count Ingest	Change Count Ingest	Prefix Count Removal	Change Count Removal
1	8,563.47	16,333.20	23,242.84	23,583.79
2	8,326.05	16,173.12	22,781.20	22,674.71

Comments on Results

The "Prefix Counting" method is quite intrusive and does have more significant impact on the system under test than the "Data Change Counting" method. For route ingestion, the "Prefix Counting" method causes the rate to go down almost 50% compared to the "Data Change Counting" method. However, it seems to have practically no effect on route removal rates after a peer disconnection.

Future improvements to testing include ingestion from several peers at once, and propagation of data between eBGP peers.

BGP Data Advertisement

Here, the play.py tool is started without any initial routes present and then connected to ODL. It is only used to count the number of BGP Update messages from ODL.

While the play.py tool is connected, ODL's app peer is filled with routes. Then the play.py tool is restarted, which makes ODL resend the data.

Finally, all data in the app peer is deleted. Time to process is measured between the start of the state change (app peer data change or play.py restart) and the end of the verification (parsing the log from play.py to see the correct number of Update messages received from ODL). During this time, the "Prefix Counting" method is used to detect whether the ODL RIB has been updated with the new app peer state, which places additional stress on ODL.

Two methods of populating the app peer data were tested. Each had two phases that differed in their use of batching. The first phase used large batches, which corresponds to the ingest of the initial generic routing strategy. The second phase used small batches, which corresponds to runtime tweaks of the routing strategy. The deletion of routes was always done by RESTCONF, where the whole app peer container was removed.

Future improvements include multiple peers; using NETCONF to add app peer data; adding tests that populate app peer without any BGP peer connected; and adding tests that delete only some data from app peer.

BGP App Peer Populated by RESTCONF

Here, RESTCONF is the bottleneck. In the first phase, a single request with 100k routes was sent. In the second phase, a sequence of 100k requests with 1 route each was sent, one request at a time. Using multiple workers to send updates would improve performance, but as the PATCH method is not supported in Beryllium (and there is no specific RPC to allow batching), RESTCONF will always be slow. See Table 4.28.

Table 4.28 Routes per Second Measured on Environment #1

Test Run	Prefix Count Ingest	Change Count Ingest	Prefix Count Removal	Change Count Removal
1	2,079.78	206.68	4,952.95*	10,009.01
2	2,096.44	209.27	4,951.48*	9,849.79

An asterisk denotes the lower bound confirmed by the test; the actual rates are presumably higher.

BGP App Peer Populated by Java

Here, a special-purpose Java bundle (not a part of Beryllium) with an MD-SAL application for adding routes to an app peer was used. The first phase still added routes in one transaction; the second phase used transactions either with 1,000 routes or with 1 route. As the time measurement in the data advertisement suite is quite granular, the scale has been increased to 1,000,000 routes per phase. See Table 4.29.

Table 4.29 Routes per Second Measured on Environment #1

Test Run	Routes per Phase	Phase 2 Batch Size	First Phase Addition	Second Phase Addition	Reconnect	Deletion
1	100,000	1,000	3,217	3,828.78	4,959.33*	9,674.45
2	1,000,000	1,000	5,991.83	10,612.11	13,742.4	13,930.497
3	1,000,000	1	5,981.22	5,655.31	20,587.15	15,252.04
4	1,000,000	1	6,101.91	6,935.73	20,931.01	14,337.43

*Denotes the lower bound confirmed by the test; the actual rate is presumably higher.

Comments on Results

Adding routes by RESTCONF one by one is slow; a batched request is 10 times faster. Java is faster still. At higher scale, ODL is generally faster, but results show higher variance. This may be caused by memory constraints, as ODL was set to use a maximum of 8 GB for heap space in all runs.

PCEP

Overview

The OpenDaylight Path Computation Element Protocol (PCEP) plugin can serve as an active stateful path computation element (PCE) capable of learning LSP state information from path computation clients (PCCs) and utilizing the delegation mechanism to update LSP parameters (update-lsp). Moreover, the PCEP plugin provides services to support dynamic creation (add-lsp) and tear down (remove-lsp) of LSPs without the need for local configuration on the PCC.

The following tests use (with small changes due to environment specifics) the Robot Framework test suites, which are also run as part of ODL's Continuous System Integration tests. Instead of real PCCs, pcc-mock is used to simulate any number of PCCs with any number of initial LSPs configured on them. Pcc-mock is a standalone Java application available from

- OpenDaylight Nexus at: https://nexus.opendaylight.org/content/repositories/opendaylight.release/org/opendaylight/bgpcep/pcep-pcc-mock/0.5.0-Beryllium/pcep-pcc-mock-0.5.0-Beryllium-executable.jar.
- Raw information about test implementation, steps to reproduce, and performance numbers are located at: https://wiki.opendaylight.org/view/BGP_LS_PCEP:Specific_Performance_Testing#Tests.

Initial Report Processing

Pcc-mock is started to simulate 1 PCC with 65,535 LSPs (maximum allowed by RSVP-TE protocol) or 512 PCCs with 128 LSPs each (65,536 LSPs total). RESTCONF is used to periodically (1 second interval) download the whole pcep-topology and to count the number of expected hop IP addresses. The "LSPs per second" value is computed as the number of LSPs divided by the time between when pcc-mock is started and when the number of visible hops is met. See Table 4.30.

Table 4.30 Results for Environment #1

Test Run	PCCs	LSPs per PCC	LSPs per second
1	1	65,535	4,620.021149
2	512	128	3,816.223141
3	512	128	4,049.932023

LSP Updating

This test continues from the moment when the initial LSPs were reported. Python utility "updater.py" is used to send Restconf RPC requests to update one hop in each LSP. Restconf calls are blocking, so when the utility finishes, all LSPs were updated already (the suite verifies pcep-topology afterward). The test is repeated several times, differing in number of (single-thread, blocking) http workers updater.py uses for sending requests.

Here, RESTCONF is the bottleneck, as there is no RESTCONF way to allow batching or asynchronous processing. NETCONF could increase performance, but of course a specific Java MD-SAL application would be the fastest. See Table 4.31.

Table 4.31 LSP Updates per Second, Measured on Environment #1

Test Run	1 (1PCCx65535LSP)	2 (512PCCx128LSP)	3 (512PCCx128LSP)
1 worker	458.2899181	478.0823017	479.0188067
2 workers	1,181.066176	1,217.598098	1,202.032244
4 workers	1,846.160347	1,898.71364	1,905.836508
8 workers	1,829.053865	1,891.971477	1,940.542461
16 workers	1,739.020831	1,913.627471	1,870.426394
32 workers	1,648.96963	1,876.370716	1,809.636891

Result Comments

Ingestion from multiple PCCs appears to be slower, but the probable reason is that pcc-mock is not quick enough at creating simulated devices.

Two workers appear to be more than twice as fast as a single worker, but that may be just JIT compilation in JVM kicking in. (Test cases were run in succession; ODL was being reinstalled only between test runs.) Multiple PCCs appear to give a slightly higher rate, perhaps because pcc-mock uses more threads in this case. For more realistic devices, the rates would be lower, because updating LSP in a real network needs considerable setup time.

Key Factors That Affect Performance

Batching, concurrency, and asynchronous client design are important to achieve good system throughput. Batching multiple flow add/modify/delete requests onto a single REST request on the northbound ODL API increases performance by a factor of five. Batching multiple flow/FIB programming requests on the southbound interface also helps performance.

The effects of batching and parallelism can be seen with NETCONF, where batching is used both on the northbound and southbound interfaces. Despite the NETCONF protocol being more chatty than OpenFlow, the RESTCONF -> NETCONF flow programming rates are much higher than the RESTCONF -> OpenFlow flow programming rates. With NETCONF, we achieved L2 / L3 prefix programming rates of up to ~200k prefixes per second (L2/L3 prefixes are equivalent to OpenFlow flows) across 16-32-64 NETCONF servers (devices). With OpenFlow, we achieved flow programming rates of ~1k to 2.5k flows per second, across all tested controllers and across 5-31-63 switches.

Batching of multiple flows into a single REST call on the northbound API improves the performance to ~9k flows per second in ODL. But the lack of flow batching in OF1.3 is one of the key factors influencing flow programming throughput of an OpenFlow system. This factor has been mitigated in OF1.5, which does support batching.

When using RESTCONF in ODL, be aware that putting data into ODL's config space means that the data is by default persisted. Persistence is a valuable attribute but can affect performance: make sure you have a fast disk system (preferably SSD, and do NOT use NFS); alternatively, if you do not need to persist data in the controller, you may want to turn off persistence on the config space entirely.

Future Work

This document focused primarily on throughput, but we will need to measure latency in future work. System designers have to strike the right balance between throughput and latency. We may also repeat the tests for clustered setup.

Additional References

Steven Noble. 2015. "Comparing SDN Controllers: OpenDaylight and ONOS." SDN Testing, June 7. https://www.sdntesting.com/comparing-sdn-controllers-opendaylight-and-onos/.

"OpenDaylight Performance Stress Test Report v1.1: Lithium SR3." Intracom Telecom SDN/NFV Lab. https://raw.githubusercontent.com/wiki/intracom-telecom-sdn/nstat/files/ODL_performance_report_v1.1.pdf.

Sridhar Rao. 2015. "SDN Series Part Eight: Comparison Of Open Source SDN Controllers." March 31. http://thenewstack.io/sdn-series-part-eight-comparison-of-open-source-sdn-controllers/.

CONCLUSION

In this chapter we explored challenges and solutions for network infrastructure. Data-intensive computing and other factors are both straining networks and catalyzing innovation. Institutions face many challenges in this area. We shared a model for secure and regulated data storage and presented a number of network advances, including InfiniBand, high-performance fabrics, NFV, and SDN. The bulk of this chapter detailed end-to-end scenarios for OpenDaylight.

NOTES

1. "Robert Metcalfe: Mathematician, Inventor." Biography.com. http://www.biography.com/people/robert-metcalfe-9542201.
2. IEEE Standards Association. "History of Ethernet." http://standards.ieee.org/events/ethernet/history.html.
3. Fibre Channel Industry Association. "FC Roadmaps." http://fibrechannel.org/fc-roadmaps/.
4. Open Networking Foundation. "Software-Defined Networking (SDN) Definition." https://www.opennetworking.org/sdn-resources/sdn-definition.
5. OpenDaylight Platform. "About the OpenDaylight Foundation." https://www.opendaylight.org/foundation/.

CASE STUDY 5: USE CASE: SUN CORRIDOR NETWORK

CASE STUDY

Jay Etchings

Sun Corridor Network is a collaboration, sponsored by the Arizona Board of Regents, of the three state universities: Arizona State University (ASU), Northern Arizona University (NAU), and the University of Arizona (UA). It was created to share high-capacity digital communications resources, network services, and applications among eligible users, joining 41 other higher education–based regional research and education networks.

Sun Corridor Network is the designated Internet2 Connector Network for the state of Arizona. The Sun Corridor is a "last mile" provider or local loop to a larger network. The SDN components will someday extend across the wide area network (WAN) and traverse such network segments. However, at this point Sun Corridor provides media handoff and basic, standard WAN protocol support and does not have SDN integration or any targeted uses for SDN.

(*Continued*)

(*Continued*)

Through our Internet2 Connector Network status, Sun Corridor Network is interconnected to over 93,000 community anchor instructions—including 80,000 schools, 300 higher-education member institutions, more than 50 leading science, education, and technology institutions such as NASA, the National Science Foundation, and the National Oceanic and Atmospheric Administration, 89 industry partners, and 100 countries.

Architecturally, we operate two redundant 100 2 peering points in Tucson and Phoenix, respectively, with diverse routing to Internet2 hubs in Los Angeles and Houston. The three universities are connected with 10 Gb redundant circuits between NAU (Flagstaff) and ASU (Phoenix), and between ASU and UA (Tucson), respectively.

Over 95% of the combined Internet traffic of the three Arizona state universities transits the Sun Corridor Network.

Two Sun Corridor Network institutions, UA and ASU, were founding members of Internet2 in 1996, providing Internet2 access to users either directly or through the Sun Corridor Network for nearly 20 years. As a stand-alone regional network, the Sun Corridor Network has been providing Internet2 Advanced Layer 1, Layer 2, and Layer 3 services since 2013.

Current Sun Corridor Network services include direct access to Internet2's research and education network, commercial peering with multiple Tier 1 Internet providers, and an advanced networking TransitRail Commercial Peering Service (TR-CPS).

TR-CPS provides strategic connectivity to portions of the public Internet and peering relationships through over 80 select entities. Internet2's commercial peering service offers a low-cost path with higher performance goals than commercial alternatives. TR-CPS provides high performance, low latency, and efficient (one-hop) access to some of the top content destinations in the world, including Google, Yahoo, Netflix, and other commercial content providers. The service supports IPv4, IPv6, and multicast.

CASE STUDY

CASE STUDY 6: USE CASE: REGULATED AND COMMODITY COMPUTE AND STORAGE, LEVERAGING INTERNET2 NEXT GENERATION

Alan Ritacco

Leveraging high-performance computing (HPC) for distributed calculations and near-real-time analytics of regulated data is no longer a nice feature but rather a requirement. Traditional or commodity HPC addresses scientific research compute and storage needs. To expand this ecosystem to include clinical PHI (protected health information) or PII (personally identifiable information) research requires secure compute and storage models and policies backed by federal grants requiring several layers of secure methodologies. Compliance layers range from traditional HIPAA (Health Insurance Portability and Accountability Act of 1996), to FISMA (Federal Information Security Management Act of 2002), and FedRAMP (Federal Risk and Authorization Management Program) compliance and policies required by federal research grants and awards. Note: There are several other policies and compliance requirements, including NIST (National Institute of Standards and Technology), that must be met in accordance with these and other guidelines.

The tracking of patient data, from emergency room visits to outpatient support for longitudinal studies and, more important, outbreak monitoring is quickly turning into a requirement that must be met according to federal and governmental standards. Clinical sample tracking of next-generation sequencing (NGS) data from infected patients is proving to be an effective method for tracking bacterial and viral infections as well as pathogen- and disease-spreading organisms. The ability to collect and track NGS data from bedside to patient records in a short time has allowed research and clinical translational sciences teams to work as one cohesive group.

To utilize this data effectively, a secure and regulated service is needed for access, compute, and storage, as noted. A workflow would be to: (1) gather the clinical repository sample(s); (2) prepare for NGS analysis; (3) sequence and align data, looking for variants as needed; (4) correlate data with clinical data repository data sets; and (5) align with tracking and PHI records. This process requires care in the tracking of PHI data during all steps, so that it is not made available to anyone without direct and prior approval.

Institutional review board (IRB) approval is typically required for those researchers or clinicians requiring access to private data. Even with this approval, a host of security-related requirements must be met. Security awareness along with certification training and handling of PHI data should be required of all users and developers (an example is CITI, the Collaborative Institutional Training Initiative). Strict change control processes along with other measures provide the building blocks for a robust and secure regulated research environment.

A security program with standards based on and drawing from measurements and guidelines set by the HIPAA and NIST security standards for the storage and management of protected health information (PHI) should be required. Data center policies should be reviewed and enforced using data standards that adhere to the security standards, such as ISO/IEC 27001:2013, AICPA SSAE16 Reporting Standards, and stakeholder trust and security principles. All administrative access to these services should require a Secure Sockets Layer (SSL) virtual private network and utilize two-factor authentication leveraging RSA tokens or similar. User access to this environment should be limited to HTTPS/SSL, and all encryption at a minimum should be 2048 bit. All data should be encrypted at rest within the secure environment, and all transport should be via secure or encrypted tunnels.

(*Continued*)

(*Continued*)

Vulnerability scan procedures and remediation methodologies should be clearly written in a policy format for compliance with data usage agreements.

A configuration for a regulated environment would require two-factor authentication, for developers and potentially all users, along with secure monitoring facilities, high-speed networking (Internet2), and firewall hardware and rules. Leveraging high-speed internet traffic to cloud services, such as Amazon Web Services (AWS), provides the needed throughput for the quantity and high level of sequence and similar data processed in commodity and regulated HPC environments. The commingling of these two environments is a new paradigm that we would like to present here.

Figure CS4.1 presents an example environment of a regulated and commodity HPC environment of tomorrow, which may consist of shared services across platforms leveraging layer-2 networking, virtual devices, and software-defined layers, including software-defined networking (SDN) and software-defined storage (SDS). Emerging technologies in SDN and SDS will allow for distribution of virtual and physical services along with shared and private storage zones. Leveraging Internet2 traffic for burst compute and storage for clinical and research computational analysis will provide the ability to work on a variety of instances while minimizing the required downloading costs of cloud storage.

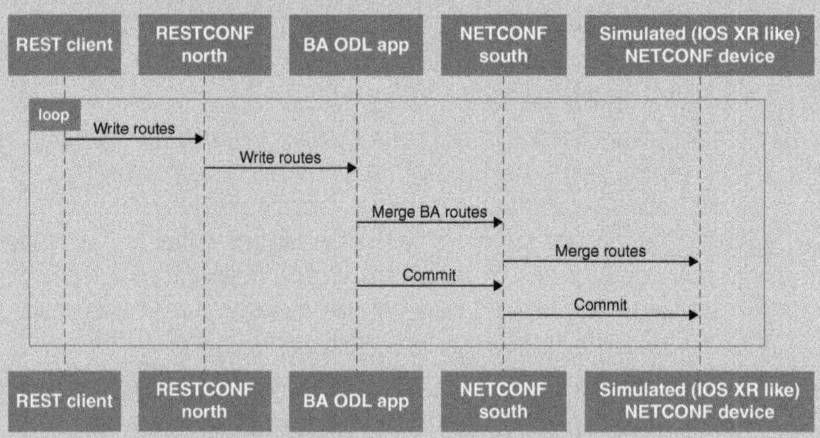

Figure CS4.1 Sample Regulated Commodity HPC Environment

Projects taking advantage of virtualized and caching storage technologies will be able to access data simultaneously and seamlessly both on premises and via in-cloud instances. Leveraging tiered storage, including archival and backup, along with smart scheduling practices, one could envision an ecosystem that provides a flexible method to deploy and implement commodity and secure high-performance computing. Working with open container–based tools can allow for flexible migrations and physical instances of compute along with storage that smartly migrates/moves data from high-speed to inexpensive cloud storage or backup media using SDS and SDN. Scheduling rules will be key in this practice.

We envision the environment shown in Figure CS4.1 to include high-speed firewall services and appropriate networking gear to filter, pass, and regulate networking flow (example: at layer-2) for the passing between the virtual and physical segments. The dynamic nature of SDN and SDS should allow for the needed virtual paths to be created and removed on the fly with minimal or no hands-on intervention. Network and security monitoring tools embedded inline will provide the needed data sources for regulatory and governmental restrictions. Networking egress points will provide access to high-speed Internet2 traffic and commodity Internet traffic. All Internet2 traffic would be encrypted point to point for both cloud compute and storage needs. Commodity Internet traffic would presumably be ratcheted down to only allow for inbound secure connections (ex: SSL/SSH) traffic, with point-to-point traffic.

CHAPTER 5

Data-Intensive Compute Infrastructures

Content contributed by Dijiang Huang, Yuli Deng, Jay Etchings, Zhiyuan Ma, and Guangchun Luo

The key element of computer design—software as well as hardware—is to manage the complexity from the lower levels of logical circuits to ever-higher levels that nest above one another. One may compare this to the number of neurons in the brain of animals from the flatworm, to a cat, to Homo sapiens, *although the history of artificial intelligence research has shown that comparing a human brain to a computer can distort as much as clarify.*

—P. E. Ceruzzi, *Computing: A Concise History*

According to many, we have now entered a new phase of science, known as fourth paradigm science. The term "fourth paradigm science" was popularized by the late Jim Gray, a Microsoft researcher who foresaw "a world of scholarly resources—text, databases, and other associated materials—that were seamlessly navigable and interoperable" [1]. Fourth paradigm science is data intensive and depends on advances in networking as well as compute power. A 2009 collection of essays published by Microsoft Research explores this new scientific methodology driven by data-intensive problems and surveys some of the exciting research in this area [2].

While the scope and nature of this paradigm shift (if indeed it is truly a paradigm shift) are open for debate, it is indisputable that the biosciences are engaging more and more deeply with big data. This trend is likely to continue for the foreseeable future. Associated with this change are substantial changes in computing and infrastructure. There are a number of ways we can chart these changes, which are still very much under way. One is the eXtreme Digital programs of the National Science Foundation (NSF), which focus on "making new infrastructure and next-generation digital services available to all researchers and educators. They'll use that infrastructure to handle the huge volumes of digital information that are now a part of their work—the results of supercomputing simulations, the data generated by large scientific instruments such as telescopes, and the existing data that can be mined from a host of public sources" [3]. Other recent NSF research priorities include:

- Approaches to parallel programming to address the parallel processing of data on data-intensive systems.
- Programming abstractions, including models, languages, and algorithms, which allow a natural expression of parallel processing of data.

- Design of data-intensive computing platforms to provide high levels of reliability, efficiency, availability, and scalability.
- Identifying applications that can exploit this computing paradigm and determining how it should evolve to support emerging data-intensive applications.

A recent NSF proposal explains that the organization's

> vision for Advanced Computing Infrastructure, which supports Cyberinfrastructure Framework for 21st Century Science and Engineering (CIF21), focuses specifically on ensuring that the science and engineering community has ready access to the advanced computational and data-driven capabilities required to tackle the most complex problems and issues facing today's scientific and educational communities [4].

Another indication of institutional interest in data-intensive computing is the Coalition for Academic Scientific Computation, a group of 86 member institutions. This organization was founded in 1989 and now focuses substantially on high-performance computing and big data capabilities. Finally, President Obama's Precision Medicine Initiative includes a $215 million investment in 2016, much of which is focused on expanding data-intensive research. Key priorities include: generating a voluntary national research cohort of a million or more volunteers to propel understanding of health and disease and drive new ways of doing research; scaling up efforts to identify genomic drivers in cancer; and developing standards for data interoperability and security.

The emergence of data-intensive computing is also leading to a shift in computing infrastructure. Traditionally high-performance computing (HPC) was all about cores, nodes, and expensive hardware. Data-intensive computing, however, is a class of parallel computing applications that utilize well-known parallelization techniques adopted from traditional HPC. Since the early 2000s this approach to large-scale data processing has been the darling of the industry, with every vendor redefining existing nomenclature and forging new terms to capture the market mystique. Everywhere we look we see big data, data intensive, and N-scale where N could equate to tera, peta, or exa. Typically, terabytes or petabytes of data for processing size would fit into the category of big data. Computing applications that devote most of their execution time to computational requirements are typically deemed compute intensive. But dealing with petascale data sets where input/output and transaction response times need to be milliseconds or perhaps microseconds is also considered data-intensive computing.

We have now indisputably entered the age of big data. Using big data in health informatics will likely provide us with enormous benefits, such as preventing disease, identifying modifiable risk factors for disease, and designing interventions for health behavior change. However, the health industry has been slow to embrace this trend due to the cost of adding analytics functions to existing electronic health records (EHRs), privacy issues, poor-quality data, and a lack of willingness to share data. Despite this, there are a number of medical big data efforts under way in the United Kingdom, including Care Coordination/Home Telehealth and the Whole System Demonstrator Program of the UK Department of Health. In the United States, companies such as Aetna Life Insurance Company, Mount Sinai Medical Center, and Microsoft HealthVault have all started their own experiments or are trying to develop some tools on medical big data, hoping to uncover useful information hidden within [5].

BIG DATA APPLICATIONS IN HEALTH INFORMATICS

Various techniques have been used to process and ingest big data in order to meet its challenges. These techniques are based on varied criteria and the applications can be classified into diverse categories.

Ross et al., in a 2014 article on big data and health records, classified data applications into three broad themes [6]:

1. Data mining
2. Data application and integration
3. Privacy and security

These classifications are helpful but unfortunately are far too rough to capture the complexity of current data practices. Other researchers divide the applications into smaller but more concentrated areas. In 2013, based on the different processing purposes in healthcare, Herland et al. classified the applications into analyzing disease patterns, clinical decision support systems, individual analytics applied for patient profiles, personalized medicine, performance-based pricing for personnel, and improving public health [7].

Within Herland et al.'s survey, big data applications have been classified into five categories based on the use case:

1. Clinical decision support system. In this field, EHRs have proved to be quite useful since they are a natural source of heterogeneous big data. Building clinical decision support system using EHRs is becoming a major trend. EHRs can be used for data mining and to make predictions based on both clinical and prior information [8, 9]. Cloud computing has been adopted in the emerging field of emergency tele-cardiology [10].

2. Disease discovery. "Disease discovery" in this context denotes research that focuses on diagnostics targeted toward disease pathology and clinical research to gain greater understanding within the domain of epidemiology. In recent years, there has been a surge in using social network data to gather information for public health research and applications.

Social media data has been used to detect the emergence of disease. Tuarob et al. combine ensemble machine learning techniques with semantic aspects of the data to identify health-related messages of social media [11]. The primary objective is to alert the public to an instance of a novel, unknown disease or acute epidemic. There has also been research dedicated to using health-related tweets for precautions [12]. A comprehensive analysis between these official and nonofficial sources can predict an early-stage outbreak. A quick reaction could be taken to address public threats, allowing an informed public to potentially prevent exposure.

3. Disease analysis. Cancer is an obvious target issue for big data to tackle. According to the World Cancer Report 2014, there were 14.1 million people who were diagnosed with cancer in 2012 [13]. For decades, people have been trying to figure out why cancer happens and how to prevent or cure it. Current big data cancer research is proceeding on a number of fronts, including giant cell [14], gastric cancer [15], breast cancer [16], and brain tumor research [17]. Researchers are also using data mining to help diagnose types of cancer and research cancer survival using tools like decision trees and other statistical methods [15, 16]. Data mining and machine learning are tools of untapped potential in the battle to decode bio-data into actionable outcomes in cancer.

4. Applications in pharmaceuticals. Pharmaceutical and drug research using big data can be divided into research focusing on drug effect analysis, drug discovery, drug repurposing, and personalized medicine or targeted therapies. For example, optimization of radiation dosage through standardized analytics could lead to many benefits, including: improved clinical outcomes, creation of data-driven best practice guidelines, opportunities for enhanced education and research, dose-reduction technology innovation, and reversal of existing commoditization trends [18]. Pharmacogenomics, the study of how genes affect a person's response to drugs, is certain to be an exciting emerging field.

5. Genomic applications. A 2014 survey on recent themes in transactional bioinformatics listed EHRs as one of four major topics in genomic studies [19]. As more researchers focus on EHR processing in genomics and pharmacogenomics, we need to consider improvements in the means of processing them. Cloud computing provided us with a solution, and it is already speeding up research that relies on algorithms [20]. We will no doubt be seeing large-scale utilization of cloud computing in future genomic studies.

To these five areas we would add information visualization.

6. Information visualization. Visualization has proven to be helpful in discovering relationships among data through visual means, driving complex analysis. There are currently many opportunities for cutting-edge visualization techniques to efficiently interpret the available information. Numerous data visualization tools offer different visualization methods to represent various types of data. Visualization techniques can be classified as follows: (1) two-dimensional/three-dimensional standard figure [21]; (2) geometric transformations [22]; (3) display icons [23]; (4) methods focused on the pixels [24]; and (5) hierarchical images [25].

Big data analysis and mining offers new research opportunities in real-time, interactive, visual analytics, hybrid-reality environments, and rich-application communities. Visualization is dynamic and interactive. Integrated with the TerraFly map application programming interface (API) and JavaScript, the query results of spatial object can be shown on a much better interface, including both map and object lists.

SOURCES OF BIG DATA IN HEALTH INFORMATICS

Data is the most important component when developing applications or conducting research. To determine what kind of methodologies to use, one needs to understand where the data comes from and what it does or should look like. In this section, we discuss the sources of big data in health informatics. There are currently several surveys about the data source type in health informatics–related big data [26, 27]. We can classify data according to numerous criteria, including:

- Data structure (i.e., structured or unstructured); target size (molecular level, tissues, organs, individual and whole population);
- The process used to generate the data; and
- Data source (medical records, administrative data, web search logs, and social media) [7].

Figure 5.1 shows major data sources for health informatics.

Medical records or EHRs refer to the systematic collection of medical information about a disease, patient, or population. This data can be further categorized into five subtypes:

1. Demographic data
2. Laboratory data
3. Medication data
4. Diagnostic data
5. Clinical data

Data Source		Structured Data	Unstructured Data	Target Usage
Main Type	**Sub Type**			
Medical Records	Demographic	✓	✗	Decision support, personalized medicine, master patient index.
	Laboratory	✓	✓	
	Medication	✓	✓	
	Diagnostic data	✓	✗	
	Clinical notes, other notes	✗	✓	
Administrative Data	Claim data	✗	✓	Quality improvement, surveillance.
	Insurance data	✓	✓	
Web Search Log	——	✗	✓	Syndromic surveillance, adverse events detection.
Social Media	Discussion	✗	✓	Drug side effects, monitoring health belief and behavior, disease outbreak.
	Blogs	✗	✓	
	Tweets/SMS of the Internet	✗	✓	

Figure 5.1 Classification of Data Sources in Health Informatics Big Data

Demographic data contains information from large populations and potentially collections of diverse disease and pathology information. This data has the capacity of providing information to establish case studies, help perform a better diagnosis, and obtain data normally related to the utilization of decision support systems, such as the building blocks for personalized medicine.

One also often sees the the term "administrative data," which refers to information collected primarily for administrative purposes. Such data usually focuses on insurance or claims, and may include medication, diagnoses, or devices. This data is used for various studies, such as to identify patients or function in the enterprise; improve quality and patient safety; or to manage patients' protected health information. There are three main challenges to utilizing this data:

1. The large quantity of the data
2. The difficulty of creating a simple analytical file out of this data
3. Recognition that administrative data alone can be of less use to the researchers if not combined with clinical data [27]

We mention administrative data as it is of high importance to all domains and critical to biomedical informatics. Web search logs can be considered a by-product of the increasing number of people who use the Internet to seek health information. By collecting and analyzing this data, researchers may have a better way for syndromic surveillance and to analyze data to forecast disease outbreaks. As more and more people use social networks, researchers and developers are increasingly turning to this field as well. This kind of data may involve discussion boards, blogs, Twitter feeds, and other kinds of services like Short Message Service (SMS), and can be mined to identify previously unreported drug side effects and to monitor health beliefs and disease outbreaks [25, 26]. This type of analysis opens the field for emerging technologies such as "NowCasting." The JS Marshall Radar Observatory at McGill University explains:

> The term ***nowcasting*** is a contraction of "now" and "forecasting"; it refers to the sets of techniques devised to make short-term forecasts, typically in the 0 to 12 hour range. Historically, nowcasting techniques have been based on simplified heuristic approaches where the current echo pattern was tracked in the past and extrapolated into the future, sometimes with some modifications to try to account for storm development and decay and/or for decreasing predictability with time. More and more though, nowcasting techniques are becoming more sophisticated, sometimes up to the point of becoming full-fledged numerical weather prediction models [28].

Although NowCasting can also be used to make economic and health predictions, it can have its drawbacks, similar to what we have witnessed in the 24-hour news cycle, where in the race to get the news to the airwaves, there continue to be errors in consistency and accuracy. Simple searches for flu remedies could amass as search data is mulled over and algorithms suggest cold-flu remedies, making it seem like an epidemic is afoot. This is not an extreme scenario when you consider the potential to ingest data at such a speed.

In August 2014, the European Central Bank held a two-day workshop on how big data can be used for forecasting. The headline speaker, Hal Varian, chief economist at Google, spoke about the predictive power of Google Trends and Google Correlate, two of their big data tools [29]. But some caution seems to be in order. The *MIT Technology Review* notes,

> Google has accurately estimated the number of flu cases, for example in the US in 2011/12, Switzerland 2007/8, Germany 2005/6 and Belgium 2007/8. This ability to monitor flu has received widespread media attention. Less well-known are the cases where Google Trends significantly overestimated the actual number of flu cases. This occurred in the US during the winter of 2012/13, in Switzerland in 2008/9, Germany in 2008/9 and Belgium in 2008/9. Why the difference? Ormerod and co. hypothesise that people making flu-related searches fall into two categories. The first are those suffering symptoms of flu and the second group are searching merely because other people are searching too, perhaps because of strong media interest in flu for example [30].

INFRASTRUCTURE FOR BIG DATA ANALYTICS

Now that we have discussed health applications of big data and data sources, we dive into the heart of the matter: big data infrastructure. In the sections that follow, we discuss service-oriented architecture (SOA), cloud computing, and hierarchical system structures.

Service-Oriented Architecture Combined with Cloud Computing

Service-oriented architecture (SOA) offers excellent flexibility and interoperability, both of which are key for working with big data. PNWsoft defines SOA as

> a means for integrating across diverse systems. Each IT resource, whether an application, system, or trading partner, can be accessed as a service. These capabilities are available through interfaces; complexity arises when service providers differ in their operating system or communication protocols, resulting in inoperability. Service orientation uses standard protocols and conventional interfaces—usually Web services—to facilitate access to business logic and information among diverse services. Specifically, SOA allows the underlying service capabilities and interfaces to be composed into processes. Each process is itself a service, one that now offers up a new, aggregated capability. Because each new process is exposed through a standardized interface, the underlying implementation of the individual service providers is free to change without impacting how the service is consumed [31].

To meet the requirements of wireless connectivity, cloud-based, responsiveness, security, support for heterogeneity/platform-independence, scalability, and robustness, SOA-based architectures are being effectively utilized. Previous iterations of personalized healthcare were built on patients' treatment and limited to inside the hospital and to clinical care. Only recently has personalized medicine been recognized to be part of people's lives and expanded from hospital to communities and individuals. Health monitoring systems are accompanied by a variety of wireless personal vital signs monitors, like wearable devices, both for medical and suitability purposes. The applications under development focus on sensing technologies and the management of distributed nodes. The needs of customers vary and requires personalized applications in medicine and healthcare.

SOA architecture is built on five service modes:

1. Hosted service
2. Proactive service
3. Transaction processing service

4. Workflow service
5. Edge componentized service

Hosted service and proactive service are two basic modes, aimed at handling service issues. The attached hosted components, serving as containers of service, can be flexibly configured. "Containers" in this sense do not necessarily indicate docker containers. SOA is widely used for designing and developing applications with sharable, reusable services, providing high scalability.

The emergence of SOA can effectively solve the problems of *information islands* and legacy, both of which can lead to costly and difficult infrastructure incompatibilities. Service-oriented architectures are typically built upon web-driven delivery mechanisms, with the Internet and web browsers enabling ubiquitous access, easy application delivery, and seamless interoperation across platforms and systems. Cloud computing, as a new web service under the SOA architecture, can easily coexist with other web services and achieve interoperability. The applications offered in the Penguin Computing on Demand (POD) are excellent examples of HPC as a Service.

POD provides numerous intelligent and personalized services by a series of subsystems on cloud computing. The services are offered on demand online via web delivery. POD is discussed in more detail in the case study on CardioSolv at the end of Chapter 6.

SOA is a proven and effective solution to integrate heterogeneous systems and technology and to reduce cost and provide data and services to stakeholders. Emergent cloud infrastructures and platform-driven services are also a key component in maximizing the availability, elasticity, and reliability of the system, with the added benefit of reduction in infrastructure costs. Cloud services offer flexibility and expedience to production models, enabling health and research organizations to provide robust and consistent services through a service provider, delivering the organization cost savings, quicker service, reliability, availability, and extensibility.

With the combination of cloud computing technologies and SOA, services can be more cost efficient to both users and providers. Moreover, to better achieve interoperability, a unified standard should be formulated among SOA, PaaS (Platform as a Service), IaaS (Infrastructure as a Service) and SaaS (Software as a Service). We should consider these once-divergent offerings one and the same as infrastructures continue to evolve.

Hierarchical Structure of Systems

Precision medicine, big data, and data science are driving discussions among researchers to define a system structure for health big data. Table 5.1 details elements and capabilities desired in a cloud-based health record data system.

Table 5.1 Desired Elements in Big Data Cloud Storage

Desired Elements	Current Architecture	Enhanced Architecture
Scalability	Administratively provisioned with estimation before deployment.	Scalability and elasticity adopting SOA and IaaS flexible models.
Security/Privacy	Reliant on major methodology: 1. Column- or cell-level encryption 2. Distributed identifier, separated identifier fields, microsegmentation 3. Anonymization	1. Separated, distributed identifier data. 2. Additional layered authentication models (dual factor).
Cloud delivery	Offered in siloed approaches with VMWare or HyperV. Small private cloud.	SaaS, PaaS, and/or IaaS incorporated models.
Mining functionality	1. Independent of typical operations. 2. Implemented third party. 3. Lacking transparency.	1. Implemented as an extension of the SaaS model. 2. Seamless data sharing with operations and analysis
Semantic/Ontological interoperability	Generally not offered in legacy models.	Included in the additional of archetype/semantic catalog management elements.

Figure 5.2 offers a model for a National Healthcare Information Network.

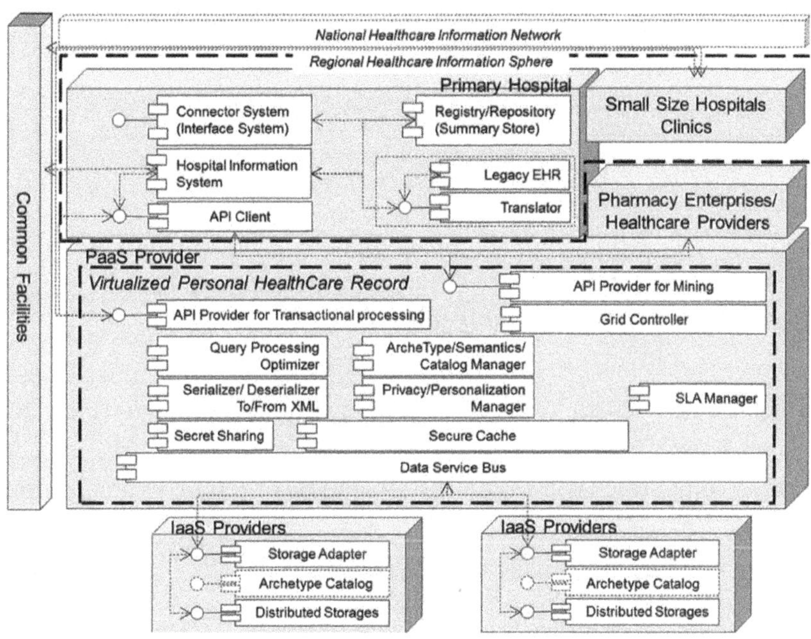

Figure 5.2 Cloud Computing–Based Model for a National Healthcare Information Network
S. Kikuchi, S. Sachdeva, and S. Bhalla, "Cloud Computing Based PHR Architecture Using Multi Layers Model," Journal of Software Engineering and Applications *5, no. 11A (2012): 903–911. doi: 10.4236/jsea.2012.531105. Used with permission.*

Figure 5.3 presents another model for a healthcare data system, this time separated out into hierarchical layers.

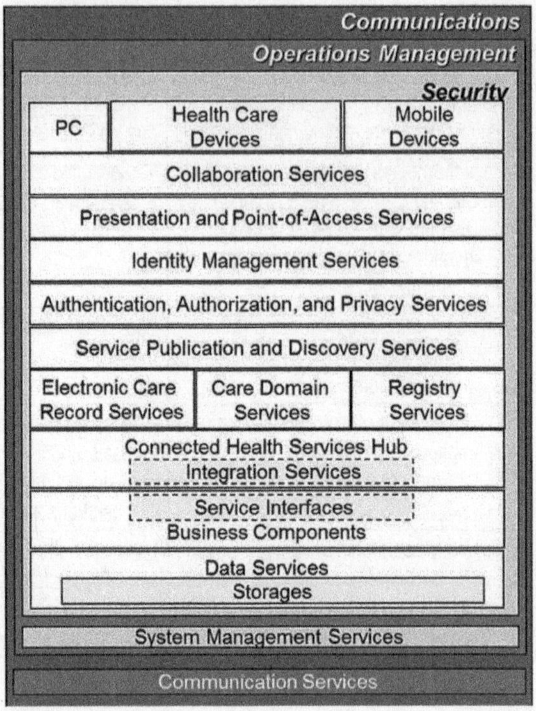

Figure 5.3 Cloud Computing–Based PHR Architecture Using Multi Layers Model
S. Kikuchi, S. Sachdeva, and S. Bhalla, "Cloud Computing–Based PHR Architecture Using Multi Layers Model," Journal of Software Engineering and Applications *5, no. 11A (2012): 903–911. doi: 10.4236/jsea.2012.531105. Used with permission.*

Through review of previous implementations and paradigms, several basic functional layers common to reported systems are proposed, as shown in Figure 5.4. The architecture mainly includes:

- Presentation layer to display user requirements;
- Application service layer to supply application servers/services to the upper layer;
- Data computing layer to run the scheduling of resources and computing tasks;
- Data storage and management layer; and
- Sensing layer.

This structure also corresponds to the classical cloud computing architecture, as loosely coupled relationships exist between each level. Each framework for the sublayers is composed of a set of modules exhibiting a set of functionalities and services. The bottom layer provides API for a cloud computing platform; the upper layer offers the open interface and user interface management; and in the layer of applications, users can share data sets and call the data mining algorithms and the visualization algorithms.

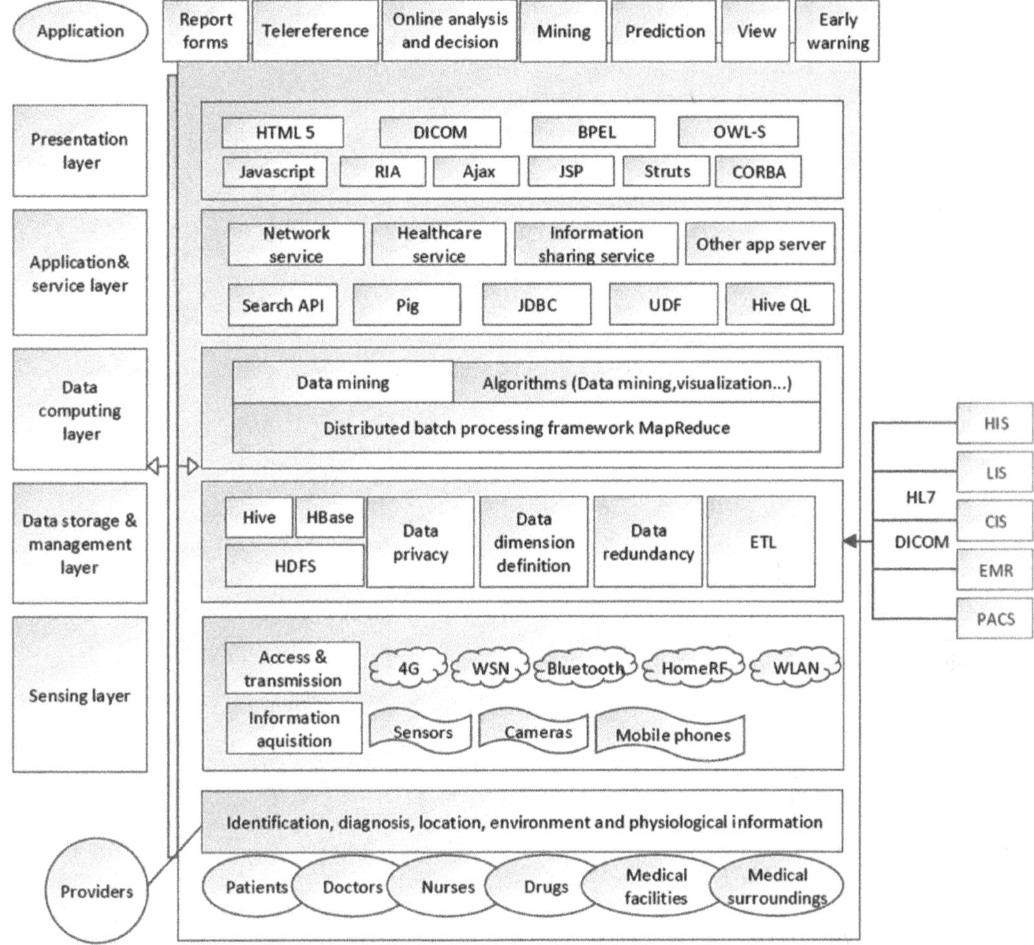

Figure 5.4 Architecture of Health Informatics Big Data Applications

Sensing Layer (Acquisition/Ingestion)

Responsible for data acquisition and data transmission, the sensing layer is divided into two sublayers, a data acquisition and an access layer. Data acquisition mainly functions as identifying information provided by patients, doctors, nurses, drugs, medical facilities, and medical surroundings, to include all that a patient may encounter and consume. This information can come from nodes that sense and capture identification parameters, as well as diagnosis, location, environment, and physiological information, captured by multiple types of sensors, cameras, and mobile phones. That information is then transmitted to the data storage layer with diverse techniques for data accessing, varying in accordance with data formats. For example, various physiological data can be collected using wireless body sensor networks. Information about outpatient charge management systems can be acquired using fixed network and radio-frequency identification (RFID)–sensor equipped mobility items such as beds, wheelchairs, and service chairs.

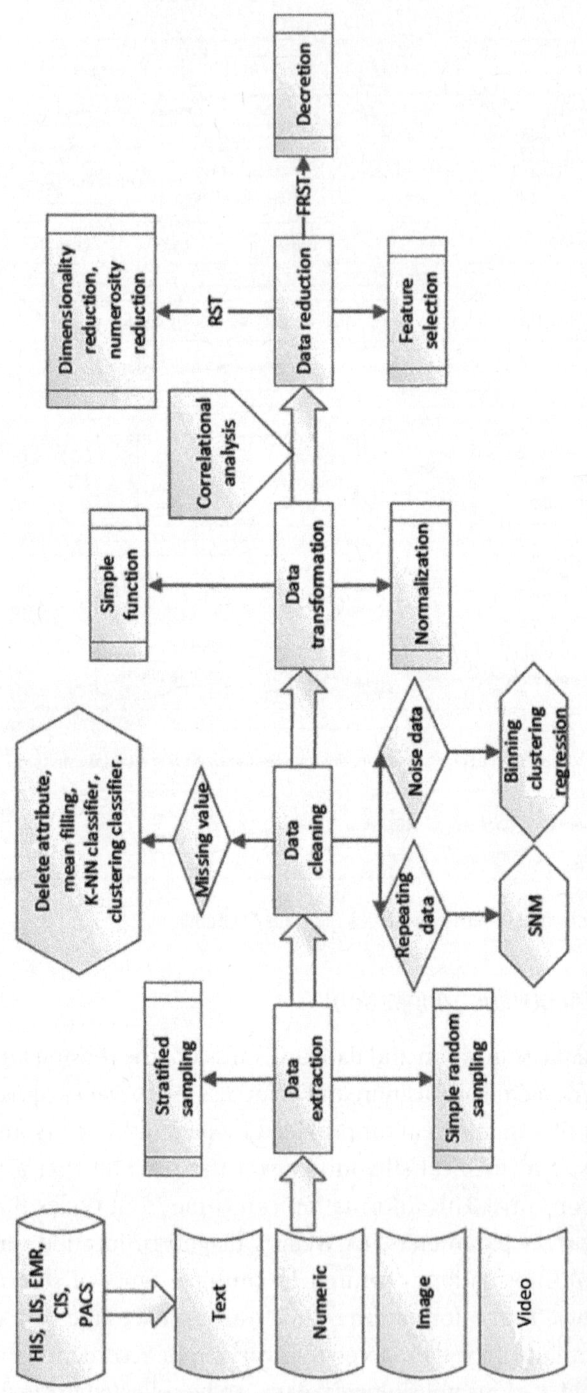

Figure 5.5 Typical Data Collection and Preprocessing Model

A typical data collection and preprocessing model is shown in Figure 5.5. As the first phase in big data utilization, data acquisition and data preprocessing are critical procedures before data analysis. Sensing and monitoring from surroundings creates large quantities of data. Collecting the data effectively is the first challenge.

In applications integrated into mobile health, for instance, data coming from varied sources could contain errors and varied formats. Therefore, a data preprocessing procedure should be an element in the collection and identification of sensor-generated data. This will reduce data payload, render data to an operable scale, and perform data cleaning while reserving and prioritizing useful data from administrative and/or debug trace data.

Health informatics can be mainly divided into four types: text, numeric, image, and video. Among them, preprocessing of medical records and web search logs is currently garnering more attention.

Preprocessing during the ingestion of clinical data, monitoring data, and web logs serves to remove noise within the data to ensure or create a higher probability of accuracy of analysis and reduce the scale of data and runtime.

Often data will differ both in format and information. It is necessary to extract required information and transform it into a proper format that is suitable or optimal for analysis. There are cases where the data itself may be invalid or vacant. Current methods of data cleaning based on the error model require effective data or accepted constraints as an assumption. To ensure data quality, data preprocessing technologies, such as data cleaning, data transformation, and data reduction, require research and are highly specific to the sensor and collection mechanism. Many sensor-driven data streams can be discarded when invalid and retransmitted or are near real time where error data is automatically discarded upon arrival. The first step is to identify the raw data, including noise, missing values, and inconsistency. Statistical classification models are utilized to find correlation, and clustering methods are used to identify outliers.

Binning methods, clustering, and regression function are applied to smooth the data [32, 33, 34]. Integration of multiple replicated database utilities solves redundancy and durability, which could be detected by correlational analysis. Unbalanced data is generally handled by the weighted support vector machines method [35, 36].

Data reduction plays an important role in data science. It can address uncertainty and missing values in the data sets. Rough Set Theory (RST) is a classic technique for this. Proposed by Zdzislaw Pawlak, traditional RST can handle nominal attributes only [37]. Fuzzy-Rough Set Theory (FRST) was proposed to solve problems of missing information during the discretization of data [38].

In 2012, Wang et al. further proved a better accuracy of FRST by constructing an attribute-based method [39]. Additional data reduction methods, such as dimensionality reduction and concept hierarchy generation, have also been widely used to address these same challenges. Feature selection combined with oversampling technique has been proposed to preprocess the imbalanced breast cancer data and has been shown to be successful in improving the performance of classifiers on specific data sets, especially decision tree analysis [40].

Data Storage and Management Layer

The data storage and management layer is responsible for integration of data gathered from the sensing layer and various medical databases. Data is ingested and then passed through an indexing layer for mass data storage.

When considering diverse data structures, the cloud health information systems technology architecture (CHISTAR) reference model extends and adapts in the Health Level 7 v3.0 to improve semantic matching [41].

A Sun Microsystems collaboration of medical service providers integrated the advanced fine-grained access control mechanism to achieve data sharing of EHR systems. This feature can also provide additional protection for patient data privacy [42]. In order to elevate the data quality, Almutiry et al. suggest a data flow framework for cloud-based health information systems that filters the existing data quality dimensions [43]. Patient-centric systems categorize the users into several security fields based on different data owners, which further simplifies the management of the data. The system model consists of Health-Service Provider, Registered User (Patient), Cloud Service Provider, and Data Access Requester. The reencryption process resides in the data management layer.

In the age of information explosion, simply increasing the number of hard disks to extend the storage capacity allowing for the growth rate of capacity, performing data backup, and assurance of data durability of file system still may not achieve performance satisfactory with application demands. Efficient and durable data storage over an extended period of time and continual management of the source shines light on new challenges in technical storage management. Distributed storage systems that leverage ephemeral disk systems or server-based storage are gaining popularity due to these relevant factors.

Figure 5.6 shows a typical distributed file system and storage model.

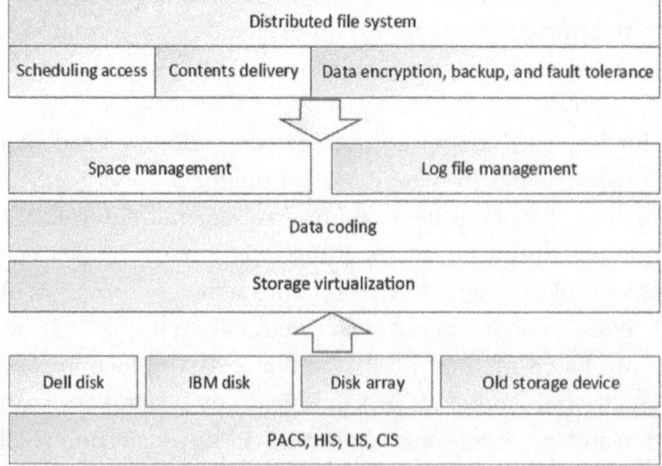

Figure 5.6 Typical Data Storage Model

File systems fixed in a location that support extension and presentation to any number of sites or multiple file systems with multiple nodes form a network file system. This also fits into the SOA or cloud models as IaaS/PaaS, depending on deployment.

Through the network communication and data transmission between nodes, each node can be distributed in different locations. Geolocated or geo-specific locality within distributed file systems removes concern for which node stores the data and permits interaction to appear as the local file system.

As depicted in Figure 5.6, data coming from different sources is stored on various hardware. Storage virtualization, in a common sense, presents the abstraction of hardware storage resources. Integrating one or more target services with additional functions provides useful and comprehensive functions in a unified way. Typical virtualization methods include: shielding complexity of the system, increasing or integrating new functions, simulation, and integration or decomposition of existing service functions.

In order to simplify the client's use, the distributed storage system provides a distributed cache system to offer the access interface as well as a local data buffer to reduce network pressure.

As an open source system, the Hadoop Distributed File System (HDFS) supports the main application scenario where it is used as the basis of parallel computing environment (graphs) components. Using master/slave architecture, a cluster consists of one namenode as master and several other datanodes. The master node serves as a management center where namespace of the system and its access are properly assigned. The datanodes are simply responsible for storing the data files. For instance, a data file is first divided into several blocks, and each block is assigned to a datanode for storing. The input data set will usually be separated into segments as independent data blocks. The output will also be stored in the file system. Current Hadoop distributions running MapReduce Version 2 (MRv2) have redundancy at the namenodes and secondary namenodes. Without going into Hadoop details, it should be noted that redundancy also exists in the data layout across the cluster as nodes in rack locations are "rack aware" and data blocks are copied to be first a node in the same rack and then a separate rack for data durability. Take a look at http://hadoop.apache.org/ or grab a copy of *Hadoop: The Definitive Guide* (3rd ed.) by Tom White: http://shop.oreilly.com/product/0636920021773.do.

As cloud computing develops, multiple workloads with different performance goals will be gathered into very large clusters. Resources stored in the large cluster demand new methods to share them. These new methods will decide the way to operate and handle the data process, aiming at accomplishing each workload goal and controlling system errors at low cost. Also, as the traditional input-output subsystem changes, conventional storage methods are insufficient to meet the demands of production and transportation. The storage optimization problem remains to be solved. Despite warehouse management, other schemes, including storage virtualization, hierarchy memory, and usage of enterprise storage, are practical ways to address mass data storage [44].

Data Computing Layer

The data computing layer is responsible for processing data on a large scale. In this layer, there are three major analysis models: batch analysis, in-database analysis, and streaming analysis.

A batch processing mode is usually used for those tasks that require data to be stored first and computed next. These tasks usually are not time critical. An example of this type of work is using EHRs to make predictions. A batch processing analysis usually involves MapReduce workflow and massive parallel processing. As shown in Figure 5.7, the data storage here serves as a buffer between MapReduce workflow and the data source. This data storage could be a data warehouse or a distributed file system. A query engine searches target data from the whole volume and passes it on to the MapReduce framework, where the data sets are further divided into smaller partitions for processing. This processing usually takes a very long time, from hours to days. The data processed is usually historical data.

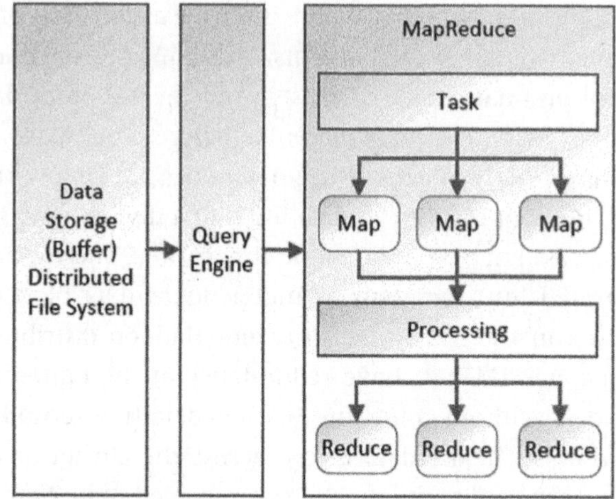

Figure 5.7 Batch Analysis

Key Points about Hadoop and MapReduce

- Hadoop/MapReduce are frameworks for automatically scaling storage and compute.
- Data and computations can be spread over thousands of nodes.
- HDFS handles Storage while MapReduce handles Compute.
- Hadoop, developed by Yahoo, is an open source implementation.
- MapReduce is Google's framework for large data computations.

Table 5.2 summarizes the benefits and challenges of Hadoop and MapReduce.

Table 5.2 Benefits and Challenges of Hadoop and MapReduce

Benefits	Challenges
Scalable, efficient, reliable	Redesigning applications
Ease of programmability	Data storage efficiency (long term)
Runs on commodity servers	Threshold to reap processing benefits
Relatively "fast" for very large jobs	Slow for small jobs (compute job time)
Fault tolerant /Durable storage	

In-Database Analysis

Traditional data mining approaches mainly focus on how to deliver analysis outside the data source. Due to the fact that large databases and data warehouses have come to use distributed file systems, an important strategy of providing timely analysis requires direct use of memory and parallel capabilities to perform analytics from specialized analytic tools or operating systems. Increasingly in-database analysis is used, which allows for computation or analysis to be done in the database rather than using complex import, extract, transform, and loading tools.

More succinctly, in-database analytics indicates a model of analysis where data processing is performed within a database to eliminate the overhead associated with moving large data sets to the analytic applications. In-database moves analytic logic into the database (RDBMS) instead of into a separate application.

Advantages of in-database analytics include parallel processing, scalability, analytic optimization, and partitioning. An example of an in-database analysis model can be seen from Figure 5.8. Some examples of this kind of analysis model may be found in Oracle in-database analytics solutions integrated with SAS In-Database Technologies like SAS Scoring accelerator or SAS Data Quality Accelerator, which is compatible across multiple database models, including DB2, Pivotal, Hadoop, Neteeza, Oracle, and SAP HANA.

Normally, this type of analysis model can be divided into three steps. First, "in-database preparation" involves data cleaning, integration, and some other preparation, depending on the analytic models. This is usually the most time-consuming step of the three. Unlike other data mining and analysis, the preparation procedures happen within the data infrastructure. The resulting data will then be stored locally or sent out for analysis.

The second step is "in-database model deployment," which consists of analytic model construction and mode deployment. In this part, algorithms embedded in the data infrastructure are used to develop and create analytic models. The resulting model may be stored in a model repository or passed out for further use. After the model is deployed in a target database, the third

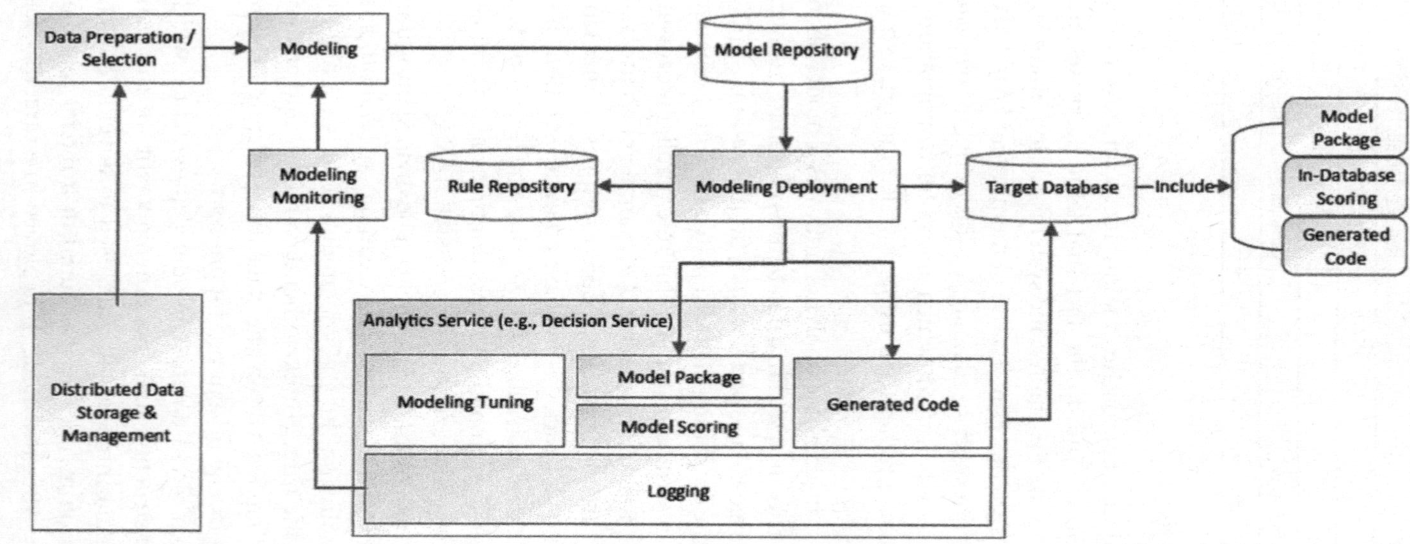

Figure 5.8 In-Database Analysis
SAS In-Database Technologies: Manage Data Where It Lives, SAS, http://www.sas.com/en_us/software/data-management/in-database-processing.html.

procedure "in-database deployment and scoring" begins. This part involves an analytic service that may vary depending on the analytic tasks. In general, this service will contain model tuning, model package, model scoring, generated code, and logging. The procedure monitors the process when generating the models, and furthermore, it turns the model into the proper form for storage that can be recalled when needed. After everything is set, the data infrastructure may also have a model package, in-database scoring, and generated code, in addition to the data itself. The additional benefits aside from the data move penalty would be fresh consistent views across data, improved data mining and IT group productivity, reduced time to insights and processing, and ease of access to excellent-quality, clean data.

In-Memory Analysis and Streaming Analysis

In-memory analytics and streaming analysis in big data, promoted by streaming computing, denotes those analysis tasks that require high real-time and high-throughput computing and/or large physical memory footprints. This kind of analysis, based on system structure, can be further divided into two types. The first one is the master-slave model. The master nodes here are responsible for global control, such as resource allocation, load balancing, and so on. Besides master nodes, there are multiple slave nodes, each of which has a special function and receives a data stream from the master node before processing the data accordingly. After that, all results are sent back to the master node.

Twitter Storm is an example of streaming analysis that uses this master-slave model to process streaming big data. Storm is a platform performing analysis on streams of data as they arrive, facilitating immediate knowledge and the potential to act on that knowledge. Figure 5.9 shows the Tweet scoring pipeline.

Figure 5.10 is a Storm cluster and is used to illustrate how the master-slave model works. In the master node there is Nimbus, which acts like Hadoop's Job Tracker. In Storm, Nimbus is responsible for distributing code around the clusters, assigning tasks to other nodes, and monitoring system status. The processing tasks are handled by the slave node, which consists of supervisors and workers. Each slave node has only one supervisor and multiple workers. The slave node listens for a work assignment and starts/stops workers when necessary. Each of these workers processes a subset of the task. Between the master nodes and the slave nodes, there is a Zookeeper cluster, which acts as a coordinator of Nimbus and supervisors. Some of the system status conditions, such as failure, will also be kept in this cluster. If the Nimbus or supervisor is down, the cluster will start backup as if nothing had happened.

Another kind of streaming analysis is the symmetric model. Figure 5.11 shows a system structure of this model, where there is only one type of node: the processing node. The right part of this figure is a demonstration of how this model works.

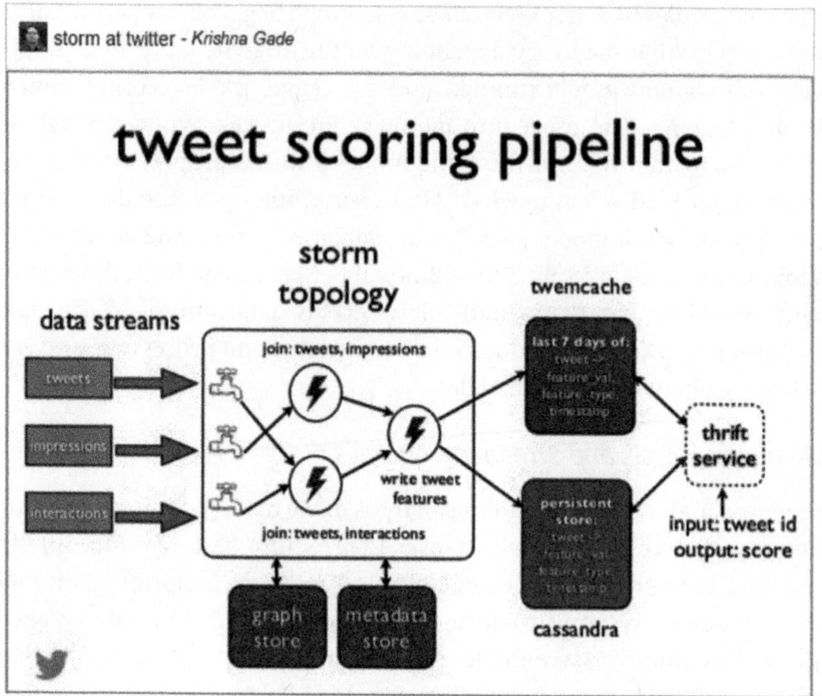

Figure 5.9 Processing 50 Billion Messages a Day with an Average Total Latency of > 50 Milliseconds
Krishna Gade from Facebook's analytics@webscale conference—krishna@twitter.com

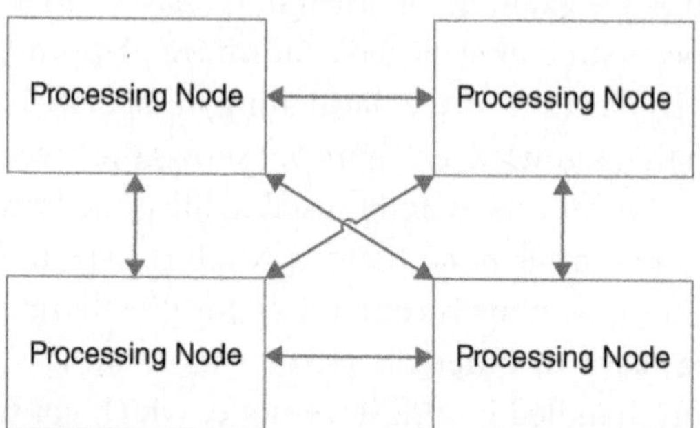

Figure 5.10 Symmetric Analysis Model, Streaming Analysis System Structure

In every processing node, there are four parts. The processing element container acts like a jobs processor, but unlike jobs these may consist of key values. As an example of symmetric analysis, Yahoo S4 uses functionality, types of events, keyed attributes, and value of key attribute as the content of the container. Besides the processing container, there are event listeners, dispatchers, and emitters. All of these components enable the processing node to communicate with other nodes by emitting and listening to events as well as dispatching events. Beneath the processing node, there is a communication layer, which

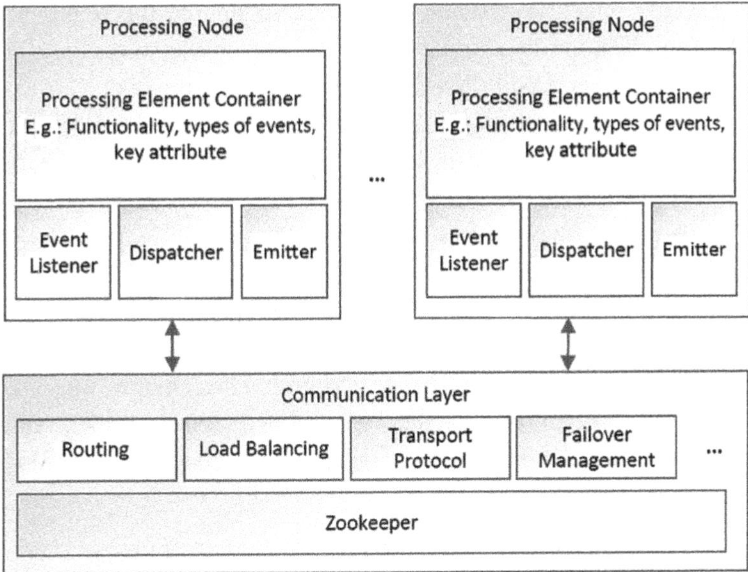

Figure 5.11 Symmetric Analysis Demonstration

serves as a bus in the system. All the events are routed to the processing node by this layer, which involves routing and transport protocols. To optimize the robustness and performance of the system, load balancing, failover management, and some other mechanisms may be included in this layer. Zookeeper is located at the bottom of the communication layer to manage the clusters that reside on this layer.

Application Service Layer

Running on the cloud platform layer, this layer consists of a series of application servers. Each application server corresponds to a business need and interacts with the computing layer through the service interface furnished by Java Database Connectivity, Universal Disk Format, and so on. It also provides users with a standard, unified service interface, dispatching the service channel. The application service layer can integrate various application servers and the load balancer. J2EE framework appears to be an effective choice with the potential to deliver an enterprise service system structured framework and multimedia middleware for distributed transaction processing. And it is flexible, to allow many hosts to join to provide more services.

Presentation Layer

The presentation layer, or external service interface layer, transfers the service and data of the system to users. It employs JavaScript, Rich Internet Application,

Ajax, JavaServer Pages, and struts framework to enable the interaction with users. Continuous study in automatic service composition techniques is added to the interoperable service of the presentation layer. Business Process Execution Language and the Web Ontology Language-Based framework of the Semantic Web are frequently used to perform service composition. However, due to the fact that they both need some preliminaries, such as connections between services, the workflow, and so on, neither is serviceable for large-scale data. To better use the most recent web techniques, MyPHR Machines consists of a Digital Imaging and Communications in Medicine (DICOM) viewer that has been programmed in HTML5 and related technologies [45]. Bagha et al. add an information service between the database and the web tier to accommodate semantic interoperability using a two-level modeling approach that separates data from clinical knowledge; the approach consists of a data storage model and an archetype model [41].

FUNDAMENTAL SYSTEM PROPERTIES

In developing applications in health big data, these are fundamental system properties:

- **Availability.** Nonintrusive ways to collect health and medical information are required. Meanwhile, all users who have different roles should have access to the platform whenever and wherever they are.
- **Instantaneity.** Response time in all operations should be as low as possible.
- **Security.** The platform should provide proven mechanisms to protect privacy of health data of all users. Also, measurement to storing and sharing should be protected all over the path. In addition to accepted security parameters, the platform should also provide fine-grained, verifiable controls to share information.
- **Interoperability.** The system should support heterogeneity, so that different health systems and databases can be integrated seamlessly.
- **Scalability.** The architecture should be scalable to support a high and increasing number of actors and applications.
- **Robustness.** The system should be able to work in extreme conditions and quickly and safely recover in emergency situations.

Recent research has focused on improvement of the interoperability, concurrency, scalability, maintainability, accessibility, disaster recovery, portability, reusability, and security, thereby increasing the inherent benefits of using the system. To achieve better maintainability and scalability, a fixed and unified architecture mode, such as unified hierarchy structure, unified configuration files (XML, attribution, constant, parameter, code style, etc.) is definitely needed. A universal API, such as string manipulation, file processing, database access, paging processing, report design, error message, and log processing, assures high reusability. To guarantee security, the basic demands are to uniformly manage and allocate authority and ensure secure interface. Chien-Hsing Wu proposed a framework coherently employing the symmetric key cryptography and identity-based cryptography that offers a secured, private, and full-access control of relevant data to the owners of personal health records, without sacrificing cloud service performance [46]. Moreover, the proposed framework is implemented as a separate cloud computing service in order to have better user trust. The system utilizes a cloud server to manage and compute.

Developers must choose appropriate deployment architectures to ensure that applications meet specified performance requirements; thus, each application class typically has its own deployment configuration of web, application, and database servers. Application developers must also consider several attributes for the deployment architecture, such as number of tiers, number of servers in each tier, each server's computational capacity, interconnections among servers in a tier, load balancing, and database replication strategies.

GPU-ACCELERATED COMPUTING AND BIOMEDICAL INFORMATICS

GPU-accelerated computing is the use of a graphics processing unit (GPU) together with a central processing unit (CPU) to accelerate scientific, analytics, engineering, consumer, and enterprise applications [47]. Bioscience/biochemistry/bioengineering applications can be used to reveal the mysteries of life and target medical treatments. GPU compute is keenly suited to computational tasks such as genomics, biology, pharmacology, proteomics, and drug discovery, among others. Many GPU-accelerated applications are being used for genomics and population genetics as well as agent-based modeling. Modeling in the biosciences is one of the key beneficiaries of the GPU revolution. Bioinformatics software suites purpose built for GPUs to analyze the function of genes as they relate to cellular function and/or the development of biomarkers, protein analysis, and gene networks, as in graph analysis, will unlock many new avenues in precision medicine.

Pioneered in 2007 by NVIDIA, GPU accelerators now power energy-efficient data centers in government labs, universities, enterprises, and small- and medium businesses around the world. GPUs are accelerating applications in platforms ranging from cars, to mobile phones and tablets, to drones and robots, and therefore should be applied to common biomedical challenges [47]. In 2012, Oak Ridge National Laboratory announced what was to become the world's fastest supercomputer, Titan, equipped with one NVIDIA GPU per CPU—over 18,000 GPU accelerators. Titan established records not only in absolute system performance but also in energy efficiency, with 90% of its peak performance being delivered by the GPU accelerators. Recently, the U.S. Department of Energy announced plans to build two of the world's fastest supercomputers—the Summit system at Oak Ridge National Laboratory and the Sierra system at Lawrence Livermore National Laboratory—which are each expected to have well over 100 petaFLOPS of peak performance and are scheduled to be completed in 2018. Although each system is unique, they share the same fundamental multi-GPU node architecture.

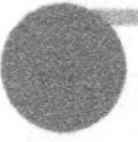

In computing, FLOPS (floating-point operations per second) is a measure of processor performance in scientific calculations that make heavy use of floating-point calculations.

$$\text{FLOPS} = \text{sockets} \times \text{cores/socket} \times \text{clock} \times \text{FLOPs/cycle}$$ [48]

See Table 5.3 for a FLOPS scale.

Table 5.3 Performance Chart

Name	Abbreviation	FLOPS Integer (floating point operations per second)
KiloFLOPS	kFLOPS	10^3
MegaFLOPS	MFLOPS	10^6
GigaFLOPS	GFLOPS	10^9
TeraFLOPS	TFLOPS	10^{12}
PetaFLOPS	PFLOPS	10^{15}
ExaFLOPS	EFLOPS	10^{18}
ZettaFLOPS	ZFLOPS	10^{21}
YottaFLOPS	YFLOPS	10^{24}

How Do Accelerators Impact Applications?

GPU-accelerated computing offers unprecedented application performance by offloading compute-intensive portions of the application to the GPU, while the remainder of the code still runs on the CPU. From a user's perspective, applications simply run significantly faster and many times parallelize more efficiently. Until recently, "Big Iron" enthusiasts believed that the application of GPU compute to large-scale analysis was inefficient and underpowered for their class of workload.

Advances in general-purpose GPUs permit the study of a new arena of problems in the biomedical sciences through computer simulations by making accessible larger systems and longer time scales. Originally, single-core processors were used for simulation. If one needed greater performance, one would simply wait until faster processors were available. Microprocessor clock rates eventually reached an asymptote, and the field turned to multicore and parallel computing solutions. This led many molecular modeling packages to port their codes to large-scale parallel computing resources, requiring users to know how to manage and operate clusters or supercomputers. While this was occurring, GPUs were evolving into hardware that can handle increasingly high-throughput, data-parallel computational workloads in order to meet the demands of the imaging and video game industry. GPUs are used for rastering and shading images and have their own graphics-oriented language. Previously, if researchers wanted to solve a computational problem using a GPU, they would have to map it to a graphics processing language. More recently, programming languages like CUDA 1.2 and OpenCL 3, which are dialects of the C language, have been developed and widely adopted by the research community, making the GPU-based software accessible to scientists, particularly in the field of computational biophysics [49, 50]. With this combination of hardware and software, GPUs now represent an option that yields both increased performance and reduced cost/performance. GPUs are hardware specifically designed for aggregate floating-point operations for highly parallel workloads on the order of TFLOPS, a high-bandwidth memory system, intra-GPU transfer rates of up to 100 gigabytes per second, and multithreading/machine instructions for complex functions often used in molecular modeling [50, 51]. With the tremendous increase in speed, simulations that once took months can now take weeks. Additionally, bigger systems can be simulated for longer time scales. Instead of using many cores on a supercomputer, simulations can now be done on a single desktop machine, increasing the performance/cost ratio. Within the biosciences, GPUs can greatly accelerate complicated molecular dynamics simulations.

CPU versus GPU*

A simple way to understand the difference between a CPU and a GPU is to compare how they process tasks. A CPU consists of a few cores optimized for sequential serial processing, while a GPU has a massively parallel architecture consisting of thousands of smaller, more efficient cores designed for handling multiple tasks simultaneously. The same analogy used to explain Hadoop could very well be applied here. Which is more efficient, pulling a load with one really large ox or with 100 small oxen? Figure 5.12 illustrates the advantage of GPU with its thousands of cores.

* Some of the text is taken from NVIDIA Newsroom, "NVIDIA GPUs Power Facebook's New Deep Learning Machine." http://nvidianews.nvidia.com/news/nvidia-gpus-power-facebook-s-new-deep-learning-machine. Used with permission.

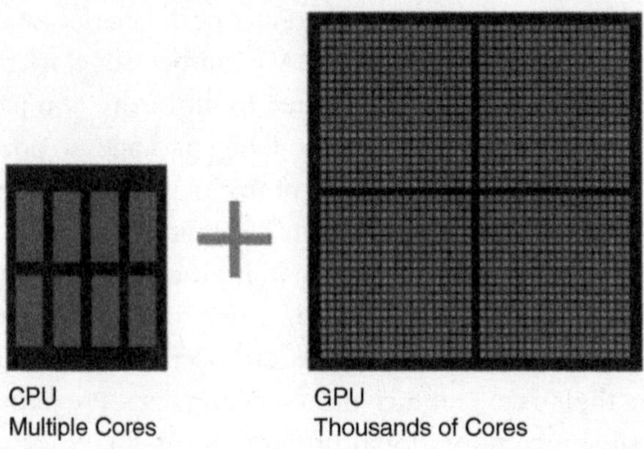

Figure 5.12 CPU versus GPU

On December 10, 2015, NVIDIA announced that Facebook would power its next-generation computing system with the NVIDIA Tesla Accelerated Computing Platform, enabling it to drive a broad range of machine learning applications.

While training complex deep neural networks to conduct machine learning can take days or weeks on even the fastest computers, the Tesla platform reduces this timeframe by 10 to 20 times. Developers can innovate more quickly and train networks that are more sophisticated, delivering improved capabilities to consumers.

Facebook is the first company to adopt NVIDIA Tesla M40 GPU accelerators to train deep neural networks. They will play a key role in the new "Big Sur" computing platform, Facebook AI Research's (FAIR) purpose-built system designed specifically for neural network training. This would mark the NVIDIA installation as the first open source artificial intelligence (AI) computing architecture. The Big Sur initiative represents the first time a computing system specifically designed for machine learning and AI research will be released as an open source solution.

Committed to doing its AI work as open source and sharing its findings with the community, Facebook intends to work with its partners to open source Big Sur specifications via the Open Compute Project. This unique approach will make it easier for AI researchers worldwide to share and improve techniques, enabling future innovation in machine learning by harnessing the power of GPU-accelerated computing.

CONCLUSION

Big data applications in health informatics are flourishing and attracting a lot of research interest. We hope that you now have a familiarity with big data applications in health informatics. Perhaps more important, you are now equipped with basic tenets of system architecture best practices as well as a layer-by-layer understanding of hierarchical system structures. Even if you follow best practices, your system can still encounter bottlenecks when dealing with big data. GPU-accelerated computing is one possible solution.

Following this chapter are two case studies. The first explores how computational modeling and scientific computing can be used to model treatment options for vascular disease. The second presents how GPU was used to study the molecular mechanisms of antibiotic resistance.

NOTES

1. Paul Ginsparg. 2009. "Text in a Data-Centric World." In *The Fourth Paradigm: Data-Intensive Scientific Discovery*, eds. Anthony Hey, Stewart Tansley, and Kristin Tolle (Redmond, WA: Microsoft Research), 185–192.
2. Anthony J. G. Hey, Stewart Tansley, and Kristin Tolle (eds.). 2009. *The Fourth Paradigm: Data-Intensive Scientific Discovery*. Redmond, WA: Microsoft Research.
3. "XSEDE | Partnerships." 2016. https://www.xsede.org/web/guest/partnerships.
4. Bob Chadduck and Anita Nikolich. 2016. "High-Performance Computing System Acquisition: Continuing the Building of a More Inclusive Computing Environment for Science and Engineering. NSF—National Science Foundation." https://www.nsf.gov/funding/pgm_summ.jsp?pims_id=503148.
5. Min Chen, Shiwen Mao, and Yunhao Liu. 2014. "Big Data: A Survey." *Mobile Networks and Applications* 19(2): 171–209. doi: 10.1007/s11036-013-0489-0.
6. M. K. Ross, W. Wei, and L. Ohno-Machado. 2014. "'Big Data' and the Electronic Health Record." *IMIA Yearbook* 9(1): 97–104. doi: 10.15265/IY-2014-0003.
7. M. Herland, T. M. Khoshgoftaar, and R. Wald. 2013. "Survey of Clinical Data Mining Applications on Big Data in Health Informatics." In *Machine Learning and Applications (ICMLA)*, 465–472.
8. J. Zhou, J. Sun, Y. Liu, J. Hu, and J. Ye. 2013. "Patient Risk Prediction Model via Top-K Stability Selection." In *Proceedings of the 2013 SIAM International Conference on Data Mining*, 55–63. http://epubs.siam.org/doi/abs/10.1137/1.9781611972832.7.
9. Leo A. Celi, Marie Csete, and David Stone. 2014. "Optimal Data Systems: The Future of Clinical Predictions and Decision Support." *Current Opinion in Critical Care* 20(5): 573–580. doi: 10.1097/MCC.0000000000000137.
10. Jui-chien Hsieh and Meng-Wei Hsu. 2012. "A Cloud Computing Based 12-Lead ECG Telemedicine Service." *BMC Medical Informatics and Decision Making* 12:77. doi: 10.1186/1472-6947-12-77.
11. Suppawong Tuarob, Conrad S. Tucker, Marcel Salathe, and Nilam Ram. 2013. "Discovering Health-Related Knowledge in Social Media Using Ensembles of Heterogeneous Features." In *Proceedings of the 22nd ACM International Conference on Conference on Information & Knowledge Management*, 1685–1690. New York: ACM. doi: 10.1145/2505515.2505629.
12. Nattiya Kanhabua, Sara Romano, Avaré Stewart, and Wolfgang Nejdl. 2012. "Supporting Temporal Analytics for Health-Related Events in Microblogs." In *Proceedings of the 21st ACM International Conference on Information and Knowledge Management*, 2686–88. New York: ACM. doi: 10.1145/2396761.2398726.
13. Bernard W. Stewart, Chris Wild, International Agency for Research on Cancer, and World Health Organization (eds.). 2014. *World Cancer Report 2014*. Lyon: International Agency for Research on Cancer.
14. Hans Petri, Alan Nevitt, Khaled Sarsour, Pavel Napalkov, and Neil Collinson. 2015. "Incidence of Giant Cell Arteritis and Characteristics of Patients: Data-Driven Analysis of Comorbidities." *Arthritis Care & Research* 67(3): 390–395. doi: 10.1002/acr.22429.
15. Arnis Kirshners, Serge Parshutin, and Marcis Leja. 2012. "Research on Application of Data Mining Methods to Diagnosing Gastric Cancer." In Petra Perner (ed.), *Advances in Data Mining*.

Applications and Theoretical Aspects, 24–37. Lecture Notes in Computer Science 7377. Berlin: Springer. http://link.springer.com/chapter/10.1007/978-3-642-31488-9_3.

16. Cheng-Min Chao, Ya-Wen Yu, Bor-Wen Cheng, and Yao-Lung Kuo. 2014. "Construction the Model on the Breast Cancer Survival Analysis Use Support Vector Machine, Logistic Regression and Decision Tree." *Journal of Medical Systems* 38(10): 106. doi: 10.1007/s10916-014-0106-1.
17. Marlene Huml, René Silye, Gerald Zauner, Stephan Hutterer, and Kurt Schilcher. 2013. "Brain Tumor Classification Using AFM in Combination with Data Mining Techniques." *BioMed Research International* (August): e176519. doi: 10.1155/2013/176519, 10.1155/2013/176519.
18. Bruce I. Reiner. 2014. "Opportunities for Radiation-Dose Optimization Through Standardized Analytics and Decision Support." *Journal of the American College of Radiology* 11(11): 1048–1052. doi:10.1016/j.jacr.2014.06.010.
19. J. C. Denny. 2014. "Surveying Recent Themes in Translational Bioinformatics: Big Data in EHRs, Omics for Drugs, and Personal Genomics." *Yearbook of Medical Informatics* 9: 199–205. doi: 10.15265/IY-2014-0015.
20. John K. Zao, Tchin-Tze Gan, Chun-Kai You, et al. 2014. "Pervasive Brain Monitoring and Data Sharing Based on Multi-Tier Distributed Computing and Linked Data Technology." *Frontiers in Human Neuroscience* 8: 370. doi: 10.3389/fnhum.2014.00370.
21. Melanie Tory, Arthur E. Kirkpatrick, M. Stella Atkins, and Torsten Moller. 2006. "Visualization Task Performance with 2D, 3D, and Combination Displays." *IEEE Transactions on Visualization and Computer Graphics* 12(1): 2–13. doi: 10.1109/TVCG.2006.17.
22. T. R. Tavares, A. L. I. Oliveira, G. G. Cabral, S. S. Mattos, and R. Grigorio. 2013. "Preprocessing Unbalanced Data Using Weighted Support Vector Machines for Prediction of Heart Disease in Children." In *2013 International Joint Conference on Neural Networks (IJCNN)*, 1–8. doi: 10.1109/IJCNN.2013.6706947.
23. Christopher G. Healey and James T. Enns. 1999. "Large Datasets at a Glance: Combining Textures and Colors in Scientific Visualization." *IEEE Transactions on Visualization and Computer Graphics* 5(2): 145–167. doi: 10.1109/2945.773807.
24. Daniel A. Keim. 2000. "Designing Pixel-Oriented Visualization Techniques: Theory and Applications." *IEEE Transactions on Visualization and Computer Graphics* 6(1): 59–78. doi: 10.1109/2945.841121.
25. Teresa A. Mesquita and André R. S. Marçal. 2013. "Hierarchic Image Classification Visualization." In Mohamed Kamel and Aurélio Campilho (eds.), *Image Analysis and Recognition*, 152–159. Lecture Notes in Computer Science 7950. Berlin: Springer. http://link.springer.com/chapter/10.1007/978-3-642-39094-4_18.
26. F. Martin-Sanchez and K. Verspoor. 2014. "Big Data in Medicine Is Driving Big Changes." *Yearbook of Medical Informatics* 9: 14–20. doi: 10.15265/IY-2014-0020.
27. N. Peek, J. H. Holmes, and J. Sun. 2014. "Technical Challenges for Big Data in Biomedicine and Health: Data Sources, Infrastructure, and Analytics." *Yearbook of Medical Informatics* 9: 42–47. doi: 10.15265/IY-2014-0018.
28. "Nowcasting." 2016. J.S. Marshall Radar Observatory. http://www.radar.mcgill.ca/science/activities/nowcasting-menu.html.
29. Paul Ormerod, Rickard Nyman, and R. Alexander Bentley. 2014. "Nowcasting Economic and Social Data: When and Why Search Engine Data Fails, an Illustration Using Google Flu Trends." *arXiv:1408.0699 [physics]*. http://arxiv.org/abs/1408.0699.
30. "The Emerging Pitfalls of Nowcasting with Big Data." 2014. *MIT Technology Review*. https://www.technologyreview.com/s/530131/the-emerging-pitfalls-of-nowcasting-with-big-data/.
31. "SOA Tutorial—Service Oriented Architecture." 2016. *PNMsoft*. http://www.pnmsoft.com/resources/bpm-tutorial/soa-tutorial/.
32. M. A. Islam, M. H. Talukder, and M. M. Hasan. 2013. "Speckle Noise Reduction from Ultrasound Image Using Modified Binning Method and Fuzzy Inference System." In *2013 International Conference on Advances in Electrical Engineering (ICAEE)*, 359–362. doi: 10.1109/ICAEE.2013.6750363.
33. S. Ramos, I. Praça, Z. Vale, T. M. Sousa, and V. Faria. 2014. "Load Profiling Tool to Support Smart Grid Operation Scenarios." In *2014 IEEE PES T&D Conference and Exposition*, 1–5. doi: 10.1109/TDC.2014.6863352.

34. Y. Aliyari Ghassabeh and F. Rudzicz. 2014. "Noisy Source Vector Quantization Using Kernel Regression." *IEEE Transactions on Communications* 62(11): 3825–34. doi: 10.1109/TCOMM.2014.2363094.

35. M. A. H. Farquad and Indranil Bose. 2012. "Preprocessing Unbalanced Data Using Support Vector Machine." *Decision Support Systems* 53(1): 226–233. doi: 10.1016/j.dss.2012.01.016.

36. Tavares et al., 2013. "Preprocessing Unbalanced Data Using Weighted Support Vector Machines for Prediction of Heart Disease in Children."

37. Zdzisław Pawlak. 1982. "Rough Sets." *International Journal of Computer & Information Sciences* 11(5): 341–56. doi: 10.1007/BF01001956.

38. R. Jensen and Q. Shen. 2007. "Tolerance-Based and Fuzzy-Rough Feature Selection." In *2007 IEEE International Fuzzy Systems Conference*, 1–6. doi: 10.1109/FUZZY.2007.4295481.

39. Xueen Wang, Deqiang Han, and Chongzhao Han. 2012. "Fuzzy-Rough Set Based Attribute Reduction with a Simple Fuzzification Method." In *2012 24th Chinese Control and Decision Conference (CCDC)*, 3793–3797. doi:10.1109/CCDC.2012.6244610.

40. J. Jojan and A. Srivihok. 2013. "Preprocessing of Imbalanced Breast Cancer Data Using Feature Selection Combined with Over-Sampling Technique for Classification." In *International Conference on Advanced Computer Science and Information Systems (ICAC-SIS)*, IEEE, 407–412.

41. Arshdeep Bahga and Vijay K. Madisetti. 2013. "A Cloud-Based Approach for Interoperable Electronic Health Records (EHRs)." *IEEE Journal of Biomedical and Health Informatics* 17(5): 894–906. doi: 10.1109/JBHI.2013.2257818.

42. J. Sun and Y. Fang. 2010. "Cross-Domain Data Sharing in Distributed Electronic Health Record Systems." *IEEE Transactions on Parallel and Distributed Systems* 21(6): 754–64. doi:10.1109/TPDS.2009.124.

43. O. Almutiry, G. Wills, and A. Alwabel. 2013. "Toward a Framework for Data Quality in Cloud-Based Health Information System." In *2013 International Conference on Information Society (i-Society)*, 153–157.

44. J. Tai, B. Sheng, Y. Yao, and N. Mi. 2014. "Live Data Migration for Reducing SLA Violations in Multi-Tiered Storage Systems." In *2014 IEEE International Conference on Cloud Engineering (IC2E)*, 361–366. doi: 10.1109/IC2E.2014.8.

45. P. Van Gorp and M. Comuzzi. 2014. "Lifelong Personal Health Data and Application Software via Virtual Machines in the Cloud." *IEEE Journal of Biomedical and Health Informatics* 18(1): 36–45. doi: 10.1109/JBHI.2013.2257821.

46. C. H. Wu, J. J. Hwang, and Z. Y. Zhuang. 2013. "A Trusted and Efficient Cloud Computing Service with Personal Health Record." In *2013 International Conference on Information Science and Applications (ICISA)*, 1–5. doi: 10.1109/ICISA.2013.6579425.

47. "NVIDIA on GPU Computing and the Difference Between GPUs and CPUs." GPU vs CPU? What Is GPU Computing? http://www.nvidia.com/object/what-is-gpu-computing.html.

48. "How to Calculate HPC Efficiency." Penguin Computing. November 1, 2012. www.penguincomputing.com/how-to-calculate-hpc-efficiency; Bojan Nikolic. "How to Easily Measure Floating Point Operations per Second (FLOPS)." www.bnikolic.co.uk/blog/hpc-howto-measure-flops.html.

49. Mark S. Friedrichs, Peter Eastman, Vishal Vaidyanathan, et al. 2009. "Accelerating Molecular Dynamic Simulation on Graphics Processing Units." *Journal of Computational Chemistry* 30(6): 864–872. doi: 10.1002/jcc.21209.

50. John E. Stone, David J. Hardy, Ivan S. Ufimtsev, and Klaus Schulten. 2010. "GPU-Accelerated Molecular Modeling Coming of Age." *Journal of Molecular Graphics & Modelling* 29(2): 116–25. doi: 10.1016/j.jmgm.2010.06.010.

51. Volodymyr V. Kindratenko, Jeremy J. Enos, Guochun Shi, et al. 2009. "GPU Clusters for High-Performance Computing." In *Proceedings—IEEE International Conference on Cluster Computing, ICCC*, 1–8. doi: 10.1109/CLUSTR.2009.5289128.

CASE STUDY

CASE STUDY 7: USING GPU TO STUDY PROTEIN EVOLUTION TO UNDERSTAND ANTIBIOTIC RESISTANCE

Avishek Kumar

Antibiotic resistance is an issue of paramount importance. Bacteria are becoming more resistant, and novel antibiotics are getting more expensive to develop, creating a dire public health issue. One solution to this problem is to understand the molecular mechanisms of antibiotic resistance by studying the evolution of enzymes that are responsible for antibiotic resistance in bacteria and leveraging this information in drug design. To this aim, we use GPU-accelerated molecular dynamics computer simulations to study the evolution of proteins known as beta-lactamases that can rapidly degrade penicillin. Interestingly, ancestral beta-lactamases that lived over 3 billion years ago were also drug resistant. A major difference between ancestral beta-lactamases and their modern counterparts is that the ancestral forms could degrade a variety of antibiotics rather than just penicillin. Through protein evolution, ancestral beta-lactamases have evolved from generalists to specialists in fighting penicillin. Thus, computer simulations of ancestral and modern beta-lactamases can provide insights into the evolution and mechanisms of antibiotic resistance. First, we describe how general-purpose graphics processing units (GPGPUs) now allow computational scientists to access a new arena of physical phenomena and time scales to study the antibiotic resistance problem. We then briefly outline our method of studying protein dynamics via molecular dynamics. Finally, we show how the evolution of protein function occurs through changes in protein dynamics.

Molecular dynamics (MD) is a computer simulation method that provides a bridge or computational microscope between the microscopic length and time scales and the macroscopic world of everyday life. MD models the individual atoms and their interatomic interactions of condensed phase materials (e.g., proteins or materials) and calculates properties that can be tested against experimental measurement. Without an understanding of how experimental measurements are connected to the atomic structure and dynamics obtained from methods like molecular dynamics, we have an understanding no better than alchemy. The far-reaching impact of molecular dynamics was recently recognized by the awarding of the 2013 Nobel Prize in Chemistry to Martin Karplus, Michael Leavitt, and Ariel Warshel "for the development of multi-scale models for complex for chemical systems" [1]. In an MD calculation, each atom is treated as a point mass and Newton's equations are used to advance the positions and velocities,

$$m_i \frac{\partial^2 r_i}{\partial t^2} = f_i \tag{1}$$

$$f_i = -\frac{\partial U(r_1, r_2, r_3, \ldots, r_{n-1}, r_n)}{\partial r_i} \tag{2}$$

Eq. 1 is simply Newton's second law,

where:

m_i = mass of atom i

r_i = position of atom i

f_i = force on atom i

$U(r_1,r_2,r_3,...,r_{n-1},r_n)$ is the potential energy that is a function of the positions of the other atoms in the system. The negative derivative of U is equal to the forces on atom i. The energy function commonly referred to as the force field is the most computationally expensive portion of the calculation and increases with increasing system size. The force field consists of a bonded portion to represent covalent bonds and nonbonded interactions to represent electrostatic and van der Waals forces. More detailed explanations of force fields and molecular dynamics can be found in the texts described in the listed notes [8, 9, 10, 11]. In MD simulations, we are typically concerned with dynamic motions occurring on the nano- to micro-time scales. To properly capture atomic motion we have to start at the fastest of atomic motions, atomic vibrations, on the femtosecond level. From the femtosecond level, we can integrate Newton's laws of motion in femtosecond time steps until we reach the nano- or micro- time scale to calculate an MD trajectory. MD is a serial algorithm, meaning that each step is dependent on the previous step. This means we have to compute ~500 million steps just to approach the microsecond. GPU(s) allow us to push the system sizes used and the time scales available due to their tremendous increase in performance. Although MD is a serial algorithm, the evaluation of each individual time step is highly parallelizable, a feature of the algorithm that has been exploited when mapping the MD algorithm to GPU hardware [4, 5, 6, 12, 13, 14]. One of the earliest successes of GPU-accelerated MD is the distributed computing project Folding@Home. Folding@Home is a distributed computing project that employs the spare cycles on participating personal computing devices to perform molecular dynamics in protein folding studies and drug design. The project currently utilizes CPUs, GPUs, Sony PlayStation 3 units, and some smartphones. In 2006, Folding@Home [15] pioneered the first GPU acceleration using DirectX to perform MD and the first distributed computing using GPUs. Subsequent versions of Folding@Home have moved onto using OpenCL [4] through the OpenMM [16] platform. Currently 87% of Folding@Home computations take place on GPUs. The Abalone, ACEMD [17], AMBER [13], CHARMM [18], DL_POLY [19], GROMACS [20], HOOMD-Blue [21], LAMMPS [22], and NAMD MD codes have now all been ported to GPUs. We are currently using the AMBER 14 [13] GPU-accelerated MD package to study the conformational dynamics of proteins.

Proteins are the workhorses of biology. They perform a vast array of functions in the cell, including, but not limited to, catalyzing chemical reactions, storing and transporting molecules in the cell, DNA replication, cell signaling, and providing structural support for a cell. This large array of functions is remarkable considering

(*Continued*)

(*Continued*)

all proteins are thought to have evolved from a common set of ancestral proteins. In light of increasing antibiotic resistance, the study of the molecular mechanisms driving protein evolution is important for public health.

The evolution of protein function can be understood through changes in a protein's conformational dynamics. Previously, protein function was understood through the sequence-structure-function paradigm. A protein's sequence is made up of a combination of 20 naturally occurring amino acids. Based on this sequence, proteins fold into a three-dimensional (3D) structure that determines the protein's function. The newer understanding of protein function is known as the sequence-structure-encoded dynamics-function paradigm. It has subsequently been found that the sequence of a protein can be mutated and it will still maintain its 3D structure; the structure is more conserved than the sequence. A protein evolves through mutations in its sequence. These mutations in the sequence lead to changes in the conformational dynamics of the protein, the accessible motion of the rotational degrees of freedom in the protein through changes in dihedral angles. Instead of considering a protein as a static 3D structure, it is more accurate to visualize a protein as an ensemble of accessible conformations. Changes in conformational dynamics lead to the acquisition of new functions; therefore, studying the changes in a protein's conformational dynamics can provide an understanding of protein evolution and the acquisition of new functions. It is now possible to obtain ancestral sequences and resurrect ancient gene sequences in the laboratory. The first crucial step is to generate accurate phylogenetic trees to show the evolutionary relationship among ancestral variants of a protein by methods such as parsimony [23], maximum likelihood [23, 24, 25, 26, 27], and Markov chain Monte Carlo–based Bayesian Inference [28]. Once we have obtained the phylogenetic tree, we can use GPU-accelerated MD to simulate the branches, ancestral variants of the protein, to obtain the conformational dynamics and analyze the relationship between protein evolution and changes in conformational dynamics.

The problem of antibiotic resistance can now be studied in weeks on a desktop machine. Our previous study of beta-lactamase [29], on which this analysis in this case study is based, took months to perform on a supercomputer. Beta-lactamases are enzymatic proteins produced by many bacteria in order to degrade beta-lactum antibiotics—the most commonly used today [30, 31, 32, 33]. TEM1 (PDB: 1BTL) is the modern-day beta-lactamase that specializes in degrading penicillin [34]. This is not a new phenomenon; antibiotic resistance has been found to be an ancient phenomenon [35, 36]. It has been shown that ancestral proteins dating back billions of years have the ability to degrade antibiotics. Modern enzymes—proteins that catalyze chemical reactions—are highly efficient specialists that efficiently degrade certain molecules. Their primordial ancestors were generalists that could degrade molecules of varying sizes and shapes and performed a variety of biological functions, known as promiscuous proteins [37, 38, 39, 40, 41]. Modern specialist proteins have evolved from their generalist ancestors into efficient specialists by acquiring new biological functions via changes in conformational dynamics [29, 42].

To understand the evolution and origin of TEM1 as a penicillin specialist, ancestors of TEM1 were resurrected and expressed, and their structures were determined PNCA (PDB: 4C6Y), GNCA (PDB: 4B88), and ENCA (PDB: 3ZDJ), respectively [29] . As shown in Figure CS5.1, each structure has a similar sequence (53%–79% sequence similarity), structure (root mean square deviation of 0.53–0.86 Angstrom) as compared to TEM1, and there are no large differences at each variant's active site, the part of the protein where enzymatic reactions occur [29]. Given that the sequence, structure, and active site are all similar, the only difference between the beta-lactamase variants is through their conformational dynamics. Changes in dynamics caused by mutations in the protein sequence lead to substrate specificity of the protein [42, 29]. Divergent evolution of the conformational dynamics best explains the evolution of the catalytic function of beta-lactamase.

We investigated how different functions arise from different conformational dynamics using GPU-accelerated MD and the dynamic flexibility index (DFI) metric. Figure CS5.1 shows ribbon diagrams for beta-lactamases.

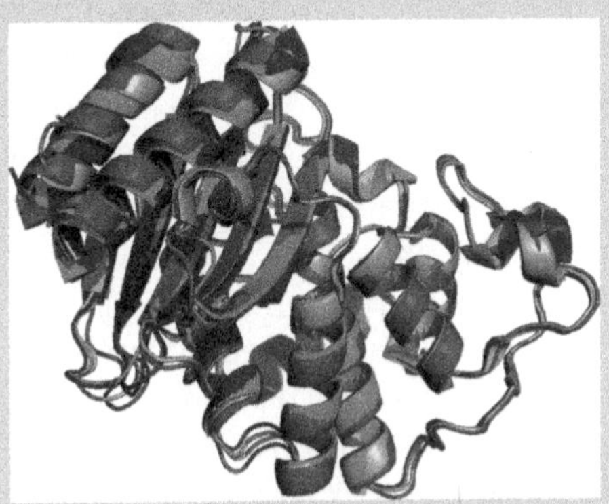

Figure CS5.1 Ribbon Diagrams of Beta-lactamases

Ancestors of the protein TEM1, a protein whose function is to degrade penicillin, were resurrected and expressed and their structures were determined—PNCA, GNCA, and ENCA. Despite having different functions, TEM1 (PDB: 1BTL, Red), ENCA (PDB: 3ZDJ, Orange), GNCA(PDB: 4B88, Green), and PNCA (PDB: 4C6Y, Blue) have similar sequences (53%–79% sequence similarity) and structures (0.53–0.84 Angstrom difference in RMSD) as compared to TEM1. Given the similarity in sequence and structure, their acquisition of divergent functions and evolution must occur through changes in the conformational dynamics—the accessible motion of internal rotational degrees of freedom.

Using GPU-accelerated molecular dynamics, we simulated the dynamics of each beta-lactamase. Our previous CPU runs [29] were run using the AMBER ff96SB force

(*Continued*)

(*Continued*)

field [43], implicit solvation [44], and a special technique known as replica exchange molecular dynamics [45], an algorithm to gain a more accurate distribution of a given protein's conformational dynamics by running multiple simulations at different temperatures. Typically, a single CPU run on a 40-core supercomputer will take months (~250ps (metric horse power)/day) when trying to simulate up to 10 nano seconds (ns) per replica giving 400 ns aggregate simulation time. This is not including hitting the wall time, the maximum time allowed to run a job on a supercomputer, resubmitting a batch job, and waiting for the job to launch in the queue, which adds a considerable amount of time. On a GPU-accelerated machine we progress at about 50 ns/day, several orders of magnitude higher. The molecular dynamics simulations were performed using the AMBER 14 package, ff14SB force field [46], TIP3P solvation model [47], with a 2 femtosecond time step. After running molecular-dynamics simulations for 200 ns (~4 days), we divided the trajectory into eight equal windows of 25 ns. For each window we calculated the covariance matrix of atomic positions and the first eigenvector, which corresponds to the lowest frequency, first normal mode, or slowest global motion of the protein. The covariance matrix calculated from an MD simulation provides information on the sequence-encoded dynamics, as MD simulations take into account long-range interactions, solvation effects, and the biochemical specificity of amino acids. We then calculated the Pearson correlation between an eigenvector of a window and the eigenvector of the previous window. The window with the highest correlation is considered to be the most equilibrated. This covariance matrix of this window was used to calculate the DFI profile of a given variant.

DFI measures the flexibility of a particular position by finding how robust the position is to a perturbation. In a crowded cell environment, a protein is exposed to many different forces exerted by surrounding macromolecules and ligands. These forces are mimicked, to a first approximation, by applying small random forces on the protein and calculating the displacement of each residue. To calculate DFI, an external random force is sequentially applied on each residue. The perturbation cascades through the residue interaction network and may introduce conformational changes in the protein. The DFI of a particular position is the total displacement of that position induced by perturbations on all other residue of the protein. A large DFI value indicates a flexible part of the protein. A small DFI value indicates a hinge part of the protein that transfers motion from one part of the protein to the other, similar to joints in a skeleton. If a protein is promiscuous, the residues around the active site should have high DFI values, indicating flexible regions. This flexibility allows the active site to deform in order to accommodate different molecules with different shapes and sizes. The DFI values of all residues form the DFI profile of the protein.

DFI has previously been able to capture conformational changes upon binding [48], identify allosteric pathways and critical residues that mediate long-range communication [49], produce an ensemble of conformations for docking studies

[50, 51, 52, 53, 54], distinguish between disease-associated and neutral mutations in protein-protein interfaces and the human proteome [55, 56], explain how disrupting hinge position in human ferritin lead to disease [57],and explain fluorescence in GFP [58].

Figure CS5.2 shows the DFI profiles of TEM1, ENCA, GNCA, and PNCA. The oldest in the lineage is PNCA, then GNCA, ENCA, and TEM1, the modern beta-lactamase. PNCA and GNCA are generalists and promiscuous proteins. TEM1 and ENCA are the most recent forms of beta-lactamase and specialize in degrading penicillin. The residue positions in the vicinity of the active site show the most pronounced change when comparing TEM1 to its ancestral forms. Upon visual inspection, there are three regions where PNCA or GNCA is more flexible than TEM1 or ENCA—region A, residues 60–80; region B, residues130–140; region C, residues 165–175; region D, residues 200–220. The increased flexibility of regions A, B, and C around the active site suggests that the increased flexibility is required to accommodate different molecules of different shapes and sizes. This also suggests that the mechanism for evolution from generalists to specialists is due to decreasing flexibility of the active site, which has previously shown in active site for cortisol. In region D, TEM1 and ENCA are more flexible than GNCA and PNCA. We conjecture that this could be due to a relationship between flexibility and rigidity of a protein. It's possible that the global flexibility of a protein is conserved; therefore, a decrease in flexibility in one part of the protein (rigidification) may correspond to an increase in the flexibility in a different part of the protein.

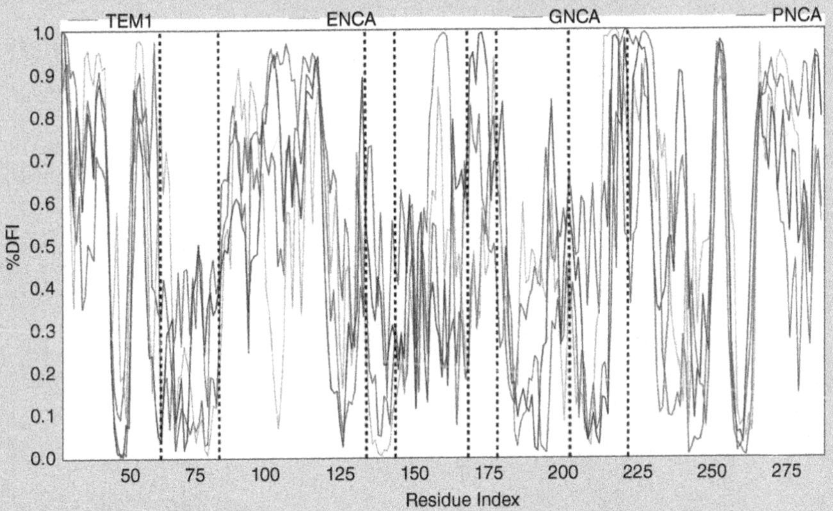

Figure CS5.2 DFI Profile of TEM1 and Ancestral Beta-lactamases, ENCA, GNCA, and PNCA

(*Continued*)

(*Continued*)

In order to further clarify the relationship between the conformational dynamics of the beta-lactamase variants, we performed a singular-value-decomposition-based clustering analysis of the DFI profiles of each variant. In Figure CS5.3 (top), we projected the DFI profiles of each variant onto the first two principal components. There is a clear separation between the pairs GNCA, PNCA and TEM1, ENCA. In Figure CS5.3 (bottom), we clustered the results using the average criterion and found that the variants cluster in the same sequence of evolution—PNCA, GNCA-ENCA, and TEM1. This provides strong evidence that the mechanism of evolution occurs through changes in conformational dynamics. The figure shows clustering analysis of DFI profiles.

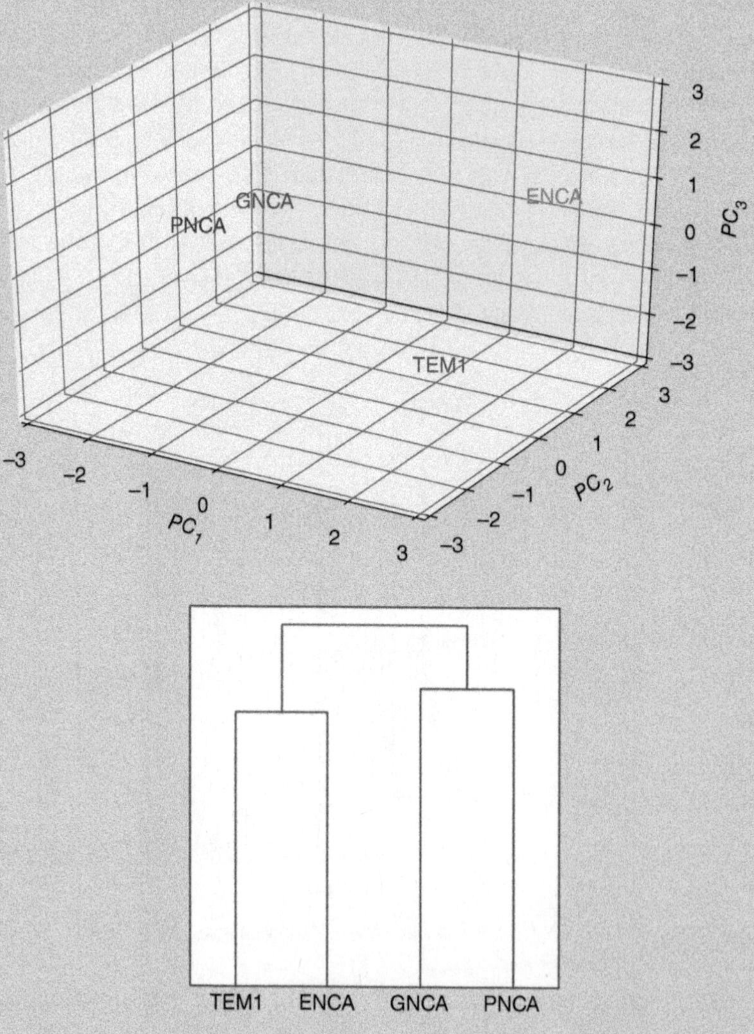

Figure CS5.3 Clustering Analysis of DFI Profiles A and B

Protein dynamics underlie the biological function of a protein. We explored the relationship between protein dynamics and protein evolution. We have found that changes in protein dynamics can explain the mechanism of protein evolution and, in this case, antibiotic resistance. With the emergence of GPU-accelerated MD, we are only beginning to scratch the surface of the problems that can be solved. Instead of only simulating four beta-lactamase variants from the phylogenetic tree, we could simulate the entire phylogenetic tree and gain a much deeper understanding of the relationship between protein evolution, protein function, and changes in conformational dynamics. It is also conceivable that proteins can be engineered through sequence mutations that lead to changes in conformational dynamics, thereby altering their function [59, 60]. These new sequences can then be rapidly simulated and tested in days using GPU-accelerated molecular dynamics rather than waiting for months on shared supercomputer resources. Additionally, understanding the molecular mechanisms of resistance can provide information at the molecular level on how to prevent resistance. The opportunities afforded by GPU(s) open up a new and exciting arena of study.

NOTES

1. Martin Karplus. "Development of Multiscale Models for Complex Chemical Systems from H H2 to Biomolecules." Nobel Lecture. https://www.nobelprize.org/nobel_prizes/chemistry/laureates/2013/karplus-lecture.html.
2. Sanders, J., and Kandrot, E. *CUDA by Example: An Introduction to General-Purpose GPU Programming.* (Addison-Wesley, 2011).
3. NVIDIA. *NVIDIA: CUDA C Programming Guide* (NIVIDA, 2007).
4. Stone, J. E., Gohara, D. and Shi, G. OpenCL: A parallel programming standard for heterogeneous computing systems. *Comput. Sci. Eng.* 12, 66–73 (2010).
5. Friedrichs, M. S., et al. Accelerating molecular dynamic simulation on graphics processing units. *J. Comput. Chem.* 30, 864–872 (2009).
6. Stone, J. E., Hardy, D. J., Ufimtsev, I. S. and Schulten, K. GPU-accelerated molecular modeling coming of age. *J. Mol. Graph. Model.* 29, 116–125 (2010).
7. Kindratenko, V. V., et al. GPU clusters for high-performance computing. In 1–8 (IEEE, 2009). doi:10.1109/CLUSTR.2009.5289128.
8. Frenkel, D., and Smit, B. *Understanding Molecular Simulation: From Algorithms to Applications* (Academic Press, 2002).
9. Leach, A. R. *Molecular Modelling: Principles and Applications* (Prentice Hall, 2001).
10. Tuckerman, M. E. *Statistical Mechanics: Theory and Molecular Simulation* (Oxford University Press, 2010).
11. Zuckerman, D. M. *Statistical Physics of Biomolecules: An Introduction* (CRC Press/Taylor & Francis, 2010).
12. Narumi, T., Sakamaki, R., Kameoka, S. and Yasuoka, K. Overheads in accelerating molecular dynamics simulations with GPUs. In 143–150 (IEEE, 2008). doi:10.1109/PDCAT.2008.68.
13. Salomon-Ferrer, R., Götz, A. W., Poole, D., Le Grand, S. and Walker, R. C. Routine microsecond molecular dynamics simulations with AMBER on GPUs. 2. Explicit solvent particle mesh Ewald. *J. Chem. Theory Comput.* 9, 3878–3888 (2013).
14. Götz, A. W., et al., Routine microsecond molecular dynamics simulations with AMBER on GPUs. 1. Generalized born. *J. Chem. Theory Comput.* 8, 1542–1555 (2012).

(*Continued*)

(*Continued*)

15. Marianayagam, N. J., Fawzi, N. L. and Head-Gordon, T. Protein folding by distributed computing and the denatured state ensemble. *Proc. Natl. Acad. Sci.* 102, 16684–16689 (2005).

16. Eastman, P. and Pande, V. OpenMM: A hardware-independent framework for molecular simulations. *Comput. Sci. Eng.* 12, 34–39 (2010).

17. Harvey, M. J., Giupponi, G. and Fabritiis, G. D. ACEMD: Accelerating biomolecular dynamics in the microsecond time scale. *J. Chem. Theory Comput.* 5, 1632–1639 (2009).

18. Brooks, B. R., et al. CHARMM: The biomolecular simulation program. *J. Comput. Chem.* 30, 1545–1614 (2009).

19. Smith, W., Yong, C. W., and Rodger, P. M. DL_POLY: Application to molecular simulation. *Mol. Simul.* 28, 385–471 (2002).

20. Van der Spoel, D., and Hess, B. GROMACS—The road ahead. Wiley Interdiscip. *Rev. Comput. Mol. Sci.* 1, 710–715 (2011).

21. Nguyen, T. D., Phillips, C. L., Anderson, J. A., and Glotzer, S. C. Rigid body constraints realized in massively-parallel molecular dynamics on graphics processing units. *Comput. Phys. Commun.* 182, 2307–2313 (2011).

22. Morozov, I. V., et al. Molecular dynamics simulations of the relaxation processes in the condensed matter on GPUs. *Comput. Phys. Commun.* 182, 1974–1978 (2011).

23. Kolaczkowski, B., and Thornton, J. W. Performance of maximum parsimony and likelihood phylogenetics when evolution is heterogeneous. *Nature* 431, 980–984 (2004).

24. Pollock, D. D., Taylor, W. R., and Goldman, N. Coevolving protein residues: Maximum likelihood identification and relationship to structure. *J. Mol. Biol.* 287, 187–198 (1999).

25. Tuffley, C., and Steel, M. Links between maximum likelihood and maximum parsimony under a simple model of site substitution. *Bull. Math. Biol.* 59, 581–607 (1997).

26. Yang, Z. PAML: A program package for phylogenetic analysis by maximum likelihood. *Comput. Appl. Biosci. CABIOS* 13, 555–556 (1997).

27. Gaut, B. S., and Lewis, P. O. Success of maximum likelihood phylogeny inference in the four-taxon case. *Mol. Biol. Evol.* 12, 152–162 (1995).

28. Huelsenbeck, J. P., and Ronquist, F. MRBAYES: Bayesian inference of phylogenetic trees. *Bioinformatics* 17, 754–755 (2001).

29. Zou, T., Risso, V. A., Gavira, J. A., Sanchez-Ruiz, J. M., and Ozkan, S. B. Evolution of conformational dynamics determines the conversion of a promiscuous generalist into a specialist enzyme. *Mol. Biol.* Evol. 32, 132–143 (2015).

30. Cantón, R., and Coque, T. M. The CTX-M beta-lactamase pandemic. *Curr. Opin. Microbiol.* 9, 466–475 (2006).

31. Levy, S. B., and Marshall, B. Antibacterial resistance worldwide: Causes, challenges and responses. *Nat. Med.* 10, S122–129 (2004).

32. Livermore, D. M. β-Lactamases in laboratory and clinical resistance. *Clin. Microbiol. Rev.* 8, 557–584 (1995).

33. Pitout, J.D.D., and Laupland, K. B. Extended-spectrum beta-lactamase-producing Enterobacteriaceae: An emerging public-health concern. *Lancet Infect.* Dis. 8, 159–166 (2008).

34. Risso, V. A., Gavira, J. A., Mejia-Carmona, D. F., Gaucher, E. A., and Sanchez-Ruiz, J. M. Hyperstability and substrate promiscuity in laboratory resurrections of Precambrian β-lactamases. *J. Am. Chem. Soc.* 135, 2899–2902 (2013).

35. Allen, H. K., Moe, L. A., Rodbumrer, J., Gaarder, A., and Handelsman, J. Functional metagenomics reveals diverse beta-lactamases in a remote Alaskan soil. *ISME* J. 3, 243–251 (2009).

36. Toth, M., Smith, C., Frase, H., Mobashery, S. and Vakulenko, S. An antibiotic-resistance enzyme from a deep-sea bacterium. *J. Am. Chem. Soc.* 132, 816–823 (2010).

37. Babtie, A., Tokuriki, N., and Hollfelder, F. What makes an enzyme promiscuous? *Curr. Opin. Chem. Biol.* 14, 200–207 (2010).

38. Copley, S. D. Enzymes with extra talents: Moonlighting functions and catalytic promiscuity. *Curr. Opin. Chem. Biol.* 7, 265–272 (2003).

39. Garcia-Seisdedos, H., Ibarra-Molero, B., and Sanchez-Ruiz, J. M. Probing the mutational interplay between primary and promiscuous protein functions: A computational-experimental approach. *PLoS Comput. Biol.* 8, e1002558 (2012).

40. Khersonsky, O., and Tawfik, D. S. Enzyme promiscuity: A mechanistic and evolutionary perspective. Annu. Rev. Biochem. 79, 471–505 (2010).

41. Khersonsky, O., Roodveldt, C., and Tawfik, D. S. Enzyme promiscuity: Evolutionary and mechanistic aspects. *Curr. Opin. Chem. Biol.* 10, 498–508 (2006).

42. Glembo, T. J., Farrell, D. W., Gerek, Z. N., Thorpe, M., and Ozkan, S. B. Collective dynamics differentiates functional divergence in protein evolution. *PLoS Comput. Biol.* 8, e1002428 (2012).

43. Pearlman, D. A., et al. AMBER, a package of computer programs for applying molecular mechanics, normal mode analysis, molecular dynamics and free energy calculations to simulate the structural and energetic properties of molecules. *Comput. Phys. Commun.* 91, 1–41 (1995).

44. Onufriev, A., Bashford, D., and Case, D. A. Modification of the generalized Born model suitable for macromolecules. *J. Phys. Chem. B* 104, 3712–3720 (2000).

45. Sugita, Y., and Okamoto, Y. Replica-exchange molecular dynamics method for protein folding. *Chem. Phys. Lett.* 314, 141–151 (1999).

46. Maier, J. A., et al. ff14SB: Improving the accuracy of protein side chain and backbone parameters from ff99SB. *J. Chem. Theory Comput.* 11, 3696–3713 (2015).

47. Sun, Y., and Kollman, P. A. Hydrophobic solvation of methane and nonbond parameters of the TIP3P water model. *J. Comput. Chem.* 16, 1164–1169 (1995).

48. Gerek, Z. N., and Ozkan, S. B. Change in allosteric network affects binding affinities of PDZ domains: Analysis through perturbation response scanning. *PLoS Comput. Biol.* 7, e1002154 (2011).

49. Gerek, Z. N., Keskin, O., and Ozkan, S. B. Identification of specificity and promiscuity of PDZ domain interactions through their dynamic behavior. *Proteins* 77, 796–811 (2009).

50. Bolia, A., Gerek, Z. N., Keskin, O., Banu Ozkan, S., and Dev, K. K. The binding affinities of proteins interacting with the PDZ domain of PICK1. *Proteins Struct. Funct. Bioinforma.* 80, 1393–1408 (2012).

51. Bolia, A., Gerek, Z. N., and Ozkan, S. B. BP-Dock: A flexible docking scheme for exploring protein–ligand interactions based on unbound structures. *J. Chem. Inf. Model.* 54, 913–925 (2014).

52. Bolia, A., et al. A flexible docking scheme efficiently captures the energetics of glycan-cyanovirin binding. *Biophys.* J. 106, 1142–1151 (2014).

53. Bolia, A., et al. The binding affinities of proteins interacting with the PDZ domain of PICK1.

54. Bolia, A., et al. A flexible docking scheme efficiently captures the energetics of glycan-cyanovirin binding.

55. Nevin Gerek, Z., Kumar, S., and Banu Ozkan, S. Structural dynamics flexibility informs function and evolution at a proteome scale. *Evol. Appl.* 6, 423–433 (2013).

56. Butler, B. M., Gerek, Z. N., Kumar, S., and Ozkan, S. B. Conformational dynamics of nonsynonymous variants at protein interfaces reveals disease association: The role of dynamics in neutral and damaging nsSNVs. *Proteins Struct. Funct. Bioinforma.* 83, 428–435 (2015).

57. Kumar, A., Glembo, T. J., and Ozkan, S. B. The role of conformational dynamics and allostery in the disease development of human ferritin. *Biophys. J.* (2015). doi:10.1016/j.bpj.2015.06.060.

58. Kim, H., et al. A hinge migration mechanism unlocks the evolution of green-to-red photoconversion in GFP-like proteins. *Structure* 23, 34–43 (2015).

59. Kazlauskas, R. J. Enhancing catalytic promiscuity for biocatalysis. *Curr. Opin. Chem. Biol.* 9, 195–201 (2005).

60. Nobeli, I., Favia, A. D., and Thornton, J. M. Protein promiscuity and its implications for biotechnology. *Nat. Biotechnol.* 27, 157–167 (2009).

CASE STUDY

CASE STUDY 8: COMPUTATIONAL MODELING OF ENDOVASCULAR PROCEDURES: A NEW APPROACH SAVING LIVES AND REDUCING COSTS

M. Haithem Babiker and Robert S. Green

INTRODUCTION

Vascular disease is common in 14% of the population and is a leading cause of death in the United States. Until recently, treatment required surgery excavating to the problem site. For example, in order to treat a cerebral aneurysm (CA), a dangerous bulge developing in a blood vessel in the brain, surgeons would excavate through the skull. Now surgeons can treat the aneurysm endovascularly (i.e., from inside the affected vessel) using a catheter and one or more stents and/or related devices. However, the precision with which this remarkable minimally invasive therapy is used has lagged. For example, there are a multitude of device types, sizes, and insertion techniques available but no method to select the optimum treatment scenario. Until now the technique and equipment used were primarily determined by an individual practitioner's prior training and experience as well as generalized conventions and even trial and error. This shortcoming is costly and adversely affects quality of care.

To improve treatment planning capabilities, EndoVantage, LLC, has developed the EndoVantage Interventional Suite (EVIS). EVIS is a novel computer simulation platform that enables pretreatment planning of endovascular procedures. This technology sits in the cloud and utilizes real patient data, state-of-the-art finite element analysis, and computational fluid dynamics to simulate treatment for each unique patient case. Simulation results are then used to evaluate the outcomes of different treatment options. This treatment planning capability can drastically reduce procedure time, treatment costs, and the high retreatment rates associated with endovascular treatments.

EVIS

The EVIS platform involves a three-step process for simulating treatment, as shown in Figure CS5.4. In the first step, the patient's image data (magnetic resonance or computed tomography) are segmented and reconstructed to form an accurate 3D computational model of the patient's anatomy. In the second step, the patient's computational model is used to simulate treatment using device-specific modeling approaches. One or more appropriate medical devices to be considered for treatment are selected from a library of rigorously validated finite element device models. These devices are then virtually deployed into the patient's anatomy using the clinical deployment procedure specific to that device, as shown in

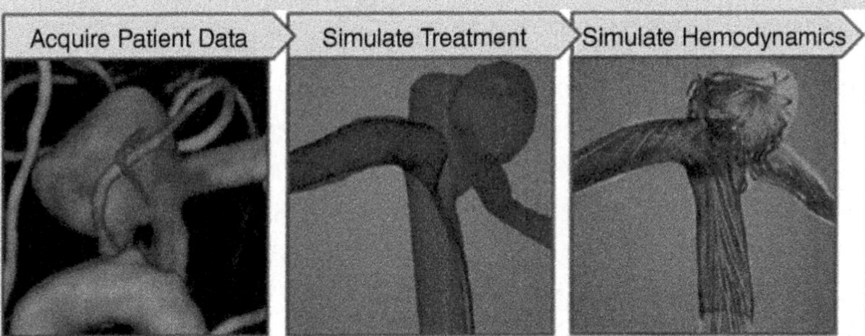

Figure CS5.4 EVIS Steps

Figure CS5.5. Virtual deployment first considers navigation of the device to the treatment site using a simulated clinical guide-wire. Device unsheathing from the delivery catheter is then simulated using an algorithm that optimizes the delivery of the device into the vessel. Finally, in the third step, computational fluid dynamics simulations are performed to predict changes in blood flow brought about by the device. EVIS's deployment and blood flow simulations provide practitioners with a better understanding of how well the outcome of each treatment scenario will meet specific posttreatment goals. Figure CS5.4 depicts the general EVIS workflow. Figure CS5.5 shows finite element deployment of a neurovascular stent in a cerebral aneurysm.

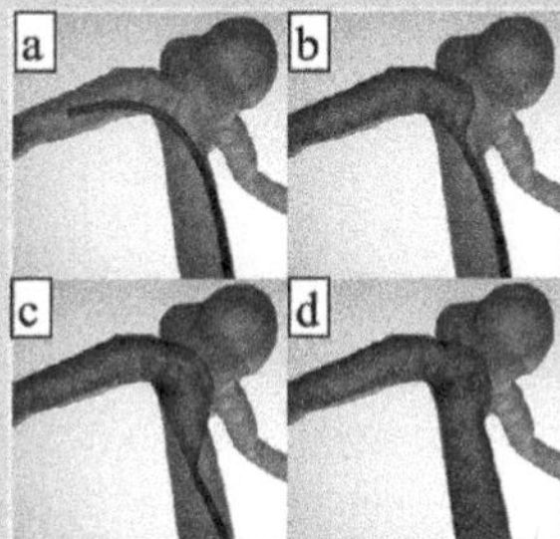

Figure CS5.5 Finite Element Deployment of a Neurovascular Stent in a Cerebral Aneurysm

SCIENTIFIC COMPUTING

In order to simulate device deployment, the equation of motion (Eq. 1) is solved in EVIS using an explicit central difference integration scheme. Millions of iterations are required for solving the entire deployment procedure, which can

(*Continued*)

(*Continued*)

lead to very lengthy simulation times. To ensure simulation times are compatible with clinical workflows, the simulation domain is decomposed into many domains on a high-performance cluster, and the equations of motions are solved at each domain using a parallel finite element solver and message passing interface. Simulation times are further reduced by dynamically decomposing the solution domain and adjusting the size of each domain at specific time points during the simulation. This dynamic approach to domain decomposition greatly reduces simulation times.

$$[M]\ddot{u}+[C]\dot{u}+[K]u=F_{ext} \tag{1}$$

To simulate changes in blood flow after treatment, the blood volume is discretized into millions of control volumes or mesh elements. The patient's vascular geometry and established flow conditions are used to assign boundary conditions to the simulation. A simplified form of the Navier Stokes governing equations (Eqs. 2–3) is then solved at each mesh element using a finite volume solver. To reduce computation time, the mesh is further decomposed into fixed domains, and a message passing interface is used to parallelize the Navier Stokes solver on a high-performance cluster.

$$\nabla u=0 \tag{2}$$

$$\rho\left(\frac{\partial v}{\partial t}+v\cdot\nabla v\right)=-\nabla P+\mu\nabla^2 v \tag{3}$$

Highly parallelized finite element and finite volume solvers and advances in high-performance computing hardware have allowed EVIS's simulation times to fit within clinical workflows (typically 0.5 to 3 days). In the near future, further advances in scientific computing may allow for the prediction of patient treatment scenarios in a matter of minutes and the application of EVIS for emergency cases.

VALIDATION

EVIS has been validated through a rigorous multistep verification and validation process. First, device geometry is validated against micro–computed topography and high-magnification images. Second, the mechanical behavior of the finite element device models is validated against radial and axial bench-top experimental measurements, as shown in Figure CS5.6. Third, device apposition, diameter, and length after deployment are validated against bench-top and clinical device deployments. Examples of bench-top and clinical deployment validations for a neurovascular flow diverter are presented in Figure CS5.7 and Figure CS5.8. A

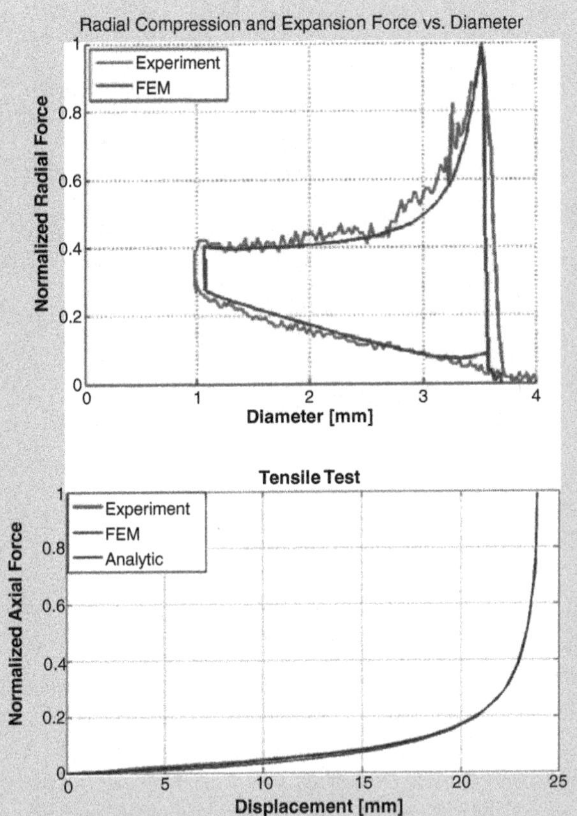

Figure CS5.6 Validation of Flow Diverter Radial and Axial Force

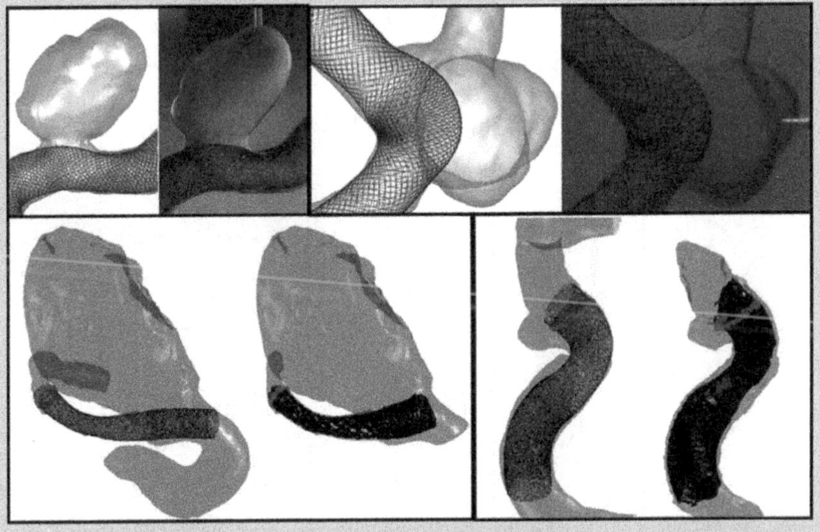

Figure CS5.7 Validation of Flow Diverter Deployment Simulations against Bench-Top (top row) and Clinical (bottom row) Deployments

(*Continued*)

(*Continued*)

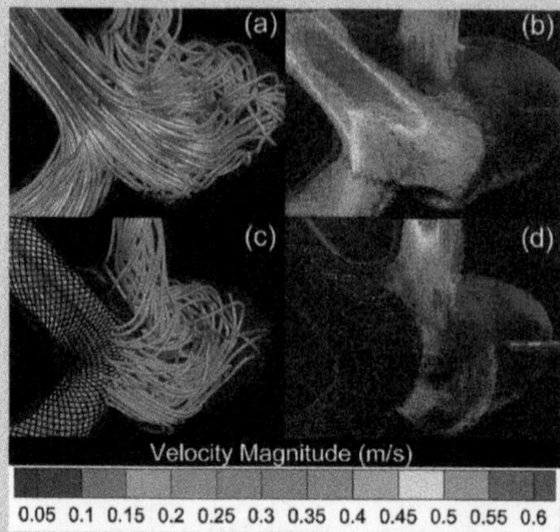

Figure CS5.8 Comparison between CFD and PIV Results for an Anatomical Basilar Tip Aneurysm

recent study that compared EVIS simulated flow diverter deployments and clinical deployments showed that simulations correctly predicted postdeployment device length and regions where the device bulges, becomes stenosed, and poorly apposes to the vessel wall. Minimal difference in postdeployment device length was observed between simulated and clinically deployed devices in 10 patient cases. Simulated and physical device diameters were also compared at multiple cross-sections along each vessel's center line. Results also showed a minimal difference in device diameter along the vessel center line. CFD results were also validated against particle-image velocimetry (PIV) data, as shown in Figure CS5.9.

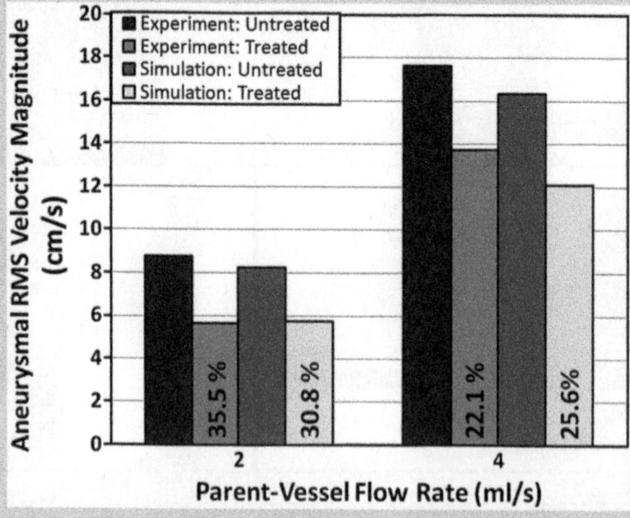

Figure CS5.9 Aneurysmal RMS Particle Velocity Magnitude

MEDICAL DEVICE DEVELOPMENT

In addition to patient-specific pretreatment planning, EVIS offers an innovative approach to medical device development. Using the same modeling and simulation techniques, medical devices are subjected to robust testing not currently possible, including simulating devices virtually in hundreds of patients. EndoVantage currently houses over 100 different patient anatomies, each one quantified in terms of many different shape-based metrics. With EVIS design defects and potentially dangerous scenarios can be detected early, saving development time and preventing potential deaths and product recalls. In addition, EVIS is used to generate data for Food and Drug Administration submissions and for use in sales, marketing, and training. In time EVIS will be used to conduct virtual clinical trials of medical devices, dramatically reducing time to market while avoiding potential patient harm.

CONCLUSION

Although computational simulation techniques have been used by aerospace, auto, and other industries for some time, their application in the medical field is recent. EVIS combines sheer computational power, cutting-edge simulation software, and novel medical techniques to dramatically change the practice of medicine and development of medical devices.

CHAPTER 6

Cloud Computing and Emerging Architectures*

* Some of this chapter is taken from Jay Etchings, @hpcwire. "New Models for Research, Part IV — Delivering Research as a Service." HPCwire New Models for Research Part IV Delivering Research as a Service Comments. 2015. https://www.hpcwire.com/2015/04/27/new-models-for-research-part-iii-delivering-research-as-a-service. Used with permission.

The proliferation of the broadband commodity Internet, the growing presence of Internet2 in higher education, and widespread adoption of virtualization technologies have enabled cloud computing to jump from a niche technology to a mainstream and widespread one. Cloud computing represents a major paradigm shift in the industry, rapidly displacing brick-and-mortar data centers. Enabling ubiquitous, on-demand global access to a shared pool of configurable computing resources while lowering operational as well as capital expenditures, cloud computing is projected to reach $106 billion in 2016, and the global cloud computing service market will reach $127 billion by 2017 [1]. Cloud computing is clearly here to stay. Our focus here is on research data management, which is distinctly different from enterprise data management. So you can expect some contrast in the way the challenges are defined, unpacked, and addressed. Research data management poses its own set of unique challenges, even though the advent of big data is being felt by both enterprises and research institutions.

While computing power and commodity hardware continue to decline in cost, the costs and obstacles to owning and operating a large data center continue to grow. Combined with the emerging costs of becoming compliant, these factors are pushing many organizations to outsource data center physical infrastructure and operations entirely. During my consulting work I often asked stakeholders about their research and objectives and noted what parts of their answer focused on data center management. Typically, this is an afterthought for many research teams as they are focused on the science, not the underlying components. If that is the case, then cloud computing might be an especially good fit.

Like many terms in technology, "cloud computing" could mean a variety of things to different stakeholders. Much of this confusion is due to vendors' rush to define the buzzword du jour to be synonymous with their products. I am quite sure there are still plenty of people who think that Cloudera has something to do with cloud computing. When the Hadoop distribution Cloudera was formed in 2008, it was decided that the term "cloud" was hot and thus Cloudera was born. In 2014 Cloudera announced Cloudera Director, which enabled users to deploy and manage Hadoop in cloud environments. This is just one of the many examples of vendor-driven obfuscation or buzzword du jour jacking. Thankfully the National Institute of Standards and Technology (NIST), which is part of the U.S. government, has defined the term "cloud computing" in its guide 800-145 [2] [3].

Those readers familiar with the NIST frameworks for cloud computing can bypass the "Cloud Basics" section and move on to "Challenges Facing Cloud Computing" and "Hybrid Campus Clouds." After this we examine Research as a Service (RaaS), a key component of some versions of cloud computing, and also consider federated access. From there we examine Zeta Architecture, an emergent architecture that is used by Google that offers better hardware utilization, fewer moving parts, and greater responsiveness and flexibility. Zeta and other emerging architectures are catalyzed by limitations on one-size-fit-all enterprise architectures. Following this chapter is a case study on using on-demand computing for biomedical research on ventricular tachycardia.

CLOUD BASICS

The NIST definition of cloud computing is an excellent starting point.

> *Cloud computing* is a model for enabling ubiquitous, convenient, on-demand network access to a shared pool of configurable computing resources (e.g., networks, servers, storage, applications, and services) that can be rapidly provisioned and released with minimal management effort or service provider interaction. This cloud model is composed of five essential characteristics, three service models, and four deployment models [3].

Essential Characteristics*

On-demand self-service A consumer can unilaterally provision computing capabilities, such as server time and network storage, as needed automatically without requiring human interaction with each service provider.

Broad network access Capabilities are available over the network and accessed through standard mechanisms that promote use by heterogeneous thin or thick client platforms (e.g., mobile phones, tablets, laptops, and workstations).

Resource pooling The provider's computing resources are pooled to serve multiple consumers using a multitenant model, with different physical and virtual resources dynamically assigned and reassigned according to consumer demand. There is a sense of location independence in that the customer generally has no control or knowledge over the exact location of the provided resources but may be able to specify location at a higher level of abstraction (e.g., country, state, or data center). Examples of resources include storage, processing, memory, and network bandwidth.

Rapid elasticity Capabilities can be elastically provisioned and released, in some cases automatically, to scale rapidly outward and inward

---

* This section, "Service Models," and "Deployment Models" are taken from Peter Mell and Tim Grance, "The NIST Definition of Cloud Computing," October 7, 2009, https://www.nist.gov/sites/default/files/documents/itl/cloud/cloud-def-v15.pdf.

commensurate with demand. To the consumer, the capabilities available for provisioning often appear to be unlimited and can be appropriated in any quantity at any time.

Measured service Cloud systems automatically control and optimize resource use by leveraging a metering capability at some level of abstraction appropriate to the type of service (e.g., storage, processing, bandwidth, and active user accounts). Resource usage can be monitored, controlled, and reported, providing transparency for both the provider and consumer of the utilized service.

Service Models

Software as a Service (SaaS) The capability provided to the consumer is to use the provider's applications running on a cloud infrastructure. The applications are accessible from various client devices through either a thin client interface, such as a web browser (e.g., web-based e-mail), or a program interface. The consumer does not manage or control the underlying cloud infrastructure, including network, servers, operating systems, storage, or even individual application capabilities, with the possible exception of limited user-specific application configuration settings.

Platform as a Service (PaaS) The capability provided to the consumer is to deploy onto the cloud infrastructure consumer-created or -acquired applications created using programming languages, libraries, services, and tools supported by the provider. The consumer does not manage or control the underlying cloud infrastructure, including network, servers, operating systems, or storage but has control over the deployed applications and possibly configuration settings for the application hosting environment.

Infrastructure as a Service (IaaS) The capability provided to the consumer is to provision processing, storage, networks, and other fundamental computing resources where the consumer is able to deploy and run arbitrary software, which can include operating systems and applications. The consumer does not manage or control the underlying cloud infrastructure but has control over operating systems, storage, and deployed applications and possibly limited control of select networking components (e.g., host firewalls).

Deployment Models

Private cloud The cloud infrastructure is provisioned for exclusive use by a single organization comprising multiple consumers (e.g., business units). It may be owned, managed, and operated by the organization, a third party, or some combination, and it may exist on or off premises.

Community cloud The cloud infrastructure is provisioned for exclusive use by a specific community of consumers from organizations that have shared concerns (e.g., mission, security requirements, policy, and compliance considerations). It may be owned, managed, and operated by one or more of the organizations in the community, a third party, or some combination of these, and it may exist on or off premises.

Public cloud The cloud infrastructure is provisioned for open use by the general public. It may be owned, managed, and operated by a business, academic, or government organization, or some combination of these. It exists on the premises of the cloud provider.

Hybrid cloud The cloud infrastructure is a composition of two or more distinct cloud infrastructures (private, community, or public) that remain unique entities but are bound together by standardized or proprietary technology that enables data and application portability (e.g., cloud bursting for load balancing between clouds).

CHALLENGES FACING CLOUD COMPUTING APPLICATIONS IN BIOMEDICINE

Biomedicine faces several challenges in shifting to cloud computing, including those listed next.

- Large-scale biological and biomedical databases are typically large "mobile" data sets.
- Data integration and ontologies in biology and medicine are requirements.
- Integration and analysis of molecular and clinical data require security considerations.
- Visualization and exploration of omics and clinical data require big data components.
- Visualization (parallelized) and analysis of biomedical images require heavy lifting.
- Computing environments for at-scale collaboration with grid computing are foreign to biomedicine.
- Workflows in bioinformatics and biomedicine (pipelines) lack maturity and uniformity.
- Emerging architectures and programming models for bioinformatics and biomedicine and new and dynamic.
- Privacy issues for cloud-based biomedical applications will continue to evolve.
- Web services (portals) for bioinformatics and biomedicine must be commonplace.

Development has been progressing in the realm of cloud-based bioinformatics tools. Figure 6.1 shows many cloud-specific applications.

Program	Description	URL
	Sequence Alignment	
Cloud-Coffee	Multiple sequence alignment	http://www.tcoffee.org/
USM	MapReduce solution to sequence comparison	http://usm.github.io/
	Sequence Mapping and Assembly	
CloudBurst	Reference-based read mapping	http://cloudburst-bio.sourceforge.net/
CloudAligner	Short read mapping	http://cloudaligner.sourceforge.net/
SEAL	Short read mapping and duplicate removal	http://biodoop-seal.sourceforge.net/
Crossbow	Combine sequence aligner Bowtie and the SNP caller SOAPsnp	http://bowtie-bio.sourceforge.net/crossbow/
Contrail	*De novo* assembly	http://contrail-bio.sourceforge.net/
Eoulsan	Sequencing data analysis	http://transcriptome.ens.fr/eoulsan/
Quake	Quality-aware detection and correction of sequencing errors	http://www.cbcb.umd.edu/software/quake/
	Gene Expression	
Myrna	Differential expression analysis for RNA-seq	http://bowtie-bio.sourceforge.net/myrna/
FX	RNA-seq analysis tool	http://fx.gmi.ac.kr/
ArrayExpressHTS	RNA-seq process and quality assessment	http://www.ebi.ac.uk/services
	Comprehensive Application	
BioVLab	A virtual collaborative lab for biomedical applications	https://sites.google.com/site/biovlab/
Hadoop-BAM	Directly manipulate NGS data	http://sourceforge.net/projects/hadoop-bam/
SeqWare	A scalable NoSQL database for NGS data	http://seqware.sourceforge.net
PeakRanger	Peak caller for ChIP-seq data	http://ranger.sourceforge.net/
YunBe	Gene set analysis for biomarker identification	http://tinyurl.com/yunbedownload/
GATK	Genome analysis toolkit	http://www.broadinstitute.org/gatk/
Cloud BioLinux	A virtual machine with over 135 bioinformatics packages	http://cloudbiolinux.org/
CloVR	A virtual machine for automated sequence analysis	http://clovr.org/

Figure 6.1 Enabling Large-Scale Biomedical Analysis in the Cloud
Cloud-based informatics tools. http://www.hindawi.com/journals/bmri/2013/185679/tab1/.

HYBRID CAMPUS CLOUDS

Many academic and research institutions are adopting hybrid clouds for their campuses. Hybrid clouds enable resource aggregation, rapid elastic scale, and tremendous flexibility. Cloud-oriented architectures (COAs) substantially increase the life span of a data center asset, but, more important, let researchers focus on research and discovery of public value rather than wrestling with the problems of legacy platforms. The COA should not be confused with service-oriented architecture (SOA) concepts and cloud provider services as those typically only cover distributed computing items such as middleware. The university hybrid cloud model, COA, represents an amalgamation of clouds, living both in the private and public space. On-premise clouds are used for preprocessing of massive amounts of raw source data, and off-premise public clouds, both private and public, are where metadata and collaborative data lives.

Few standards exist yet for cloud interoperability. We envision a type of cloud service aimed at giving researchers and developers everything they need to develop applications, access RaaS, whose subcomponents are IaaS, PaaS, and bare-metal (nonvirtualized) IaaS, removing the administrative overhead of dealing with lower-technology stack layers and reducing development overhead. Collections of software tools and libraries are installed, preconfigured, integrated, and bundled into self-service options. Within the cloud management platform there is great flexibility in tool sets for the creation of a cloud service allowing true XaaS ("XaaS" is the hip collective term representing a number of things, including X as a Service, anything as a service, or everything as a service). The COA model, synonymous with the hybrid cloud in this writer's mind, unites PaaS—sharing of infrastructure between many researchers through secure multitenant delivery, including virtual private cloud (VPC). This offers a lightweight alternative to a private cloud for remote collaboration where hybrid cloud resources exist within the secure network.

This model adopted by the university and greater research computing initiative opens the door to on-demand resources, consumption metering, and self-service to the performance computing world with functional automation of the whole technology stack.

Figure 6.2 shows the logical architecture of the COA stack and RaaS components.

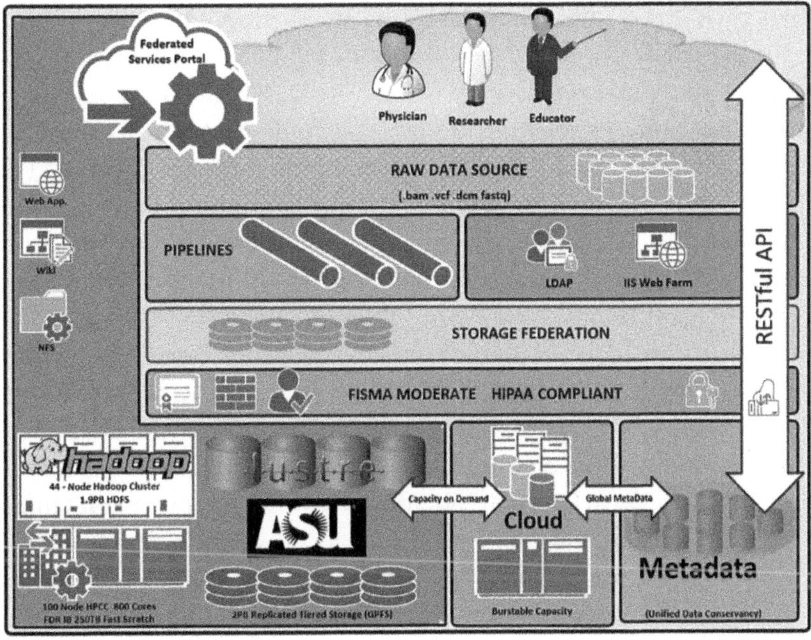

Figure 6.2 Research as a Service Schema
Jay Etchings, Director, Research Computing Operations, Arizona State University

RESEARCH AS A SERVICE

As far back as the inception of the cloud with applications like Salesforce in 1999 and Amazon Web Services in 2002, health informatics applications and data in the cloud have existed. Early attempts at health informatics in the cloud or as a service were challenged by security and privacy issues that truly prevented their adoption. As a former Medicaid-Medicare recovery audit contractor, I can attest that the audits were nothing short of brutal and founded on technologies a decade old. At the time just the thought of a virtual local area network (VLAN) or a storage area network (SAN) where the same physical devices were shared broke policy. Many technical healthcare professionals have long recognized cloud computing benefits in terms of elasticity, flexibility, and potential cost reduction in both capital and operational outlay. Considerations such as data security, patient privacy, network performance, and economics have led to a hybrid cloud model adopted even unknowingly by many large-scale operations. Research and healthcare applications will naturally migrate to this cloud model as it matures and becomes more widely available. A shift to the cloud will also be driven by the increase in data-intensive analytics that is, in part, a function of the burgeoning Internet of Things.

An important component of the hybrid campus cloud is RaaS. RaaS leverages the XaaS model, Internet2 Innovation Platform, workload deterministic provisioning, and open big data. A significant challenge throughout the history of research compute has been what is known as the Tragedy of Reproducibility in Science, or more aptly named the Tragedy of Irreproducibility in Science. With the advent of the Internet, research scientists have benefited from new avenues for potential peer reviews. One of the stumbling blocks RaaS aims to overcome has more to do with the physical components in the experiment rather than the science. In the years I have been involved in biomedical informatics, I have personally dedicated many hours to replicating an experimental environment so that a specific test could be validated. With technology's life cycle ranging from months to a couple of years, the rapid changes generate additional unplanned obstacles.

RaaS at its core is a collection of containerized components that perform a research task. Then as a validated, saved, archived project, the software layer can be shared for peer review or more pragmatically utilized within a pipeline to meet a larger holistically defined goal. With discrepancies around the operating system, kernel version, libraries, network, and other configurations removed, the debates can focus on the science, which is where our bright minds are best exercised.

Hadoop is a fundamental component in the offering in both physical and virtual instantiations graphical management layers available to researchers. Hadoop delivered in this manner allows for elasticity of the compute component of the Hadoop cluster (since it is decoupled from the storage) and we support multitenant access to the underlying Hadoop Distributed File System (HDFS), which is owned and managed by the greater data nodes.

The service also includes access to graphics processing units (GPUs) for computation called GPGPU (general-purpose GPU) and enterprise-class and virtualized workloads. The overall demand may dictate the need for popular high-end GPU cards. For researchers interested in Xeon Phi, there is a single test bed in near line production. Intel Xeon Phi is currently known *not* to work with ESX in pass-through (VM Direct Path input/output [I/O]) mode. Work is ongoing in this area and preliminary results look very good. Virtualization being extended to support GPU compute capacity promises to open yet again new computational opportunities for researchers wishing to move to the cloud and realize its benefits.

FEDERATED ACCESS WEB PORTALS

Federated application services coupled with single sign-on capabilities are a much-sought-after component to any business in the cloud services application space. A once "nice to have" has become a requirement for access controls, compliance, and ease of use. Internet2 supplies Shibboleth access packages for single sign-on, preserving both privacy (identity management) and security (asset management). Shibboleth is a standards-based, open source software package for web single sign-on across or within organizational boundaries. It allows sites to make informed authorization decisions for individual access of protected online resources in a privacy-preserving manner. The logical workflow is depicted in Figure 6.3.

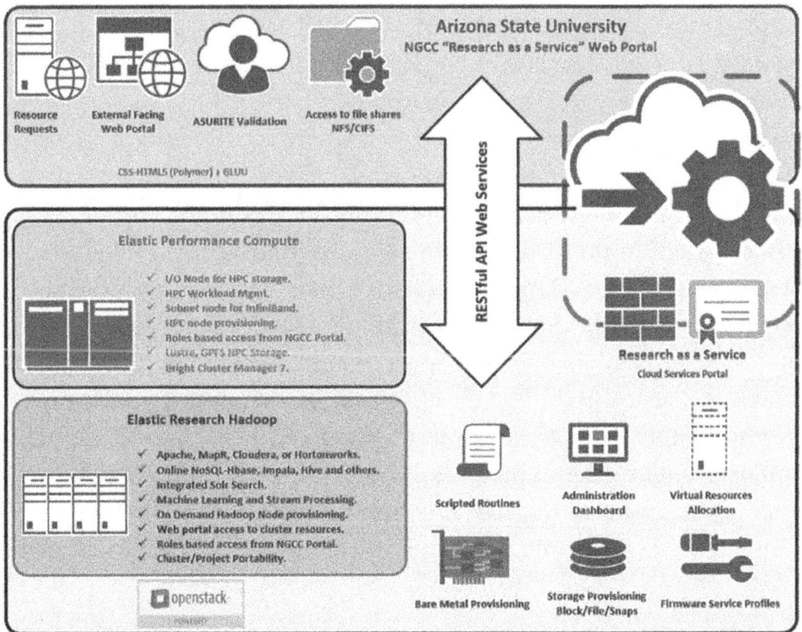

Figure 6.3 Federated Access Web Portal Workflow

The web portal supplies cloud-based access to the complete portfolio of tools and recipes for researchers to quickly access, build, deploy, and reset if desired. As web service relies on some of the same underlying Hypertext Transfer Protocol (HTTP) and web-based architecture as common web applications, it is susceptible to similar threats and vulnerabilities. Web services security is based on several important concepts, including those listed next.*

Authorization The permission to use a computer resource, granted, directly or indirectly, by an application or system owner.

Identification and authentication Verifying the identity of a user, process, or device, often as a prerequisite to allowing access to resources in an information system.

Integrity The property that data has not been altered in an unauthorized manner while in storage, during processing, or in transit.

Nonrepudiation Assurance that the sender of information is provided with proof of delivery and the recipient is provided with proof of the sender's identity, so neither can later deny having processed the information.

CLUSTER HOMOGENEITY

The standard high-performance compute cluster is a group of computers that work together sharing interprocess communication (IPC) to act as a team to solve a problem. It consists of no fewer than two computers, a master and a slave in some cases, or two workers with a master scheduler. The purposes of a cluster could vary from large-scale computational (high-performance cluster [HPC]), data storage (storage cluster with ephemeral storage), to next-generation grid computing solutions like Hadoop or Apache Spark, which share memory on each individual node to create a single pool where transactions run in memory. Apache Spark is a fast general engine for large-scale data processing and has made a splash in bioinformatics boasting up to 100 times faster speeds than Hadoop MapReduce or 10 times faster on disk transactions. Even many HPC traditionalists have moved their workloads to Spark with great results.

Large-scale clusters inherently have a new level of complexity. However, one best practice is to ensure some level of homogeneity within the hardware stack. Having like-for-like adapters on an InfiniBand fabric or maintaining consistent Ethernet adapters throughout a cluster can help to avoid communication problems and ease provisioning through the usage of templates.

Once again, ensuring some level of homogeneity within the hardware stack is a best practice and is application and operating system specific. Certainly we

* The definitions are taken from NIST IR 7298, Glossary of Key Information Security Terms, and NIST SP 800–100.

may architect clusters with homogeneous or heterogeneous architectures, as Hadoop is well known to be tolerant of differential architectural components, as is the distributed object storage system Swift. HPCs with homogeneous architecture and identical configurations, including memory, central processing unit (CPU), and disk size and type and so forth, will perform better and make the debugging of workload distribution issues smoother.

Programmers creating message passing interface programs write their applications with a distributed workload in such a way that all nodes will complete steps in approximately the same time and return a consistent result. A homogeneous cluster design addresses that objective and provides a "rule-out" step in debugging issues. Additionally, there is a robust scalability component, as seen in the Open Compute Project, which leverages the same robustness. As nodes fail (plan for this, as they always will), with a homogeneous cluster you can have a cold spare ready to plug in with minimal downtime or impact to production.

EMERGING ARCHITECTURES (ZETA ARCHITECTURE)

As systems grow and as use cases become more differentiated, new emerging architectures are being developed and refined. These architectures diverge from one-size-fits-all approaches offered by some vendors. Zeta Architecture is one example of a promising emergent architecture for bioinformatics. Zeta Architecture is an enterprise architecture, documented by Jim Scott of MapR, that enables new approaches to research data processes and defines a scalable way for increasing the speed of integrating data into use-inspired research. Zeta Architecture can extend private and public capacities to support entry into the cloud with cloud hybridization. Scott has borrowed concepts from Google's Borg to create a hybrid solution leveraging the cloud for scale-out analytics. Before exploring Zeta Architecture in more detail, we examine the history and some limitations of enterprise architecture.

A Brief History of Enterprise Architectures

There will be no successful path to the future without understanding and appreciating history, which is why it is of the utmost importance to understand how the current state of enterprise architectures has come about. While building out a data center, resources are often thought about as pools of servers where each pool will meet the needs of a specific use case. Lines are created between the pools of servers, resulting in static partitions. They are static in the sense that the resources cannot grow dynamically. The growth in any particular partition over time has no direct effect on the other partitions. This partitioning model simplifies troubleshooting to identify when something fails within one of those static partitions.

Static partitioning provides a simplified way to calculate the theoretical maximum throughput of the software running in that partition, which means that capacity planning is pretty straightforward. Engineering teams are usually pretty concerned about understanding the capacity of the software. The information technology (IT) operations team usually needs to understand where to add capacity for future growth. This information will give you a maximum for your volume, for your compute, and for your memory. Most use cases will never realize complete utilization of resources in all given pools, and this is due in part to the workload imbalance created by static partitioning. Resource isolation is a big deal, and as nearly every engineer will attest to, fast troubleshooting is very important. Production or IT operations, development, and quality assurance (QA) all need mechanisms to isolate issues so they may understand where a problem originates. They also want to understand if it is one or multiple issues. Their goal is to quickly track down and identify an issue, deploy a fix, and ensure that the problem has been resolved.

Business continuity encompasses the topics of what keeps your business in business. We've got to make sure that we don't forget about things like backups and the schedules that come along with these. Disaster recovery plans should be in place not only for peace of mind but to ensure that businesses can continue in the face of the unexpected. Backup plans are generally defined against each of the static partitions, which tend to include how to recover from a single server lost to the entire data center. Most of these plans, which include plans for recovery, will have different levels of outage preparedness, going from hours to days of downtime. Clearly every business can benefit from having rock-solid plans and processes for outages.

Isolated Workloads Come at a Cost

One of the most notorious issues of isolated workloads is wasted capacity and wasted energy. Think about a common use case like web servers. Take an instance where a business uses 10 web servers running at 5% utilization (very normal for web servers), delivering web content with a load balancer sitting in front so it can handle traffic spikes. If utilization is nearly always below 10%, that leaves 90% as constantly wasted resources. Not only is there a capital cost for the 10 web servers, but when factoring in the energy costs, it becomes an even bigger deal. It would be nice to get better utilization of capital for the business. Isolation of resources isn't free, because every server needs to be monitored. Underutilized hardware consumes more than just energy; it also consumes time to manage them by keeping them secure and up to date.

Processes to move data from servers generating information to servers processing information tend to be rather complicated to set up and manage. Beyond the processes, they normally require people to monitor them around the clock. These jobs typically sit in a very high-profile position in a business workflow; if they are tied to revenue generation and if any of them fails, you may have to answer to your customers. In any good agile deployment process, there is a desire to promote software between any number of environments to support the business. Promoting software between environments is tricky, because environments tend to come in different shapes and sizes and usually do not contain the name number of servers per pool in a development environment as they would in a production environment. Given three servers in QA and 100 servers in production, is there a guarantee that the code that was tested is going to act the same way in production? Most assuredly not. Most people have probably lived through this scenario when going into a production environment. This is perhaps one of the most difficult and least fun things to troubleshoot.

Goals with a New Approach

The first goal with a new enterprise architectural approach should be the ability to leverage all existing hardware in the data center. This would enable resources to be put on any business problem at any time. There is still a need to maintain some form of isolation that meets the needs discussed in the current model. The requirements for moving software between environments need to be understood, and the processes need to be able to accommodate the new architecture and deliver more than what already exists. Backing up data for point-in-time recovery, or from tape or any other form of backup, needs to be improved in terms of what exists today. Too many architectures do not deliver any real added benefits for disaster recovery, and the restoration processes for a serious disaster could take weeks. The goal of this new approach should be to support real-time business continuity. This would mean that in the face of a disaster, recovery—if any—should be able to be accomplished within a time frame in line with high availability expectations (e.g., 99.9% or better). That is to say, this architecture will deliver the ability, but the onus is still on the implementer to know how many nines are necessary for the business. A cohesive security and compliance model including authorization and authentication should be considered to make management of systems easier and less prone to error. All the components have to be able to work with the same security controls. Users, jobs, and data need to be secured. We must ensure that even the most stringent regulatory environments are able to use this architecture.

The high-level component view is intended to support the goals defined for this new architecture. It is not intended to dictate which specific software or project, open source or otherwise, must be used. As we continue through this section, it's important to understand that the approach is one of efficiency and simplicity. At times it sounds too simple. Indeed, in the vendor-agnostic world of enterprise architectures, the physical infrastructure components need to have a degree of ease. However, it's not quite as clear as this formula: "Need a distributed fault-tolerant file system? Use HDFS. Need a distributed/fault-tolerant message-queue? Use Kafka. Need to coordinate between your worker processes? Use Zookeeper. Need to run it on a flexible grid of computing resources and handle failures? Run it on Mesos." It is not this simple because the overarching application layer reliant on physical resources adds framework to the model. There are seven pluggable components of this new enterprise architectural approach, and all the components must work together:

Deployment/container management system Having a standardized approach for deploying software is important. All resource consumers should be able to be isolated and deployed in a standard way.

Distributed filesystem Utilizing a shared distributed filesystem, all applications will be able to read and write to a common location, which enables simplification of the rest of the architecture.

Dynamic and global resource management Allows dynamic allocation of resources to enable the business to easily accommodate whatever task is the most important that day. As we look at what technologies can fit in here, we're basically going to start right in the middle. Mesos is a data center–wide resource manager; YARN is a resource manager for functionality that lives in the Hadoop ecosystem. When used alone, they create silos of clusters. To get around this, project Myriad can be utilized. Myriad enables Apache Mesos to manage YARN. When combined, these resource management tools bring all the resources into a single cluster.

Enterprise applications In the past, enterprise applications would drive the rest of the architecture. However, in Zeta Architecture, there is a shift. The rest of the architecture now simplifies these applications by delivering the components necessary to realize all of the business goals defined for this architecture.

Pluggable compute model/execution engine Different groups within a business have different needs and requirements for meeting the demands put upon them at any given time, which requires the support of potentially different engines and models to meet the needs of the business.

Real-time data storage This supports the need for high-speed business applications through the use of real-time databases.

Solution architecture This focuses on solving a particular business problem. There may be one or more applications built to deliver the complete solution. These solution architectures generally encompass a higher-level interaction among common algorithms or libraries, software components, and business workflows. All too often, solution architectures are folded into enterprise architectures, but there is a clear separation with the Zeta Architecture.*

Figure 6.4 shows the resources and technologies that are part of the Zeta Architecture.

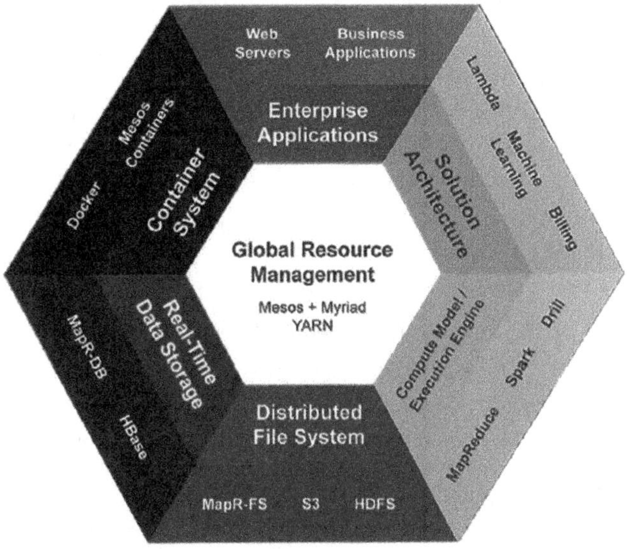

Figure 6.4 Example Technologies That Fit into the Zeta Architecture

There is flexibility available within the area of the distributed file system. If running on a cloud provider like Amazon, there is S3. Within a private data center, there is MapR-FS or HDFS. What is important to understand is that these functionalities and capabilities are going to be the foundation of the rest of this architecture. While MapR-FS implements all of the application programming interfaces (APIs) supported by HDFS, it delivers far more functionality than is available within HDFS. Real-time applications require guarantees on data retrieval and storage. This will include technologies like MapR-DB, which fully implements the HBase APIs as well as HBase. While this is the area of which Cassandra, an open source distributed database system, and MongoDB, an open source database, would be a part, they are not referenced in this architecture because they do not support running on distributed file systems like MapR-FS or HDFS. While it is conceivable that they could be adapted to run here, their self-limitation is what prevents them from participating in this architecture.

The compute model/execution engine is where the biggest opportunity shows up from an analytics and streaming perspective. In general, more than one at a time will be used to cover multiple use cases, and they need to support the distributed file system to leverage all of the compute power. This

*All definitions are taken from Jim Scott. "Zeta Architecture—What's in the Name?" https://www.mapr.com/blog/zeta-architecture-whats-in-a-name. Used with permission.

enables problem solving with multiple technologies, including using Hadoop MapReduce, Apache Drill, Apache Spark, or any others than can work with this distributed file system.

The containers portion of this architecture is significant, as it delivers a type of isolation that is important in certain use cases. The isolation provided by containers gives the ability to move software more easily from development to QA to production. Mesos ships with its own container system, but it also supports Docker and Kubernetes. This provides a better process model, which helps to ensure consistent software between environments. In the solution architecture space, there are concepts like machine learning, recommendation engines, or even the Lambda architecture. These are solution architectures that are going to leverage this platform, and you need to be able to describe them in a way that is more specific than the enterprise architecture itself. The simplest example of an enterprise application that could be used here is a web server. Take an Apache web server deployed in a container that is configured to write its logs straight through to the distributed file system. This bypasses log shipping and allows for the data to be processed or analyzed immediately, without delay.

The Google Example

Doug Cutting, the founder of Hadoop, once declared that "Google is living a few years in the future and sends the rest of us messages" [4]. We tend to agree, so we will take a moment to look at Google's architecture. Figure 6.5 shows Google's architecture. This architecture will allow anyone who implements it to run at Google scale.

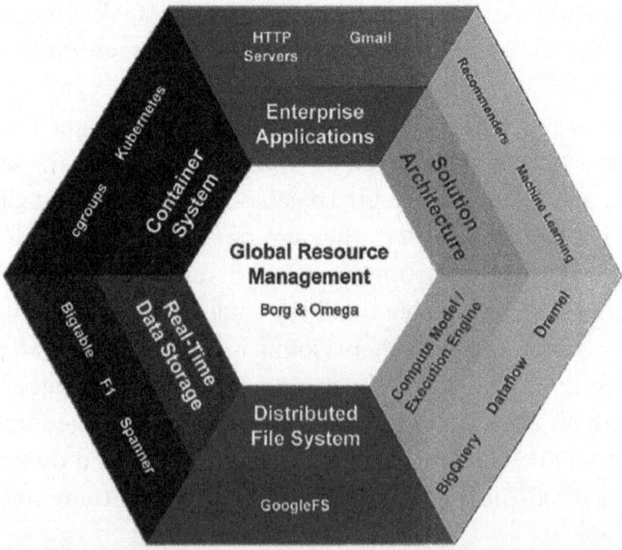

Figure 6.5 Technologies Google Leverages Laid over the Zeta Architecture

Let's take a look at a few interesting points regarding Google's technologies in this diagram: Borg is sometimes referred to as the "project that is unnamed" within Google, but outside of Google it's called Borg. Borg is

> a cluster manager that runs hundreds of thousands of jobs, from many thousands of different applications, across a number of clusters each with up to tens of thousands of machines. It achieves high utilization by combining admission control, efficient task-packing, over-commitment, and machine sharing with process-level performance isolation. It supports high-availability applications with runtime features that minimize fault-recovery time, and scheduling policies that reduce the probability of correlated failures. Borg simplifies life for its users by offering a declarative job specification language, name service integration, real-time job monitoring, and tools to analyze and simulate system behavior. [5]

Omega is Google's scheduler, and it is defined as the crux of the entire distributed processing platform, as it figures out where and when to place jobs. From a solution architecture perspective, Gmail conceptually operates on top of a recommendation engine. The machine learning concepts in general are delivered in many of Google's product offerings. Take a step back for a moment to understand all of the components that comprise a familiar application. It is probably implemented with many of these same concepts. The question is: Does the application leverage all of these in a heterogeneous way?

Integration of the Zeta Architecture

All processes running in the data center should be broken into two groups. The first group are those processes that offer resources. Global resource manager (CPU and memory) and the distributed file system (disk space and I/O) offer resources. The second group are those processes that consume resources. Web servers, Apache Drill, and Apache Spark, among others, are all resource consumers. Resource consumers should be containerized, whereas those offering resources should never be containerized.

Integrating business applications into this architecture requires plugging into standard APIs. Many custom adapters have been written to work with the HDFS API; however, most integrations require some sort of custom plugin to be able to fully utilize HDFS. On MapR-FS, there is native Network File System (NFS) support. In this case, any application that can read/write to an NFS mount can plug into this architecture. The added benefit of this approach is that when the application plugs in with these standards, the data is automatically replicated by the distributed file system. A pluggable security model is required, as applications come in many varieties, and it is unrealistic to expect them all to implement the same security model. Linux pluggable authentication modules are very convenient in most cases, as there is a tremendous amount of flexibility. Kerberos is an option here, but it is not a perfect solution for long-running jobs.

While many relational database management systems have the potential to work in this model, most do not openly support these distributed file systems. Some have their own, but those are explicitly for that product's use. Some will work just fine over a native NFS adapter, while others may not. If the relational database management system of choice supports this, there is a great opportunity if the data format can be read by the analytics execution engine. Historically, data analytics teams usually get the short straw when it comes to getting resources. They do not typically get access to production systems. Generally they have to get data dumps and have access to less than adequate compute resources. This model allows data analytics teams to participate in this new type of isolation and have dynamic access to the globally managed resources.

Zeta and Application Architectures

Nearly every application architecture needs to concern itself with many different things, including data protection schemes, how to back up data, recovery from failures, and running multiple instances of software. The Zeta Architecture simplifies those application architectures because it delivers many of those pieces, which means there's less stuff to go wrong. Fewer moving parts means fewer potential failure points. Better hardware utilization means less to operate and lower operational costs. The business is then capable of leveraging a global set of resources to solve any problem based on what is most important right now. Priority number one can change quickly in any business. Resilience is extremely important in an application architecture. The Hadoop ecosystem components help to protect against disk and server failure. However, they don't protect against people making mistakes. With a statically partitioned model, backups are usually completely performed only once per week, with partials performed nightly. Recovering from failures and mistakes takes significant time. In this new model, recovery is easier to plan for and more resilience is present in the system because of the availability of near-real-time backups and utilization of the features of the distributed file system.

Streaming Applications

Occasionally there is a need to stream data in as opposed to waiting for some periodic interval of time before processing the data. If an application architecture calls for acting on each and every event that may occur in a log file in real time, then streaming should be considered. This would fall into the pluggable compute model/execution engine portion of the Zeta Architecture and it may or may not be considered "analytics" based. For this use case, there are a few options available. The first is to set up the stream processing engine with a source that tails the log file from the distributed file system. The second approach is for the application generating the logs to write the log information to some type of agent that can persist the log to disk and send it to the streaming processing engine simultaneously. The last approach is to skip the disk altogether and send the information directly to the stream processing engine or some queue sitting in front of it. Each of these approaches is going to have varying benefits/trade-offs, all of which should be considered before making a selection.

CONCLUSION

In this chapter we explored the basics of cloud computing and RaaS, both of which are becoming increasingly important and widely used in the field of biomedicine. As systems and use cases become more complex, new architectures are emerging. We focused on Zeta Architecture, which Google relies on. Google performs over 2 billion container deployments per week and operates a highly complex and efficient system. Containers will help deliver the isolation needed to be able to move into the future. This architecture gives many companies or organizations that use it a competitive advantage. Zeta Architecture will become the traditional way of thinking about building and deploying software in the data center, whether on premise or hosted. This is the model to create an as-it-happens organization—one that can sense and respond in real time. At the end of this chapter is a case study on CardioSolv and how it uses on-demand computing to conduct research into ventricular tachycardia.

NOTES

1. Louis Columbo. 2015 "Roundup of Cloud Computing Forecasts and Market Estimates, 2015." *Forbes Online*. http://www.forbes.com/sites/louiscolumbus/2015/01/24/roundup-of-cloud-computing-forecastsand-market-estimates-2015/.
2. "Final Version of NIST Cloud Computing Definition Published." 2011. NIST *Tech Beat*, October 25. http://www.nist.gov/itl/csd/cloud-102511.cfm.
3. Peter Mell and Tam Grace. 2009. "The NIST Definition of Cloud Computing." Version 15. National Institute of Standards and Technology, Information Technology Laboratory, October 7. https://www.nist.gov/sites/default/files/documents/itl/cloud/cloud-def-v15.pdf.
4. Jim Scott. 2014. "5 Google Projects That Changed Big Data Forever." MapR. https://www.mapr.com/blog/5-google-projects-changed-big-data-forever.
5. Abhishek Verma, Luis Pedrosa, Madhukar R. Korupolu, David Oppenheimer, Eric Tune, and John Wilkes. 2015. "Large-Scale Cluster Management at Google with Borg." *Proceedings of the European Conference on Computer Systems (EuroSys)*, ACM, Bordeaux, France. http://research.google.com/pubs/pub43438.html.

CASE STUDY

CASE STUDY 9: CARDIOSOLV USES PENGUIN'S RESEARCH CLOUD FOR ON-DEMAND COMPUTE

Brock Tice

LARGE-SCALE SIMULATIONS IN THE CLOUD WITH CARDIOSOLV AND PENGUIN COMPUTING

CardioSolv Ablation Technologies utilizes proprietary software and algorithms to reconstruct heart and infarct morphology using preoperative imaging, conduct an analysis of ventricular tachycardia (VT) circuits and filaments, and predict locations and extent of ablation targets, register model geometry and predicted ablation target with the image of the heart, and employ CardioSolv's patient-specific model in guidance of VT ablation therapy. CardioSolv partners with Penguin Computing On-Demand (POD). POD's cluster dramatically decreases processing time without CardioSolv having to invest in on-premise infrastructure. This lets CardioSolv focus on biomedical research rather than IT.

Ventricular tachycardia (V-tach or VT) is a type of tachycardia, or a rapid heartbeat, that arises from improper electrical activity of the heart presenting as a rapid heart rhythm. VT associated with myocardial infarction is a life-threatening arrhythmia that poses challenging clinical problems. Catheter ablation is a possible treatment for those with recurrent VT. However, this is an invasive surgical procedure that typically is prescribed once pharmacological options have been exhausted. The innovative CardioSolv software solution can reduce time and cost related to VT ablation procedures but, more important, improve patient outcomes for those who undergo VT ablation procedures. The software runs complex simulations in parallel, making many of the current methods obsolete.

The current methods have reached levels of modest success and have driven development for CardioSolv's innovation. Head of Technologies at CardioSolv Brock Tice and his team diligently supported both production and research and development environments for the large-scale simulations and began to exhaust local resources. Outgrowing their on-premise data center, staying current with processor families, and the costs associated with these factors caused them to seek alternative solutions in the public cloud.

> Cloud computing is a model for enabling ubiquitous, convenient, on-demand network access to a shared pool of configurable computing resources (e.g., networks, servers, storage, applications, and services) that can be rapidly provisioned and released with minimal management effort or service provider interaction.
>
> *—NIST Special Publication 800-145, "The NIST Definition of Cloud Computing," http://csrc.nist.gov/publications/nistpubs/800-145/SP800-145.pdf.*

"We need to run very large simulations with relatively low frequency (0–8 times per month, generally closer to 0 or 1 so far), using upward of 6,000 core-hours. We have neither the financial resources at this early startup stage to purchase the required number of compute nodes, nor the space, power, or cooling to house them," remarks Tice as he discusses the decision to sell senior leadership on the bold move. A careful examination of the options led the team back to Penguin Computing and its POD solution. POD provides seamless access to a state-of-the-art high-performance cluster without all the up-front investment and ongoing upkeep costs. When an innovator like CardioSolv can bypass large capital expenditures and ongoing bloated operational expenditures, that revenue can be returned to research and development, creating a new paradigm for VT ablation, reducing procedure times, and improving patient outcomes.

While companies are well aware of competing cloud computing options such as Linode, Amazon EC2, and Rackspace, many of these aim their offerings toward operationalized IT infrastructures, such as Microsoft Exchange, SharePoint, or database applications. Research computing and health informatics at this scale require ultra-low-latency infrastructure needed to properly parallelize a 256-core or greater simulation run. Scaling on many other cloud providers is suboptimal despite their boasts of 10-Gigabit Ethernet as an internode communication medium.

The simulation workloads run at CardioSolv predict ablation lesion sites for patients suffering from infarct-scar-related monomorphic VT. Our innovative suite creates a model of a patient's heart from a magnetic resonance imaging scan and then runs it through a series of rigorous simulations on the POD cluster to pinpoint the location in the patient's heart where electrical problems are occurring. We use those results to advise physicians on where they might ablate to stop the electrical problems. We also use a proprietary analysis of the activation patterns to find those ablation sites, which is being run on POD rather than locally. It can take all day to run on a very robust workstation. With POD it takes less than an hour. Figure CS6.1 shows simulation output.

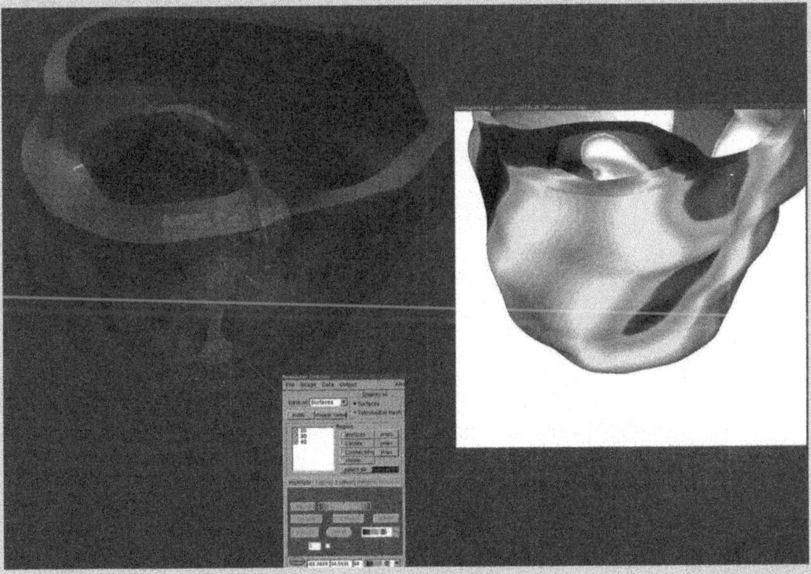

Figure CS6.1 Simulation Output

(Continued)

(*Continued*)

As a company we have never run these simulations at the desired scale; before POD, we were simply unable to. Our 8-node Nehalem development cluster takes more than a week to run one patient. With POD as a partner, we can have it done in less than 12 hours.

IMPROVED OUTCOMES + REDUCED PROCEDURE TIMES

Our POD partnership also allows us to have the same access and robust reporting we had with our on-premise solutions without the operational maintenance costs. Figure CS6.2 shows our Penguin Computing (POD) interface.

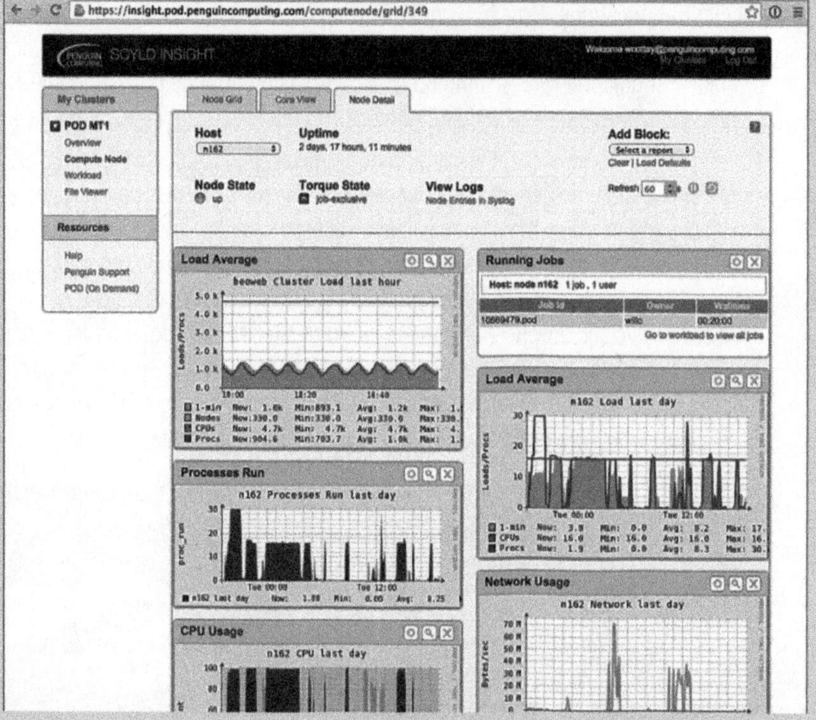

Figure CS6.2 Penguin Computing on Demand Interface

HIGH-PERFORMANCE COMPUTING ON DEMAND AS A SERVICE

POD allows organizations to utilize a high-performance, bare-metal, HPC computing environment in the cloud without having to invest in on-premise infrastructure. Nor do organizations have to deal with multitenant cloud environments and the performance, scalability, and security challenges associated with shared infrastructure. Figure CS6.3 shows the Account management portal on POD.

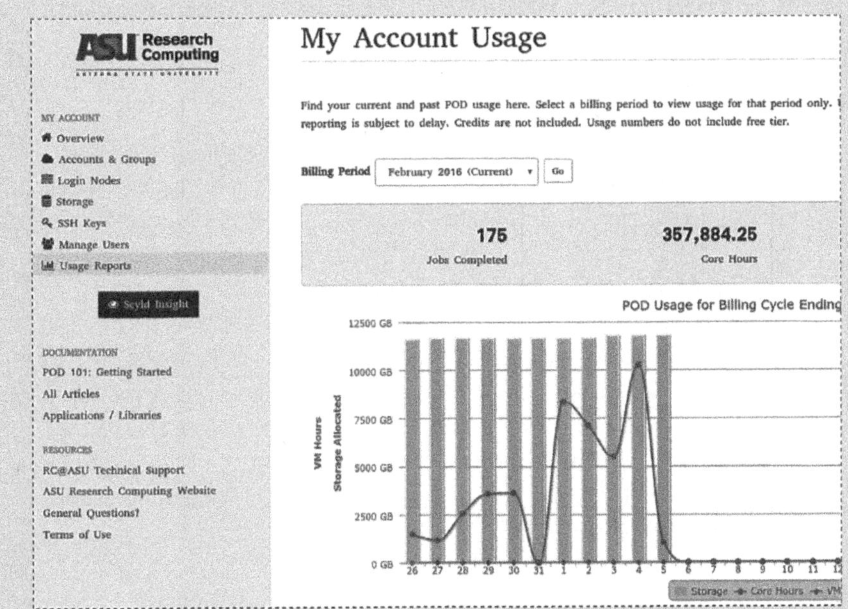

Figure CS6.3 Account Management Portal on POD

Computational jobs are easy to submit and monitor from either a traditional Linux command line interface (CLI) environment, or through the use of an intuitive and secure web portal. POD's HPC cluster is ready to run with hundreds of applications preinstalled, eliminating much of the complexity of building, managing, and scaling HPC environments. This efficiency and economy of scale saves both capital and operational costs while ensuring a clear, predictable pricing model.

POD's bare-metal, InfiniBand on-demand HPC compute cluster is ideal for organizations in manufacturing, biosciences, research, energy, design, and finance—or any organization with high-performance computing needs.

SUPPORT BY HPC EXPERTS

Penguin Computing has well over a decade in optimizing HPC environments and applications. As a user of POD, we provide you with free support from our HPC experts who can assist you in running applications, managing workflows, and getting the best experience out of POD.

Penguin Computing has a long history of supplying and supporting HPC customers. With this history comes significant expertise in the HPC market, which is the foundation of the POD offering. HPC experts are part of the POD service team and have experience in a wide range of HPC domains. The architects of the POD infrastructure are experienced in designing systems for customers and thus all POD servers are Penguin Computing designed.

(*Continued*)

(*Continued*)

SUMMARY

The POD cloud offering has been designed for HPC professionals by HPC professionals with years of experience. As cloud computing has gained a strong foothold in companies of all sizes for developer and enterprise applications, the uptake of the cloud for HPC use has been lacking. By using years of experience and focusing on the HPC market, the POD offering is what HPC users have come to expect in terms of application performance, while reducing both capital expenditures and operating expenditures. Users can easily upload data, perform calculations, and visualize the results in an integrated, cost-effective manner. CardioSolv Ablation Technologies' innovative technology, licensed from Johns Hopkins University, is based on years of research by leaders in the academic field of cardiac modeling. The Penguin Computing–CardioSolv partnership enables better patient outcomes delivered through the cloud.

■■■

CardiSolv LLC is a private scientific services and consulting company specializing in predictive cardiac modeling and simulation for academic researchers, clinicians, and industrial research personnel.

CHAPTER 7

Data Science

Now that we have so much more data and this data is being stored longer and in more accessible formats, data scientists are increasingly in demand. Demand for data scientists is growing sharply across many fields and sectors. The term "data scientist" can refer to specific training and background (with more and more advanced degree programs cropping up), but for the purposes of this discussion, let's assume that data scientists are those who are being asked to extract insight, draw conclusions, and make predictions from data. Data scientists work with data, analyzing, transforming, and building models and databases. Sometimes those acting in data science capacities have relatively little formal training in data science. We certainly hope that everyone engaged in data science has a sufficient understanding of statistics so as not to employ dubious methods or arrive at erroneous conclusions.

We covered some tools specific to genomic analysis in Chapter 2. In this chapter we explore NoSQL database offerings and statistical tools for 21st-century data science. Data science is a vast topic that we will not be able to cover exhaustively in this chapter. If you'd like more information, I would suggest consulting:

- Nathan Marz and James Warren, *Big Data Principles and Best Practices of Scalable Real-Time Data Systems*. Shelter Island, NY: Manning Publications, 2015.
- Sandy Ryza, Uri Laserson, Sean Owen, and Josh Wills, *Advanced Analytics with Spark: Patterns for Learning from Data at Scale*. Sebastopol, CA: O'Reilly, 2015.

One way and perhaps the most common way of thinking about contemporary data science is as a sort of laundry list of tools. Data scientists usually need to be familiar with Hadoop, Hive, HBase, Pig, MapReduce, and other Hadoop ecosystem components and/or non-Structured Query Language (NoSQL) databases such as Cassandra, MongoDB, CouchDB, MarkLogic, and RedShift. Data science often engages with data warehouses and is concerned with business intelligence (BI) and ETL tools (Extract, Transform, Load). And, of course, knowledge of relational database management system (RDBMS) data modeling and Structured Query Language (SQL), Python, and R is essential. This list could go on, and it will change as rapidly as technology itself.

But as important as all these building blocks are, they are simply sets of tools. A data scientist worth his or her snuff needs to have a strong foundation in statistics and likely some proficiency with applied mathematics. Many, indeed most, of the statistical and mathematical underpinnings of contemporary data science are quite old and have stood the test of time. For those of you who are less familiar with statistics or would like a refresher, this chapter is followed by an appendix, "A Brief Statistics Primer." The chapter begins with an overview of NoSQL approaches to biomedical data science. Then we explore (later in this chapter) how Splunk, which can collect and analyze high volumes of machine-generated data, can be used in healthcare analytics. A detailed section on using Hadoop for genomic analysis (expression quantitative trait loci [eQTL]) also covers Apache Spark, Hive tables, and MapReduce. The parallelization afforded by Hadoop enables you to get your results faster. Following this chapter is a case study on the Hortonworks Data Platform at University of California Irvine Health.

NOSQL APPROACHES TO BIOMEDICAL DATA SCIENCE

A section on data science for biomedicine would be incomplete without a discussion of NoSQL approaches and the multiple special-purpose offerings available. Medical records, images, X rays, and clinical data are central to biomedicine and key to precision medicine for the future. NoSQL database offerings are enabling new and promising work. In 2006 Google published its now-famous "Bigtable" paper, which was followed closely by Amazon's 2007 debut of DynamoDB [1]. The concepts from these pioneering efforts led to 225 NoSQL database offerings as of 2016. Our focus, as always, is the open source offerings, such as HBase, Cassandra, MongoDB, and others built within Facebook, LinkedIn, Twitter, and other companies. For an up-to-date count of NoSQL players, please check http://nosql-database.org/.

As discussed in previous chapters, NoSQL was originally thought to represent "No SQL" as a descriptor for nonrelational databases. Now, because many nonrelational database–like systems provide SQL interfaces and compatibility for interoperation, NoSQL has transmogrified into "Not Only SQL." The nosql-database.org defines NoSQL as:

> Next Generation Databases mostly addressing some of the points: being non-relational, distributed, open-source and horizontally scalable. Often more characteristics apply such as: schema-free, easy replication support, simple application programming interface (API), eventually consistent/BASE (not ACID), a huge amount of data and more.

NoSQL could actually be classed as four different types of databases:

1. Key value/tuple stores, such as Redis, Riak, or Amazon DynamoDB
2. Wide column stores or column-families, such as HBase and Cassandra
3. Databases geared toward documents, such as Elasticsearch and MongoDB
4. Graph databases, such as Neo4j, Graphbase, and Onyx.

Consider these the four pillars of the NoSQL family for data-intensive compute.

We discuss a couple of these options in this section, but certainly not all 225!

MongoDB (Humongous) is an open source cross-platform document-oriented database. Classified as a NoSQL database, MongoDB avoids the traditional table-based relational database structure in favor of JSON-like documents with dynamic schemas, making the integration of data in certain types of applications easier and faster. MongoDB is developed by MongoDB Inc. and is free and open source, published under a combination of the GNU Affero General Public License and the Apache License. As of July 2015, MongoDB was the fourth most widely mentioned database engine on the web and the most popular for document stores.

- Current version 3.2
- License: AGPL (Drivers: Apache)
- Protocol: Custom, binary (BSON), written in C++
- **Pluses:** Schema-less; greater performance over a wide range of features; maps files to memory for data storage; journaling; geospatial indexing out of the box; auto failover with master/slave replication; and built-in sharding.* Convenient web interface. Still probably the best successor to EMC Centera for large document repositories. Free, with free online classes at MongoDB University. (https://university.mongodb.com/exams)
- **Minuses:** An empty database uses about 200 megabytes; JavaScript dependent; experts and/or qualified folks are still pricey. Not really SQL, although many features are retained. Data wrangling and ETL from your legacy infrastructure require considerable planning. Not super-fast due to MapReduce reliance (although faster than others); no joins and eats up memory depending on the task.
- URL: https://www.mongodb.com.

CouchDB (self-described as a database for the web) completely embraces the web and stores gobs of data with JSON documents. Provides document access and index queries via HTTP or a simple web browser. Index, combine, and transform your documents with JavaScript for access from most web-driven

* Sharding, MongoDB explains, is the process of storing data records across multiple machines and is MongoDB's approach to meeting the demands of data growth. As the size of the data increases, a single machine may not be sufficient to store the data nor provide an acceptable read and write throughput. Sharding solves the problem with horizontal scaling. With sharding, you add more machines to support data growth and the demands of read and write operations.

mobile devices and apps. CouchDB comes with a suite of features, such as on-the-fly document transformation and real-time change notifications, and an easy to use web administration console. CouchDB is highly available and partition tolerant, but is also eventually consistent.

- Current version 1.6.1
- License: Apache
- Protocol: HTTP/REST API driven, written in Erlang.
- **Pluses:** Consistent DB across geo-diverse architectures; great for large accumulations of occasionally changing data where canned queries need to be executed with regularity; attachment aware; supports master-master replication; supports multisite deployments; versioning ready; JSON friendly; and MapReduce ad hoc queries are not too slow due to the deep indexing capacity of CouchDB.
- **Minuses:** Best for CRM apps; hides embedded MapReduce at a performance hit; requires regular compacting; and not quite as SQL-like in the sense that users need to create "views" and ad hoc queries on a regular basis. Issues cited by users in the environment include: joins and multistep processes require one-off trial and error; and too many temporary views are created as a stopgap.
- URL: http://couchdb.apache.org/.

Cassandra (Apache Cassandra database) offers scalability and high availability without compromising performance. With linear scalability and proven fault tolerance running on commodity hardware and/or public cloud infrastructure, Cassandra is a good platform for mission-critical data as multi–data center replication is in-built and optimized to reduce latency, even during a regional outage. CERN (European Organization for Nuclear Research), Comcast, GitHub, Netflix, and 1,500 more companies run on Cassandra.

Current version 3.7

- License: Apache
- Protocol: CQL3 (Cassandra Query Language) and Thrift, written in Java
- **Pluses:** Huge data sets can be stored in "near or almost" SQL; CQL 3 addresses issues in CQL 2 and Thrift (Thrift is all but dead and gone, which should be a plus); cross-site replication can be trusted, making Cassandra scalable and robust; puts a friendly face on large data sets and makes them easier to navigate and mine results from; good support for denormalization and materialized views; and decent built-in caching capacity to kick up performance.

- **Minuses:** The Thrift API can be confusing in terms of how rows and columns are mapped; thankfully, you would only run across Thrift in a legacy install; read and write ratios should be tweaked for performance (reads are disk bound); and requires tuning for replication and distribution. Facebook, Twitter, and Reddit are big Cassandra shops; however, your IT organization may lack the resources they have. Professional support is available from third parties.
- URL: https://cassandra.apache.org/.

HBase (Apache HBase, Hadoop standard) may be the correct solution if the task is random; needs real-time read/write access to data-intensive structures (big data); produces very large tables with potentially billions of rows times millions of columns; and needs to run on commodity hardware clusters. HBase is an open source, distributed, versioned, nonrelational database modeled after Google's Bigtable. Just as Bigtable leveraged the distributed data storage provided by the Google File System, HBase provides Bigtable-like capabilities on top of the Hadoop Distributed File System (HDFS).

- Current version 1.1.5
- License: Apache
- Protocol: HTTP/REST, JVM, written in Java
- **Pluses:** Supports XML; Protobuf; binary; JIRB Shell (Jruby-based); rolling restarts for configuration changes and incremental upgrades; billions of rows and millions of columns; and rolled in with all packaged distributions of Hadoop. It is widely supported and understood.
- **Minuses:** Hadoop is probably still the best way to run MapReduce jobs on huge data sets; best results are obtained if you already run the Hadoop/HDFS stack. However, this means you are still impacted by potential MapReduce latency and/or batchlike operational output. Plan ahead and remember the GIGO (garbage in, garbage out) principle. It is not the best RDBMS replacement. HBase is memory and CPU intensive and can eat up the cluster components. Save yourself issues and tune the garbage collection and watch heap size or pay later.
- URL: https://hbase.apache.org.

Accumulo (Bigtable with cell-level security) is a sorted, distributed key/value store with robust, secure, scalable data storage and retrieval that is built on top of Hadoop. Featuring improvements on the Bigtable design in the form of cell-based access control for highly improved security and multitenancy, improved compression, and a server-side programming mechanism for modification of key/value pairs at various points in the data management process. It was created in 2008 by the U.S. National Security Agency (NSA) and contributed to the Apache Foundation as an incubator project in September 2011.

- Current version 1.6.5
- License: Apache
- Protocol: Thrift, written in Java and C++
- **Pluses:** Good performance; cell-level security; scalable master; FATE fault-tolerant executer; server-side programming mechanism to encode functions such as filtering and aggregation; cell labels and namespaces. Developed by the NSA.
- **Minuses:** Another Bigtable clone; also runs on top of Hadoop; supports larger rows than memory allows, which can be problematic; reliant on Hadoop underpinnings like Zookeeper. Accumulo was built to remain in a single secure data center, and replication is a new feature. Accumulo relies heavily on ZooKeeper for distributed lock management and state. Due to the consistent nature of ZooKeeper and its protocol, wide area network replication is not optimal for Accumulo.

A couple of favorite emergent model databases that we have experimented with for research data management and integrated into targeted funding opportunities in biomedicine are discussed next. The databases described next are not 100% open source and have varied license structures. We indicate the license and terms in the descriptions.

Graph Databases

Graph databases are not necessarily new; however, their usage in biomedicine is emergent. A graph database is an online database management system with Create, Read, Update, and Delete (CRUD) operations working on a graph data model. Graph databases are generally built for use with transactional (online transaction processing; OLTP) systems. Accordingly, they are normally optimized for transactional performance and engineered with transactional integrity and operational availability in mind. Unlike other databases, relationships take first priority in graph databases. This means your application doesn't have to infer data connections using foreign keys or out-of-band processing, such as MapReduce.

Due to their ability to store data and create relationships between multiple diverse data points, graph databases have the potential to unlock discovery of public value in our understanding of cancer. An example would be creating a relationship between type of cancer (glioblastoma multiforme), tumor cell population, treatment-resistant mutations, drug therapy, optimal dosage level, treatment success rate, effectiveness against mutations, and date brought to market. In the graph database, an entirely new set of relationship-based questions can be asked, which could open new possibilities. If we apply this methodology to cancer research and treatment, it could enable research oncologists to ask new and interesting questions, allowing for tailored treatments and delivery of precision medicine.

Neo4J (world's leading graph database) is a highly scalable, native graph database purpose-built to leverage not only data but also its relationships. With a native graph storage and processing engine, Neo4J can deliver constant, real-time performance that would strain traditional relational database models. Neo4j is an open source project, whose source and copyright is owned and maintained by Neo Technology. Graph-style, with rich or complex interconnections between data elements, makes Neo4J very promising in the evaluation of biomarker discovery.

- Current version 3.0.3
- License: Creative Commons 3.0 (GPL)
- Other Licenses: Enterprise, Commercial, Evaluation, Educational and Community/Open Source, and cool options for startups. See: https://neo4j.com/licensing/
- Protocol: REST-HTTP Java Embedded, API for a host of languages, written in Java
- **Pluses:** Two editions (Community and Enterprise) of Neo4j to choose from to make kicking the tires before a commitment a possibility; full ACID conformity and transactionality; high availability for billions of entities; horizontal read scalability; cool web-driven admin tools; online backup; advanced monitoring; support for advanced path finding (path determination) with multiple algorithms.
- **Minuses:** A high level of mathematics is required to build complex relationship graphs. Domain knowledge experts should be engaged to validate data outputs to massage graph relationships.

NeoJ4 is fully ACID compliant, meaning that is has the following transactional characteristics comprising the ACID acronym:

Atomicity: Each transaction is "all or nothing." Two states {indivisible (Atomic) OR aborted (Failed)}.

Consistency: Ensures that any transaction will bring the database from one valid state to another.

Isolation: Ensures the concurrency of transactions as if they were executed serially.

Durability: Ensures that once a transaction has been committed, it remains so, under any event.

Elasticsearch (search and analyze in real time) combines the speed of search, powerful analytics, high availability, and full text search in a schema-free, developer-friendly format with RESTful API. Interactively search, discover, and analyze your Hadoop data with ES-Hadoop, a two-way connector that solves the real-time search challenge within any Hadoop deployment.

- Current version 2.3.3
- License: Apache 2 Open Source
- Protocol: HTTP/REST Flexible API and JSON Query, written in Java
- **Pluses:** Robust advanced searching; real-time analytics; automatic and configurable sharding; multitenancy; distributed; document oriented; schema-free; RESTful API makes Elasticsearch developer friendly.
- **Minuses:** Deployments could require custom implementations and custom Lucene development. Stores as JavaScript Object Notation documents. Still reliant on a small development shop.
- URL: https://www.elastic.co/.

MarkLogic Server (enterprise NoSQL database) fuses database internals, search-style indexing, and application server behaviors into a unified system. It utilizes XML documents as a data model, storing documents within a transactional repository and indexing the words and values from each of the loaded documents, as well as the document structure. Because of its unique Universal Index, MarkLogic does not require advance knowledge of the document structure (its "schema") nor complete adherence to a particular schema. Through its application server capabilities, it's programmable and extensible.

- Current version 8.0
- License: Developer and commercial models (http://www.marklogic.com/what-is-marklogic/pricing/). Free developer edition is not a stripped-down version.
- Protocol: HTTP/REST Flexible API and REST Query, written in C++
- **Pluses:** Full text search and structured query: XPath; XQuery; range; and geospatial. Biotemporal concurrency; shared-nothing cluster; Multiversion concurrency control; petabyte-scalable elasticity; ACID + XA transactions (XA, or eXtended Architecture, is a standard that preserves ACID properties); auto-sharding; failover; master-slave cluster replication; replication; high availability; disaster recovery with full and incremental backups; government-grade security at the document level; robust developer community; decent free version for developers.

- **Minuses:** With Fortune 500 companies and healthcare.gov as clients, Marklogic may be too large and enterprise focused for engagements in research and education.
- URL: http://www.marklogic.com.

USING SPLUNK FOR DATA ANALYTICS

Splunk captures machine-generated data and enables searching, monitoring, and analysis through a web-style interface. Splunk holds great potential for healthcare data analytics.

The Healthcare Challenge

The healthcare industry is experiencing unprecedented change as it struggles to meet the demands of an increasingly interconnected, digital world where improving healthcare delivery and patient outcomes is paramount. With the advent of medical devices, sensors, mobile apps, and expanding healthcare delivery models (like virtual care), the lines between physical and digital are blurring.

Healthcare organizations have much more to do in order to make healthcare seamless to patients, providers, and payers.

However, the complexity of the healthcare ecosystem, the regulatory environment, and recent high-profile security breaches make it extremely challenging for any healthcare organization to effect meaningful, transformative change, especially given limited budgets and resources.

Data Analytics in Healthcare

Many healthcare organizations are investing in big data and analytics to tackle these issues, but so far the return on investment is unclear.

Traditional analytics tools and techniques are insufficient for current needs, where an estimated 80% of healthcare data is unstructured. Data remains locked in silos within healthcare organizations and throughout the healthcare ecosystem; manual processes, paper trails, and legacy IT are endemic. These systemic issues prevent healthcare organizations from achieving true interoperability and reaping all of its purported benefits.

Healthcare organizations need a way to analyze structured and unstructured data together, in order to have a holistic view of everything they are trying to address. The data needs to be freed and democratized so that anyone—data scientists, IT personnel, business users—can analyze and ask any question of the data.

Turning Data into Operational Intelligence

Splunk provides a platform that can collect and index unstructured and semi-structured data in real time, providing visualizations and dashboards that enable healthcare organizations to gain a full-picture view of their entire operations. The Splunk platform provides the scalability to handle massive live data streams across an entire infrastructure and the power to provide deep drill-down, statistical analysis as well as real-time, custom dashboards for anyone in an organization. No schema or upfront cleansing of data is required.

Splunk enables data aggregation from multiple sources to create end-to-end solutions that address key strategic initiatives within healthcare. Any clinical system recording access audit data can be consumed by the Splunk platform, including electronic health records (EHRs), pharmacy data, radiology, scheduling, patient-owned device data, and so on. Figure 7.1 details major Splunk capabilities, while Figure 7.2 summarizes how Splunk differs from many other offerings.

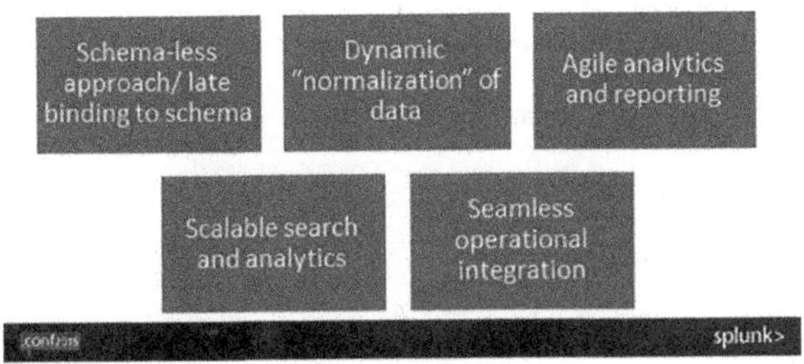

Figure 7.1 Splunk's Central Capabilities

	Without Splunk	With Splunk
Data Collection	Manual extraction from discharge reports, simulate test data	Actual event data and event metadata (logs)
Data Types	Data must be structured in a pre-defined schema	Structured, semi-structured, un-structured data; no fixed schema needed for data access
Visualization Methods	Excel and schema-based BI tools	Augment with big data visualization and analytics techniques
Analytics Methods	Descriptive analysis (counting, etc.)	Augment with machine learning and relevant data visualizations
Usage in Operations	Monthly; once or twice a year	Near real time (hourly, daily, weekly)

conf2015 splunk>

Figure 7.2 Splunk's Key Differences

With Splunk, healthcare organizations can shift from a reactive stance to one that is proactive, where they can make prescriptive recommendations to address key challenges.

Example 1: Improving Healthcare Delivery Operations with Process Mining

Healthcare delivery workflows vary widely, with multiple steps involving patient intake and scheduling, lab tests, counseling, consultations, and more. The difficulty in mapping these steps together has caused delays or gaps in care, redundancies, incorrect billing, and other errors.

However, each step generates an event that can be correlated and used to create a more realistic view of how a business process is performing. Devices, medication, and even patients can have radio-frequency identification tracking, which can be a data source for correlating events. By using process mining, healthcare organizations can analyze observed behavior from event data and metadata to discover patterns, monitor compliance, and optimize workflow. Unlike traditional as-is analysis of business processes (which can be biased based on the opinion of a process expert), the data doesn't lie. The data shows actual behavior, based on millions of correlated events. Figure 7.3 lists event types and attributes for healthcare data.

Event type (activity)	Attribute
Sign on selective medical service	Case ID, Activity completion time, Resource ID, Resource department code
Referral registration	Case ID, Activity completion time, Resource ID, Resource department code
Outside image registration	Case ID, Activity completion time, Resource ID, Resource department code
Payment	Case ID, Activity completion time, Resource ID, Resource department code
Test registration	Case ID, Activity completion time, Resource ID, Resource department code, Test code, Type of test, Scheduled test date
Test	Case ID, Activity completion time, Resource ID, Resource department code, Test code, Type of test, Scheduled test date
Consultation registration	Case ID, Activity completion time, Resource ID, Resource department code, Patient type, Department code, Appointment method, Appointment Date
Consultation	Case ID, Activity completion time, Resource ID, Resource Department code, Patient type, Department code, Appointment method, Appointment Date
Consultation scheduling	Case ID, Activity completion time, Resource ID, Resource department code, Patient type, Practitioner ID, Scheduled department code, Scheduled consultation date
Test scheduling	Case ID, Activity completion time, Resource ID, Resource department code, Test code, Type of test, Scheduled test date
Admission scheduling	Case ID, Activity completion time, Resource ID, Resource department code
Outside-hospital prescription printing	Case ID, Activity completion time, Resource ID
In-hospital prescription receiving	Case ID, Activity completion time, Resource ID, Resource department code
Certificate issuing	Case ID, Activity completion time, Resource ID, Resource department code
Treatment	Case ID, Treatment start date, Resource ID, Resource department code, Treatment code

Case ID: unique ID for identification of outpatient patients of the day, Resource ID: unique ID for identification of someone or something that performed the specific activity, Resource department code: unique code for identification of the resource ID's departments.

Figure 7.3 Event Types and Attributes for Healthcare Data

With this knowledge, healthcare organizations can redesign processes to be more efficient and accurate, and adjust parameters or intervene more quickly, since they can measure key performance indicators (KPIs) in real time and detect deviations and bottlenecks more readily. For instance, they can improve scheduling to better reflect patient care needs; reduce waiting times; provide a surgical checklist; and reduce errors in procedures.

One healthcare organization, which oversees 514 clinics worldwide, uses Splunk to manage dental imaging for their service members, provide insight on actual service utilization by clinicians, and identify underutilized equipment for redistribution (versus new purchases and expenditures). By correlating the Digital Imaging and Communications in Medicine (DICOM) logs and 80+ other data sources (including clinical, patient, readiness, and system performance data), the organization can determine how dental services are being utilized. It tracks the number of patients seen daily, peak service times, when patients experienced long wait times, and more.

With the data analysis in hand, the organization redistributed appointments to other clinics with more availability; looked at technology usage and redistributed equipment to clinics that were busy; and tracked patient satisfaction levels with wait times and system performance. The organization estimates that it saved $2.5 million in hardware and software costs and reduced capital expenditures by $2.2 million in annual and projected costs.

Example 2: Improving Patient Outcomes and Patient Satisfaction through Care Coordination Analytics

The healthcare delivery system includes components beyond hospital settings, such as primary care, emergency care, long-term care, nursing homes, home healthcare, prescription and nonprescription medications, medical devices, and more. Care coordination can be quite complex, especially if patients receive care from multiple sources (i.e., nurse practitioner, internist, disease specialist, social worker), and healthcare organizations are looking at mobile apps and telehealth (such as home health monitoring devices) to reduce some of the burden. Patient information must be exchanged throughout the healthcare ecosystem so that patients receive proper treatment, but there are many areas where information critical to patient care may fall through. Multiple protocols, codes, and messaging formats add to the complexity.

A solution (encompassing methods, processes, and tools) that analyzes EHR data, patient-generated data (surveys), and telehealth- and mobile health–generated data can identify gaps, redundancies, and conflicts in care. The data can come from any domain—labs, medications, patient preferences/goals, home health plans, nursing care plans, physical therapy/exercise systems, nutritional counseling, and more. The method must account for the patient's social situations, preferences, and goals.

In addition, achieving interoperability through the use of standard terminology and models is critical. Adopting Fast Healthcare Interoperability

Resources (FHIR), a standard for exchanging healthcare information electronically, can serve as a robust mechanism to facilitate interoperability among legacy healthcare systems and promote better information flow among key components of the healthcare infrastructure. Entities from both inside and outside the current health IT can gain operational intelligence from FHIR-compliant data as well as from other sources of unstructured, semistructured, and structured data.

The Splunk platform supports FHIR and data interoperability through its analytics capabilities on all types of data from diverse sources. The scalable architecture allows third-party application developers to easily deploy new innovative applications in tandem with existing EHRs, data warehouses, health information exchanges, and other sources of healthcare delivery–relevant data.

Search and analytics allow for real-time queries by consumer, provider, payer, and health systems applications. The Splunk platform also facilitates system interoperability because it can connect to legacy and newer applications.

Figure 7.4 provides a high-level overview of the analytics process model. Splunk can help both in post-mortem analysis (looking at data in retrospect) and pre-mortem analysis by extracting features and applying algorithms to near real-time data.

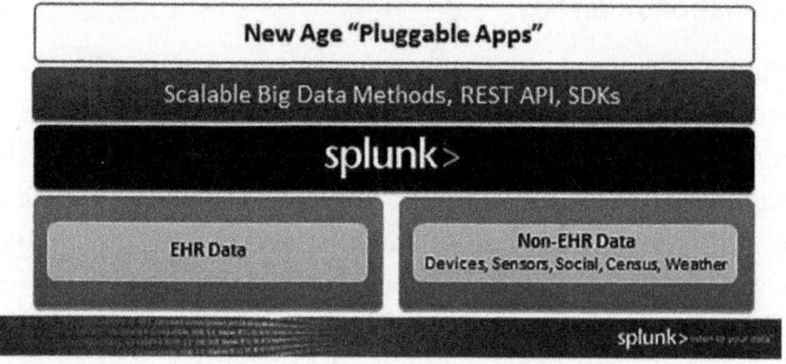

Figure 7.4 Splunk Analytics Process Model

Post-Mortem Data Analysis to Discover Knowledge

The first step is for a healthcare organization to identify a business problem or improvement opportunity, which may be discovered through the process mining of historical data. Next, all data sources that may be of potential interest must be identified. A tool that can collect data quickly from additional sources would help accelerate the cycle, as data is the key ingredient to subsequent KPI or statistical model-building exercises. Subsequently, the data may need to be normalized and transformed, or summarized for analytical questions. This step would vary for each business domain or question. For example, a caregiver for a diabetic may want different terminology for the same source data than a cardiac surgeon.

Using Splunk's dynamic normalization techniques, such as "Tagging," "Alias," and "Event Type," would help significantly, as there would be no need to apply this at the source schema level. The normalization could happen by business problem or by department. In contrast, a traditional warehouse would require the creation of multiple data marts to feed into various problems and needs. With Splunk, healthcare organizations can perform exploratory data analysis in the data preparation phase, through statistics, unsupervised learning, and visualization. They can find data quality issues and relationships among key attributes, or discover patterns in the new data, which would help prepare the right data samples for the subsequent modeling or KPI building phase. There may be unknown yet interesting and actionable patterns that can provide added insights and knowledge.

The next step would be to build KPIs or machine learning models, followed by evaluating the validity and performance of the KPI and models through consulting an expert or running the model in a limited production mode. The models could be unsupervised types, such as association rule mining or anomaly detection; or supervised types, such as classification or regression. After a couple of iterations, the KPI and models could be in production, where they would be continuously improved by feedback from operations. Figure 7.5 shows the basic process for post-mortem analysis.

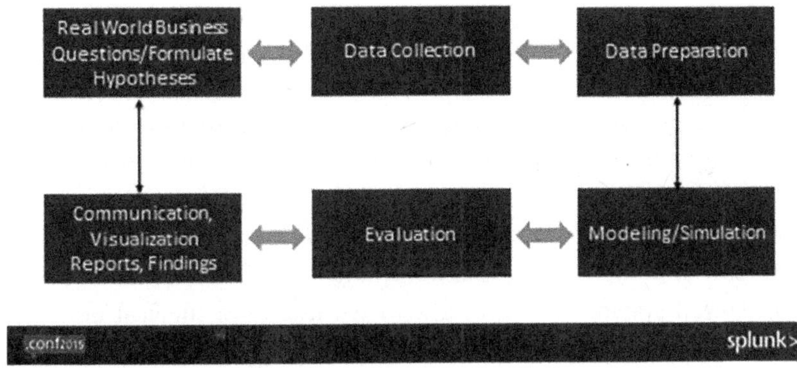

Figure 7.5 Process for Post-Mortem Analysis

Pre-Mortem Data Analysis to Apply Knowledge, Monitor Compliance, and Detect Anomalies

"Pre-mortem" refers to the cases that have not completed, where healthcare organizations have an opportunity to intervene and influence the outcome of the case, based on learnings from post-mortem analysis performed at case completion. Healthcare organizations can ingest data in near real time, extract features from the data, and apply the features to the KPI and models implemented by the post-mortem process. If the model discovers outliers or unknown patterns, it could create alerts or notable events for follow-up by an expert for corrective actions or resolution. Figure 7.6 shows the pre-mortem analysis process.

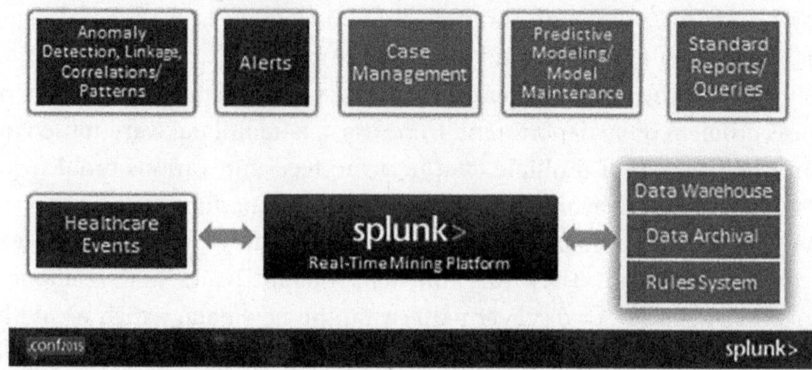

Figure 7.6 Pre-Mortem Analysis Process

Example 3: Building Resiliency into Healthcare by Monitoring Security, Privacy, and Infrastructure Reliability

Healthcare organizations rely on applications, clinical systems, and underlying IT infrastructures to deliver life-critical services. When patient records, applications, medical devices, or networks are unavailable, it can result in delays in service, diminished quality of care, and costly errors. With so many moving parts to healthcare delivery, a healthcare organization needs full, real-time visibility into the overall health of its operations.

Furthermore, patient privacy and security are essential. Emerging and advanced threats, both external and insider, have permanently changed how healthcare organizations think about cybersecurity.

Security teams at all entities within the healthcare ecosystem need an infrastructure-wide view of activities in order to identify, understand, and stop the compromise of sensitive data.

The Splunk platform provides end-to-end visibility into IT environments and their assets, by correlating and analyzing all of the relevant data sources from virtualized systems and firewalls to workstations, medical devices, and handhelds. This same data can also be used to understand a healthcare organization's security posture. Harnessing network data, endpoint data, access/identity data, and other data sources can help healthcare organizations detect contain, and remediate cyberthreats. The same data can also be used to monitor access to patient records and demonstrate compliance with healthcare regulations.

STATISTICAL ANALYSIS OF GENOMIC DATA WITH HADOOP

Since the Human Genome Project began in 2001, there has been an exponential increase in the volume of genomic data. This increase has been driven primarily by advances in sequencing technology that have brought down the price of sequencing an entire human genome from hundreds of millions of dollars to about $1,000 for a high-quality output. This increase in volume has led to considerable new demands on data storage.

The lowest-level sequencing data (fastq file format) for a single subject can occupy anywhere from 100 to 200 gigabytes (GB). With the advent of large-scale population genetics, projects like the 1,000 Genomes Project and the Cancer Genome Atlas (TCGA), sequencing and storing data for hundreds of subjects became an inevitable reality. Although the National Institutes of Health (NIH), the European Bioinformatics Institute (EMBL-EBI), and the Wellcome Trust serve as the data generators and storage hosts for these large data sets, the data sets are meant for the wider research community to download and conduct downstream analysis. Even a small subset of this data requires considerable storage space, excluding the space required for any data produced by downstream analysis. Traditionally these data sets have been stored on computing clusters at research universities using some type of parallel computing framework.

A detailed review article by Ronald Taylor explains the usefulness of Hadoop and various other distributed file systems databases in genomics [2]. Hadoop has been praised for its usefulness in terms of seamless integration on a Linux cluster, fault-tolerant system, in memory calculations that reduce I/O and therefore increase speed, and, most important, being open source.

Below we compare the two platforms, Hadoop and HPC, for efficiency and speed. Expression quantitative loci (eQTL) analysis was chosen for this comparison since this type of analysis is usually a population-scale data analysis project involving data for at least a thousand subjects.

A typical eQTL project tries to quantify the effect of genomic variation (genotype) on a quantitative trait, such as gene expression. The genotype of an individual was measured as single nucleotide polymorphisms (SNPs), which are known variable regions in the human genome. The genotype was measured for 906,600 variable regions of the genome for 1,066 cases and 111 controls. Gene expression was measured using RNA sequencing and quantification of 20,531 genes for the same number of cases and controls. eQTL analysis involves running a linear regression for each SNP and each gene combination, in this case 906,600×20,531 linear regressions. This amounts to approximately 18 billion calculations. PLINK is a population genetics tool from the Broad Institute used for this type of analysis. Optimization of this tool is achieved through parallelization techniques that require considerable manipulation of the input files and use of tools that can run parallel jobs on multiple computing nodes. The purpose of using the Hadoop framework and tools was to exclude this preprocessing requirement for input data and to achieve comparable or better efficiency.

Previously, PLINK had been used to run basic association between SNPs and gene expression on eQTL data sets. PLINK is an open source population genetics tool with capabilities for running various statistical tests on large data sets. PLINK runs on traditional HPC environments as well as any traditional computing. You can replace PLINK by utilizing Hadoop ecosystem-based tools to achieve PLINK-like functionalities and:

- Eliminate the manual work involved in "preparing" the data sets (both input for running on the HPC cores and output for analysis).
- Run faster than PLINK.
- Occupy a smaller footprint on the HDFS.
- Makes data easy to query.

The next sections provide detailed information on the steps involved in extracting the genomic data, transforming, and loading the processed eQTL data. Figure 7.7 shows the steps in the eQTL pipeline. The two primary steps in the eQTL pipeline are:

1. Extracting genomic data from online resources and transforming them to Hadoop-ready format.
2. Performing statistical analysis on the transformed data obtained from step 1 and making the output data queriable through SQL-like interfaces such as Hive.

Figure 7.7 shows the eQTL pipeline.

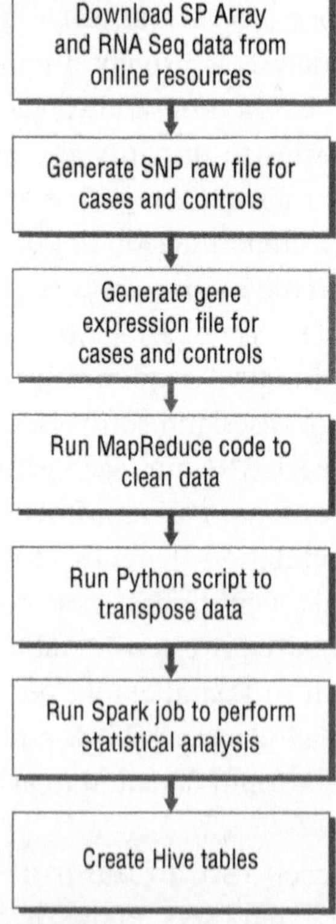

Figure 7.7 eQTL Pipeline

EXTRACTING AND TRANSFORMING GENOMIC DATA*

The filters (Disease, Data Type, Batch Number, Data Level, and Center) shown in Figure 7.8 have to be applied to download the SNP Array data. Similarly, the filters shown in Figure 7.9 have to be applied in order to download the gene expression data.

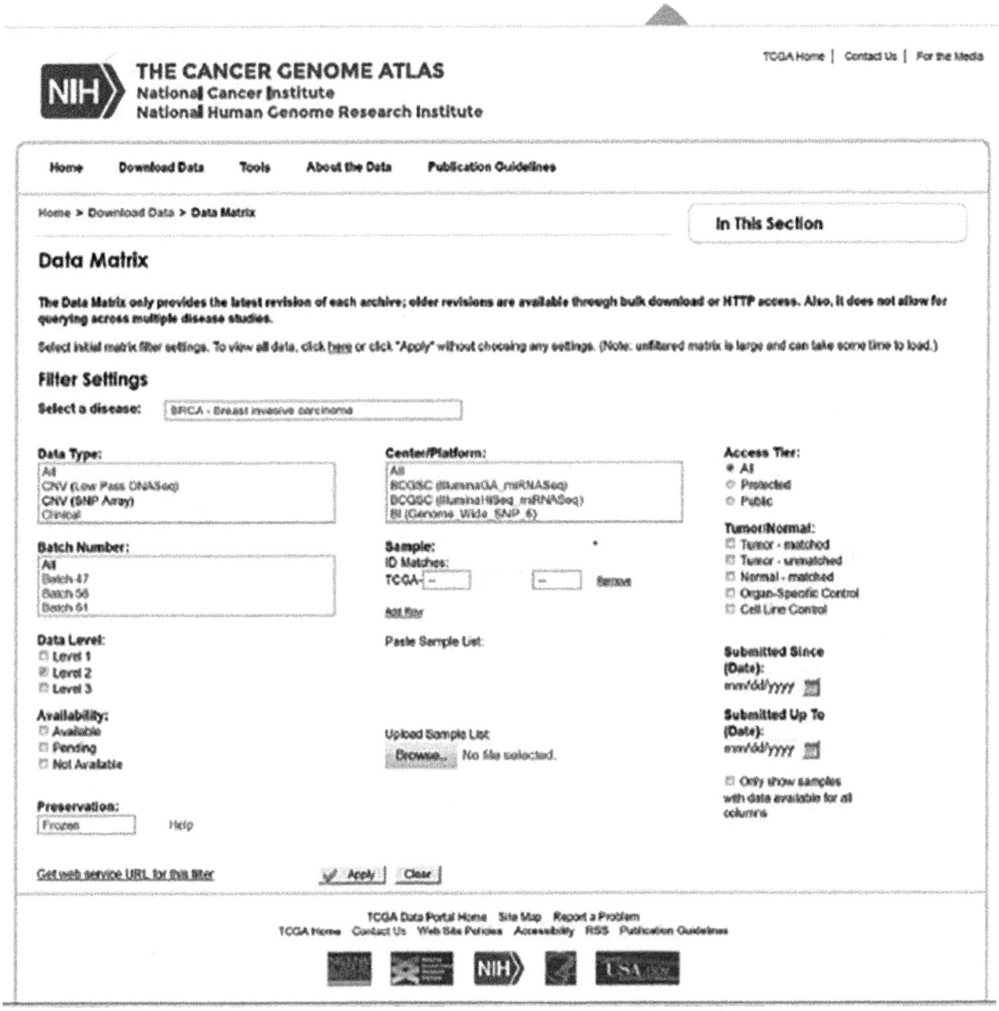

Figure 7.8 Filters Required to Download SNP Array Data

* Genomic data was downloaded from the TCGA Data Portal, https://tcga-data.nci.nih.gov/tcga/tcgaHome2.jsp.

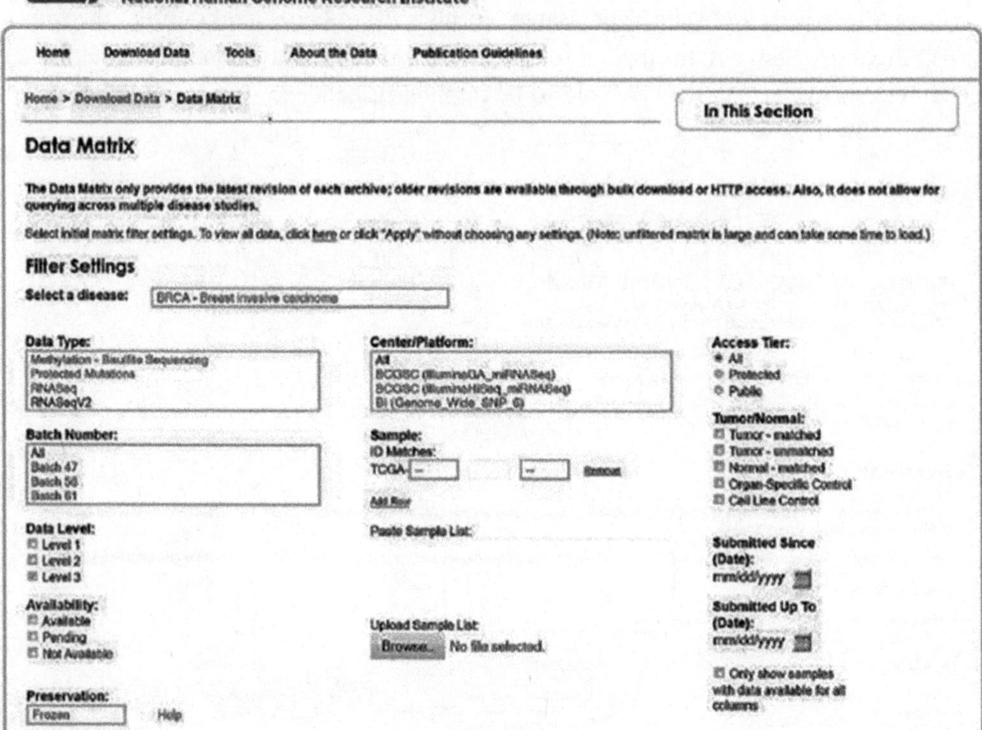

Figure 7.9 Filters Required for Gene Expression Data

The file structure of the downloaded SNP Array data and RNASeq (RNA sequencing) data is shown in Figure 7.10 and Figure 7.11, respectively.

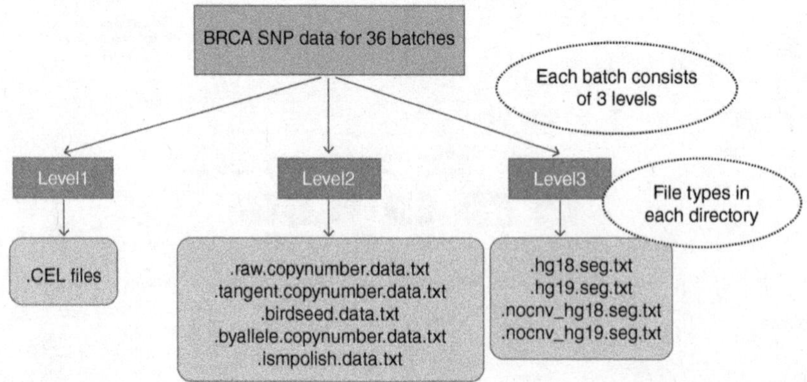

Figure 7.10 File Structure of Genotype SNP Array

The primary input data required for generating the master SNP file in a Hadoop-ready format are the files with the ".birdseed.data.txt" extension and

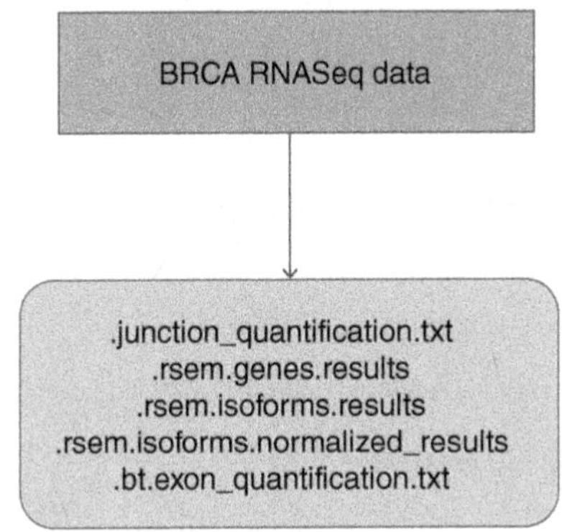

Figure 7.11 File Structure of RNASeq Data

FILE_SAMPLE_MAP.txt. The downloaded SNP Array data has 36 batches. Each batch contains files with the .birdseed.data.txt and the FILE_SAMPLE_MAP.txt. Each ".birdseed.data.txt" file contains the filename that can be cross-referenced with the filename to patient ID mapping files named in the manner of FILE_SAMPLE_MAP.txt, containing the filename to patient cross-reference records.

The primary input data required for generating the master gene expression file (controls and cases) in a Hadoop-ready format are the files with the ".rsem.genes.results" extension and the FILE_SAMPLE_MAP.txt. The counts for expression data for all patients (cases and controls) are present in the files with the .rsem.genes.results extension. The FILE_SAMPLE_MAP.txt file contains the patient IDs as columns and genes as rows, with counts for each patient under the corresponding column. Certain transformations must be performed on the FILE_SAMPLE_MAP file to extract the file name corresponding to the patient ID. The steps involved in preparation of the master SNP data and gene expression files for controls and cases are shown in Figure 7.12.

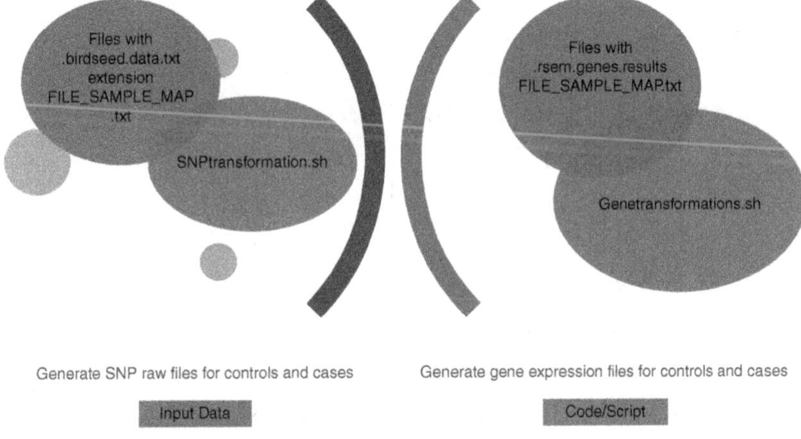

Figure 7.12 Preparation of Master SNP and Gene Expression Files for Controls and Cases

PROCESSING EQTL DATA

Input Data

The eQTL input data required for performing statistical analysis is listed next.

Controls

- SNP raw file: Size ~1.8 GB
- Gene expression size: ~37.8 megabytes (MB)
- File location: Hadoop Distributed File System (HDFS)

Cases

- SNP raw file: Size ~1.8 GB
- Gene expression size: ~361.20 MB
- File location: Hadoop Distributed File System (HDFS)

NOTE

Each patient has data for 906,600 SNPs and 20,531 gene expressions.

Software Tools

The following open source platforms and programming languages were used to process eQTL data:

- **Hadoop:** A software framework written in Java for distributed storage and distributed processing of very large data sets on computer clusters built from commodity hardware.
- **Spark:** A cluster computing framework originally developed in the AMP Lab at the University of California–Berkeley, in contrast to Hadoop's two-stage disk-based MapReduce paradigm.
- **Hive:** A data warehouse infrastructure built on top of Hadoop for providing data summarization, query, and analysis.
- **Python and Scala:** Generic high-level programming languages that can work in distributed frameworks.
- **Bash:** A UNIX shell and command language.

NGCC Hadoop Cluster Configuration

The data-intensive analysis in this example was carried out using Arizona State University's Next Generation Cyber Capability (NGCC), which includes a 44-node HDP 2.3 cluster on Dell PowerEdge 720xd servers. Each of the 40 data nodes has 128 GB RAM, 2x Intel E5–2640 12 core processors, and 22 terabytes (TB) of disk. The cluster backbone network consists of 10 Ge HA top-of-rack switching combined with Intel x520 10 Ge NICs in each server. This robust combination of server and network architecture provides the foundation for efficiently running the latest next-generation sequencing (NGS) tools and pipelines in the big data framework.

Steps to Process Data

The raw input data has to go through a set of transformations in order to use it as an input using MapReduce programs. Figure 7.13 shows the steps involved in processing the eQTL genomic data before the statistical analysis calculations.

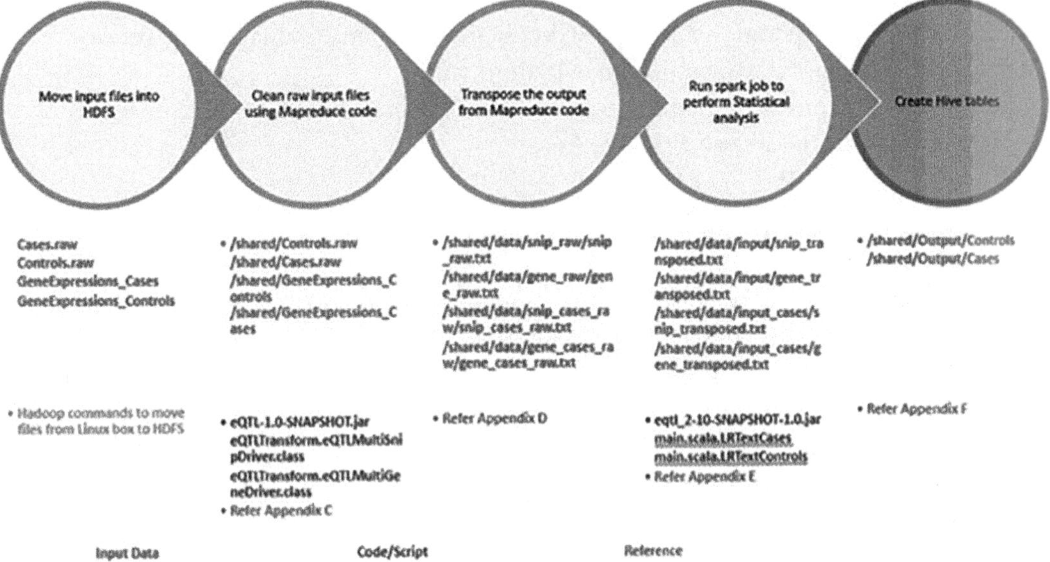

Figure 7.13 Steps Involved in the eQTL Process

Cleaning Raw Data Using MapReduce

The jar that contains the map reduce code is eQTL-1.0-SNAPSHOT.jar.

1. Remove all the patients who are not present in the gene expression file.
2. Remove all the patients from the gene expression file who are not present in the SNP file.

The output of the first step contains two files:

- SNP Header, which contains the header of the original SNP
- SNP Data, which contains the data of patients who are also present in the gene expression file

The SNP header file and SNP data file can be combined into a single file using the "cat" command in Linux. The output of the second step contains two files:

- Gene Header, which contains the header of the original gene expression file

- Gene Data, which contains the data of patients who are only present in the original SNP file

The Gene Header file and the Gene Data file can be commanded using the "cat" command in Linux.

More information on the input file formats and the code used to submit MapReduce jobs on the Hadoop cluster can be found below in the section "Cleaning Raw Data Using MapReduce."

Data Transpose Using Python

The snp_raw.txt and the gene_raw.txt obtained from the data cleaning process as described are transposed using a Python script.

The Python script used to perform data transpose can be found below in the section "Transpose Data Using Python."

Statistical Analysis in Spark

The transposed SNP and Gene files obtained from the previous step are used as inputs to the Scala code to perform statistical analysis using Spark.

The jar that contains the Scala code is eqtl_2.-10-SNAPSHOT-1.0.jar. The jar can be either in the local file system or in the HDFS. The Scala code collects the SNP data for each individual (cases or controls) and maps it to each gene expression of the corresponding individual, thus generating approximately 18 billion combinations of SNP and Gene. Once this mapping is done, statistical analysis is performed on each (SNP + Gene) combination across all patients to generate these statistics:

- Single nucleotide polymorphisms (SNP)
- Gene expression (Gene)
- Beta1 for linear regression
- Beta0 for linear regression
- Coefficient of determination (R2)
- Standard error of Beta1 (StdErrBeta1)
- Standard error of Beta0 (StdErrBeta0)
- Total sum of squares (SSTO)
- Error sum of squares (SSE)
- Sum of squares (SSR)
- Sample size
- p-value (yet to be implemented in the code)

The input file formats used in the Spark job and the code used to submit Spark jobs on the cluster for both cases and controls can be found below in the section "Statistical Analysis Using Spark."

Create Hive Tables

Hive tables are created for high-speed querying of the statistical results. The Hive tables are partitioned at the gene expression level. The Apache Tez (https:// tez.apache.org/) execution engine provided significant performance gains over MapReduce. Parquet tables were utilized to reduce storage overhead and are common to other distributed genomic software products. The Apache Tez project is aimed at building an application framework that allows for a complex directed-acyclic graph of tasks for processing data. It is built atop Apache Hadoop YARN.

GENERATING MASTER SNP FILES FOR CASES AND CONTROLS

The steps involved in transforming the downloaded SNP Sequence data into individual expression files for controls and cases are shown next.

SSH to hadoop.ngcc.asu.edu and type:

- cd /home/project/SNPtransformation/
- ./SNPtransformation.sh (./ should not be ignored)

The primary inputs required for generating the SNP expressions file for controls and cases are:

- Files with .birdseed.data.txt extension
- FILE_SAMPLE_MAP.txt

Input Data Format

A sample input from files with extension "birdseed.data.txt" is shown in Figure 7.14.

```
Hybridization REF        GAMMA_p_TCGA_b103_104_SNP_N_GenomeWideSNP_6_B03_755950   GAMMA_p_TCGA_b103_104_SNP_N_GenomeWideSNP_6_B03_755950
Composite Element REF    Call     Confidence
SNP_A-2131660    1       0.0020
SNP_A-1967418    2       0.0026
SNP_A-1969580    2       0.0049
```

Figure 7.14 Sample Input

Sample lines from files with extension ".birdseed.data.txt" are shown in Figure 7.15.

```
filename          barcode(s)
GAMMA_p_TCGA_b103_104_SNP_N_GenomeWideSNP_6_B03_755950.CEL      TCGA-BH-A1EV-11A-24D-A134-01
GAMMA_p_TCGA_b103_104_SNP_N_GenomeWideSNP_6_B04_755920.CEL      TCGA-C8-A1HI-01A-11D-A134-01
GAMMA_p_TCGA_b103_104_SNP_N_GenomeWideSNP_6_B05_755900.CEL      TCGA-BH-A1F0-01A-11D-A134-01
GAMMA_p_TCGA_b103_104_SNP_N_GenomeWideSNP_6_B06_755792.CEL      TCGA-C8-A1HF-10A-01D-A134-01
```

Figure 7.15 Sample Map

Note:

- **SNPtransformation.sh** contains the script to transform the SNP Expression data into Hadoop-ready format.
- The arguments marked in **bold** in the "SNPtransformation.sh" file are user-defined and should contain the .birdseed.data.txt and FILE_SAMPLE.MAP.txt.

- The total time taken for this process to complete in the distributed environment is **approximately** 3 hours.
- The final output files from the above "SNPtransformation" process are **Cases.raw** and **Controls.raw**.
- **Cases.raw** and **Controls.raw** files are moved into the "shared" directory on the HDFS. The user can change the location by editing the **SNPtransformation.sh.**

GENERATING GENE EXPRESSION FILES FOR CASES AND CONTROLS

The steps involved in transforming the downloaded RNA Sequence data into individual gene expression files for controls and cases are shown next.

SSH to hadoop.ngcc.asu.edu and type:

- cd/home/project/Genetransformation/
- cp/home/project/Genetransformation/Genetransformation.sh**/home/username/RNASeq/**Genetransformation.sh
- cp/home/project/Genetransformation/row_col_mapping.awk **/home/username/RNASeq/**row_col_mapping.awk
- cp/home/project/Genetransformation/transpose.awk **/home/username/RNASeq/**transpose.awk
- cd/home/username/RNASeq/
- ./Genetransformation.sh (./ should not be ignored)

The primary inputs required for generating the gene expression file for controls and cases are:

- Files with .rsem.gene.results extension
- FILE_SAMPLE_MAP.txt

Input Data Format

Files with .rsem.gene.results extension can be seen in Figure 7.16.

```
gene_id raw_count   scaled_estimate transcript_id
?|100130426 0.00    0   uc011lsn.1
?|100133144 25.01   1.10349379851693e-06    uc010unu.1,uc010uoa.1
?|100134869 60.99   1.95660236963926e-06    uc002bgz.2,uc002bic.2
```

Figure 7.16 Sample Input

FILE_SAMPLE_MAP.TXT as seen in Figure 7.17.

```
filename    barcode(s)
unc.edu.000d877f-8d03-44bc-8607-27b5ba84b5fe.1165098.junction_quantification.txt    TCGA-E9-A1RD-11A-33R-A157-07
unc.edu.000d877f-8d03-44bc-8607-27b5ba84b5fe.1167702.rsem.genes.results TCGA-E9-A1RD-11A-33R-A157-07
unc.edu.000d877f-8d03-44bc-8607-27b5ba84b5fe.1167703.rsem.isoforms.results  TCGA-E9-A1RD-11A-33R-A157-07
```

Figure 7.17 Sample Map

Note:

- **Genetransformation** contains the script to transform the RNASeq data into Hadoop-ready format.
- The arguments marked in **bold** are user-defined and should contain the .rsem.genes.results and FILE_SAMPLE.MAP.txt.
- The total time taken for this process to complete in the distributed environment is ~10 minutes.
- The final output files from the **"Genetransformation"** processes are **GeneExpression_Cases** and **GeneExpression_Controls**.
- GeneExpression_Cases and GeneExpression_Controls files are moved into the "shared" directory on the HDFS. The user can change the location by editing the Genetransformation.sh.

CLEANING RAW DATA USING MAPREDUCE

The MapReduce code accepts two input files:

- Controls or cases raw file
- Gene expression file
- See Table 7.1: Input Data

Table 7.1 Input Data

Type	SNP Input	Number of Individuals	Gene Expression Input	Number of Individuals
Controls	/shared/Controls.raw	1,078	/shared/GeneExpression_Controls	111
Cases	/shared/Cases.raw	1,078	/shared/GeneExpression_Cases	1,066

Input Data Format

A sample input SNP data for both case and control subjects is shown in Figure 7.18.

```
FID SNP_A-8282305_A SNP_A-8282305_A ....
A1IH-01 0 0 ......
A1IH-02 0 0 .....
```

Figure 7.18 SNP Data—Sample Inputs

Figure 7.19 shows the gene expression file.

```
FID  ZDHHC17_23390 RND2_8153
A1RC-01  5.30037944695518 3.05356813862792
A8OP-01  5.41801393515548 1.84499104774585
```

Figure 7.19 Gene Expression File—Sample Inputs

Note:

- The location of the input files on the HDFS is user-defined.

MapReduce Code: Controls

SSH to hadoop.ngcc.asu.edu and type:

- hadoop jar eQTL-1.0-SNAPSHOT.jar eQTLTransform.eQTLMultiSnipDriver **/shared/Controls.raw**
- **/shared/GeneExpression_Controls** /shared/data/snip_raw
- Output Files: snipHeader-r-00000 & snipData-r-00000

The output files can be combined into one file using the next script:

```
hadoop fs -cat /shared/data/snip_raw/snipHeader-r-00000
/shared/data/snip_raw/snipData-r-00000 | hadoop fs -put -
/shared/data/snip_raw/snip_raw.txt
```

- hadoopjareQTL-1.0-SNAPSHOT.jareQTLTransform.eQTLMultiGeneDriver/ **shared/Controls.raw**
- **/shared/GeneExpression_Controls** /shared/data/gene_raw
- Output files: geneHeader-r-00000 & geneData-r-00000

The output files can be combined into one file using the next script:

```
hadoop fs -cat /shared/data/gene_raw/geneHeader-r-00000
/shared/data/gene_raw/geneData-r-00000 | hadoop fs -put -
/shared/data/gene_raw/gene_raw.txt
```

Note:

- The total time taken for this process to complete in the distributed environment is ~2 minutes.
- The user should strictly comply with the order in which the arguments (input and output) are specified in the preceding scripts.

Cases

SSH to hadoop.ngcc.asu.edu and type:

- hadoop jar eQTL-1.0-SNAPSHOT.jar *eQTLTransform.eQTLMultiSnipDriver* /shared/Cases.raw /shared/GeneExpression_Cases
- /shared/data/snip_cases_raw
- Output Files: snipHeader-r-00000 & snipData-r-00000

The output files can be combined into one file using the next script:

```
hadoop fs -cat /shared/data/snip_cases_raw/snipHeader-r-00000
/shared/data/snip_cases_raw/snipData-r-00000 | hadoop fs -put -
/shared/data/snip_cases_raw/snip_cases_raw.txt
```

- hadoopjareQTL-1.0-SNAPSHOT.jareQTLTransform.eQTLMultiGeneDriver/ **shared/Controls.raw**
- **/shared/GeneExpression_Controls** /shared/data/gene_cases_raw
- Output files: geneHeader-r-00000 & geneData-r-00000

The output files can be combined into one file using the next script:

```
hadoop fs -cat /shared/data/gene_cases_raw/geneHeader-r-00000
/shared/data/gene_cases_raw/geneData-r-00000 | hadoop fs -put -
/shared/data/gene_cases_raw/gene_cases_raw.txt
```

Note:

- The argument (after Hadoop jar) is the jar file.
- The argument in *italics* is the main driver class.
- The arguments marked in **bold** are the input files and the filenames can be user-defined.
- The user should strictly comply with the order in which the arguments (input and output) are specified in the preceding scripts.
- The argument underlined is the output directory and the directory name can be user-defined. The output file for both cases and controls should only contain data for patients who are present in both the SNP file and the gene expression file.
- The total time taken for this process to complete in the distributed environment is ~5 minutes.

TRANSPOSE DATA USING PYTHON

The combined SNP files and gene expression files for both cases and controls are used as input files to the scripts written in Python.

Controls

SSH to hadoop.ngcc.asu.edu and type:

- hadoop fs -get **/shared/data/snip_raw/snip_raw.txt** snip_raw.txt
- python -c "import sys; print('\n'.join(' '.join(c) for c in zip(*(l.split() for l in sys.stdin.readlines() if l.strip()))))" < snip_raw.txt | tail -n +7
- | hadoop fs -put—/shared/data/input/snip_transposed.txt

Figure 7.20 shows sample output from a transposed SNP file.

```
SNP_A-8282305_A 0 0 0 0
SNP_A-8282312_G 0 1 0 0
```

Figure 7.20 Sample Output from Transposed SNP File

- hadoop fs -get /shared/data/gene_raw/gene_raw.txt gene_raw.txt
- python -c "import sys; print('\n'.join(' '.join(c) for c in zip(*(l.split() for l in sys.stdin.readlines() if l.strip()))))" < gene_raw.txt | tail -n
- +3 | hadoop fs -put—/shared/data/input/gene_transposed.txt

Figure 7.21 shows sample output from a transposed gene file.

```
ELMO1 1.117413333 0.430333333 0.437833333 1.141333333
CREB3L1 -0.15115 0.4445 1.88115 1.781
RPS11 1.1 -0.1 0 0.1375
```

Figure 7.21 Sample Output from Transposed Gene File

Cases

SSH to hadoop.ngcc.asu.edu and type:

- hadoop fs -get /shared/data/snip_cases_raw/snip_cases_raw.txt snip_cases_raw.txt
- python -c "import sys; print('\n'.join(' '.join(c) for c in zip(*(l.split() for l in sys.stdin.readlines() if l.strip()))))" < snip_cases_raw.txt | tail -n +7 | hadoop fs -put—/shared/data/input_cases/snip_cases_transposed.txt
- hadoop fs -get **/shared/data/gene_cases_raw/gene_cases_raw.txt** gene_cases_raw.txt
- python -c "import sys; print('\n'.join(' '.join(c) for c in zip(*(l.split() for l in sys.stdin.readlines() if l.strip()))))" < gene_cases_raw.txt | tail -n +3 | hadoop fs -put—/shared/data/input_cases/gene_cases_transposed.txt

Note:

- The arguments marked in **bold** are the input files.
- The arguments underlined are the output directory. The output file for both cases and controls should only contain data for patients who are present in both the SNP file and the gene expression file.
- The user should strictly comply with the order in which the arguments (input and output) are specified in the preceding scripts.
- The total time taken for this process to complete in the Linux environment is ~5 minutes.

STATISTICAL ANALYSIS USING SPARK

The transposed SNP and gene expression files for both cases and controls are used as input files to the scripts written in Scala. The Scala code is executed in Apache Spark. The Scala code performs a cross join between the SNP and gene expression file in memory, as shown in Figure 7.22.

```
(SNP_A-8282305_A,ELMO1),(0,1.117413333),(0,0.430333333),(0,0.437833333),(0,1.141333333)
(SNP_A-8282312_G,CREB3L1),(0,-0.15115),(1,0.4445),(0,1.88115),(0,1.781)
(SNP_A-8282305_A,CREB3L1),(0,-0.15115),(0,0.4445),(0,1.88115),(0,1.781)
(SNP_A-8282312_G,ELMO1),(0,1.117413333),(1,0.430333333),(0,0.437833333),(0,1.141333333)
(SNP_A-8282305_A,RPS11),(0,1.1),(0,-0.1),(0,0),(0,0.1375)
(SNP_A-8282312_G,RPS11),(0,1.1),(1,-0.1),(0,0),(0,0.1375)
```

Figure 7.22 Sample Output of Cross Join between SNP and Gene Expression Data

The Scala code then performs statistical analysis on each record with the first column as key (e.g.: SNP_A-8282305_A, ELMO1). The Spark script used to run the job for controls and cases is shown later.

Launching Spark Applications

Once a user application is bundled, it can be launched using the `bin/spark-submit` script. This script takes care of setting up the class path with Spark and its dependencies and can support different cluster managers and deploy modes that Spark supports.

Some commonly used options are:

spark-submit—class <main-class>—master <master-url>—deploy-mode <deploy-mode>—conf <key>=<value> <application-jar> [application-arguments]

Where:

- spark-submit: The script used to launch applications on a cluster
- —class: The entry point for your application
- —master: The master URL for the cluster, which can be yarn-client or yarn-cluster
- —deploy-mode: Whether to deploy your driver on the worker nodes (cluster) or locally as an external client (client)
- —conf: Spark configuration property in key=value format
- application-jar: Path to a bundled jar including your application and all dependencies. The URL must be globally visible inside of your cluster—for instance, an hdfs:// path or a file:// path that is present on all nodes.
- application-arguments: Arguments passed to the main method of your main class, if any (input and output file location on hdfs).

Configuration

The next list provides a brief description of the configuration parameters typically used in submitting a Spark job.

- —driver.memory: Amount of memory to use for the driver process

- —executor.memory: Amount of memory to use per executor process, in the same format as Java Virtual Machine JVM memory strings (e.g., 512m, 2g).
- —executor-cores: Number of cores to use for the executor process (Min=1; Max=24)
- —num-executors: Number of executors to use for the Spark job (Min=1; Max=40)
- —spark.shuffle.spill: If set to "true," limits the amount of memory used during reduces by spilling data out to disk.
- —spark.shuffle.compress: If set to "true," compress map output files.

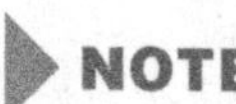

More information on submitting Spark applications and Spark configurations can be found in the latest Spark Documentation Reference at http://spark.apache.org/docs/latest/index.html.

Controls

SSH to hadoop.ngcc.asu.edu and type:

- source /etc/spark/conf/spark-1.3.1-env.sh
- spark-submit—*class main.scala.LRTextControls*—master yarn—deploy-mode client—driver-memory 2G—executor-memory 2G—executor-cores 20—conf spark.shuffle.spill=false—conf spark.shuffle.compress=true—num-executors 30 eqtl_2.-10-SNAPSHOT- 1.0.jar **"/shared/data/input/snip_transposed.txt" "/shared/data/input/gene_transposed.txt"** "/shared/Output/ Controls"

Cases

SSH to hadoop.ngcc.asu.edu and type:

- source /etc/spark/conf/spark-1.3.1-env.sh
- spark-submit—*class main.scala.LRTextCases—master yarn—deploy-mode client*—**driver-memory 2G—executor-memory 2G—executor-cores 20**—*conf spark.shuffle.spill=false—conf spark.shuffle.compress=true*—**num-executors 30** eqtl_2–10-SNAPSHOT- 1.0.jar"**/shared/data/input_cases/snip_cases_transposed.txt""/shared/data/input_cases/gene_cases_transposed.txt**" "/shared/Output/Cases"

Note:

- The argument (.jar) is the jar file.
- The argument marked in *italics* is the main driver class.

- The arguments marked in *italics underlined* **cannot be modified**.
- The arguments marked in **bold underlined can be modified**.
- The arguments underlined are the output directory. The output file for both cases and controls should only contain data for patients who are present in both the SNP file and the gene expression file.
- Parametric analyses on the driver and executor memory have indicated that the lower limit for **driver memory** and **executor memory** is 2 Gb. An upper limit of 70 Gb is recommended. The maximum memory allocated to both driver and executor cannot be higher than the maximum memory capability of the cluster, which in this case was 80G.
- The user should strictly comply with the order in which the arguments (input and output) are specified in the above scripts.
- The total run time for cases and controls depends only on the job input data size and configuration parameters, such as number of cores and number of executors.
- The greater the number of patient data present in the input files, the longer the computation time is.
- The greater the number of cores and executors used, the shorter the run time is.
- The total time taken for performing the statistical analysis on controls data using less than 10% of the cluster capacity is ~40 minutes.
- The total time taken for performing statistical analysis on cases data using less than 10% of the cluster capacity is ~6 hours.

Final Output Size

The output of the statistical analyses on controls and cases is stored in Text format. The size of the output files is shown below and in Table 7.2.

Cases: ~2.50 TB   Controls: ~2.50 TB

Table 7.2 Output Data

Sample Output						
(Controls/Cases)						
SNP_A-8282305_A RND2_8153 -0.021808512098153 53.9787064977852 53.97777641366092	2.2474332131413113 9.300841243179136E-4	1.723057451100789E-5	0.5600555170300798	0.0834881471502032		
SNP_A-8282305_A	MBNL2_10150	-0.22274966702461896	7.2014428482666535	0.005145679382640419	0.330167340351476	0.04921844113174725
18.856520722881772	18.7594911129697	0.0970296099120645				$\bar{s}$

HIVE TABLES WITH PARTITIONS

Hive tables are created from the statistical results for further high-speed analysis and queries. The tables can be created by following the steps shown next.

Controls

SSH to hadoop.ngcc.asu.edu and type:

- hive
- set hive.execution.engine=tez;
- use eqtl;
- Create an external table Controls_Text in the eqtl database

```
drop table if exists eqtl. Controls_Text;
CREATE  EXTERNAL  TABLE  if  not  exists  eqtl.  Controls_Text
(snip  STRING,  gene  STRING,beta1  Float,beta0  Float,r2
Float,stderrbeta1 Float,stderrbeta0 Float, ssto FLOAT, sse FLOAT,
ssr FLOAT)  LOCATION '/shared/Output/Controls';
```

- Create a partitioned table eqtl.TCGA_Controls_Birdseed

```
create table if not exists eqtl.TCGA_Controls_Birdseed
(snip STRING,beta1 Float,beta0 Float,r2 Float,stderrbeta1
Float,stderrbeta0 Float, ssto FLOAT, sse FLOAT, ssr FLOAT)
partitioned by (gene string comment 'gene or genotype')
STORED AS PARQUET;
```

- Insert data into the partitioned table:

```
INSERT into table eqtl. Controls partition (gene)   select snip,
beta1, beta0, r2, stderrbeta1, stderrbeta0, ssto, sse, ssr, gene
from Controls_Text distribute by gene;
```

- Pass a simple query:

```
select * from Controls where snip='rs2142791_T' and gene='ARL1_400';
```

Sample output:

```
rs2142791_T  0.045971  6.72284  0.02151577   0.0330481  0.04107084977
4.6155037  4.51619758  0.0993061  ARL1_400
```

Cases

SSH to hadoop.ngcc.asu.edu and type:

- hive
- set hive.execution.engine=tez;

- Create an external table Cases_Text in the eqtl database:

```
drop table if exists eqtl. Cases_Text;
CREATE EXTERNAL TABLE if not exists eqtl. Cases_Text (snip
STRING, gene STRING,beta1 Float,beta0 Float,r2 Float,stderrbeta1
Float,stderrbeta0 Float, ssto FLOAT, sse FLOAT, ssr FLOAT)
LOCATION '/shared/Output/Cases';
Create a partitioned table eqtl.TCGA_Cases_Birdseed drop  table if
exists eqtl. Cases;
create table if not exists eqtl.TCGA_Cases_Birdseed (snip
STRING,beta1 Float,beta0 Float,r2 Float,stderrbeta1
Float,stderrbeta0 Float, ssto FLOAT, sse FLOAT, ssr FLOAT)
partitioned by (gene string comment 'gene or genotype')
STORED AS PARQUET;
```

- Insert data into the partitioned table:

```
INSERT into table eqtl. Cases partition (gene) select snip,
beta1, beta0, r2, stderrbeta1, stderrbeta0, ssto, sse, ssr,
gene from Cases_Text distribute by gene;
```

- Pass a simple query:

```
select * from Cases where snip='rs2142791_T' and gene='ARL1_400';
```

Sample output:

```
rs2142791_T  0.051222075  7.0404625  0.005135634  0.021907581
0.025987623  310.62793  309.03256  1.5952713  ARL1_400
```

Note:

- The database in which the Hive tables are created is **eqtl** (e.g., eqtl .Controls or eqtl.Cases in the Hive script).
- The total size of the controls and cases data in the Parquet format are **1.36 TB and 780 GB**, respectively. This indicates that storing the data in the Parquet format reduces the storage footprint on the HDFS significantly.

Summary

The total time taken to complete the data processing for controls and cases, starting with cleaning the data using the MapReduce code and creating a Give table, is ~2 hours and ~7.5 hours, respectively. The transition from traditional HPC to Hadoop (MapReduce) allows greater parallelization and therefore more worker threads, reducing the time to results. The move to Apache Spark or running in memory once again provides additional performance enhancements and includes the dynamic parallelization quality.

CONCLUSION

Data science is an immense and rapidly changing field. In this chapter we hope to have oriented you to some of its statistical and mathematical underpinnings in addition to acquainting you with some widely used and very useful tools. These tools include various NoSQL offerings, Splunk, and Apache Spark. Following this chapter is a case study describing UC Irvine's Hortonworks Data Platform, which has made the university's archive of clinical data far more accessible.

NOTES

1. Fay Chang, Jeffrey Dean, Sanjay Ghemawat, et al. 2008. "Bigtable." *ACM Transactions on Computer Systems* 26, no. 2: 1–26. doi: 10.1145/1365815.1365816.
2. Ronald C. Taylor. 2010. "An Overview of the Hadoop/MapReduce/HBase Framework and Its Current Applications in Bioinformatics." *BMC Bioinformatics* 11, Suppl. 12. doi: 10.1186/1471-2105-11-s12-s1.

CASE STUDY

CASE STUDY 10: UC IRVINE HEALTH'S HORTONWORKS DATA PLATFORM

Hortonworks, Santa Clara, California

UC Irvine Health (UCIH) turned to Hadoop and Hortonworks Data Platform to improve clinical operations in the hospital and its scientific research at the medical school. Their team is building a quantified medical practice that reduces readmissions, speeds new research projects, and tracks patient vital statistics on a minute-by-minute basis.

ONE HADOOP PLATFORM FOR TWO DIFFERENT MISSIONS

The Clinical Informatics Group (CIG) at UCIH was founded in 2009 to provide high-quality information in support of the pioneering work done by researchers and clinicians at UC Irvine. The CIG began its journey toward Hadoop with an assessment of data storage.

Some data was scattered across multiple Excel spreadsheets. UCIH also had 9 million semistructured records for 1.2 million patients over 22 years, none of which was searchable or retrievable. These semistructured records included dictated radiology reports, pathology reports, and rounding notes—very valuable, in aggregate. But it was not accessible in the aggregate.

The CIG first migrated data from that "low-tech" platform to an enterprise data warehouse with integrated clinical business intelligence tools. Then it migrated again to its current modern data architecture on Hadoop, on Hortonworks Data Platform (HDP).

The single Hadoop data lake at UC Irvine Health allows the CIG to make good on its "no data left behind" doctrine and serves two different constituents: The UC Irvine School of Medicine for medical research and the UC Irvine Medical Center for the quality of its clinical practice. The medical school and the hospital have distinct big data use cases, but they are both served by a unified data platform with HDP at its core.

Charles Boicey, UC Irvine's information solutions architect, describes the efficiency of serving different stakeholders with the same comprehensive data platform:

> Hadoop is the only technology that allows healthcare to store data in its native form. If Hadoop didn't exist we would still have to make decisions about what can come into our data warehouse or the electronic medical record (and what cannot). Now we can bring everything into Hadoop, regardless of data format or speed of ingest. If I find a new data source, I can start storing it the day that I learn about it. We leave no data behind.

Now back to those 9 million semistructured legacy records. They are now searchable and retrievable in the Hadoop Distributed File System (HDFS). This allowed the UCIH team to turn off their legacy system that was used for view only, saving them more than $500,000.

SOLUTIONS FOR CLINICIANS

The CIG has already launched two new data-driven programs, one to reduce patient readmittance and another to monitor patient vitals in real time.

Predictive Analytics to Reduce Readmittance

One of UCIH's goals is to predict the likelihood of hospital readmittance within 30 days after discharge. Patients with congestive heart failure have a tendency to build up fluid, which causes them to gain weight. Rapid weight gain over a one- to two-day period is a sign that something is wrong and that the patient should see a doctor.

UCIH collaborated with medical device integration partner iSirona to develop a program that sends those heart patients home with a scale and instructions to weigh themselves once daily. The weight data is wirelessly transmitted to Hadoop, where an algorithm determines which weight changes indicate risk of readmittance. The system notifies clinicians about only those cases. All home monitoring data will be viewable in the electronic medical record via an API to Hadoop.

UCIH chose Hortonworks over competitors like Cloudera and MapR because of its commitment to 100% open source Hadoop. This openness makes collaboration with systems partners like iSirona easier. The group also appreciated HDP's unique Windows compatibility. "Healthcare is cost conscious so a proprietary Hadoop infrastructure with unclear future costs will not work for us. Hortonworks was healthcare friendly from the first phone call."

(*Continued*)

(*Continued*)

Real-Time Surveillance for Rapid Response

In a typical hospital, nurses manually measure patient vital signs every few hours. The health of their patients may change in the hours between two vital sign measurements.

In January 2015, the medical center began piloting a new technology called SensiumVitals to monitor and transmit patient vital signs *every minute*. Patients in the pilot wear a SensiumVitals patch that monitors and wirelessly transmits heart rate, respiratory rate, and temperature. Nurses are alerted if any of a patient's vital signs cross certain risk thresholds, so the staff can attend to the patient immediately.

From a long-term perspective, this sensor data enables something much more profound: predictive analytics that can allow caregivers to respond before a patient's vital signs ever cross a dangerous threshold.

Most of those minute-by-minute snapshots of vital signs will be unremarkable, but the data points they generate (4,320 per patient per day) are the building blocks for algorithms that can predict near-term outcomes with an ever-increasing degree of certainty. Like the previous example with heart patients, this data reduces average time to insight for important medical decisions the staff needs to make.

This is because an increased temperature, heart rate, or respiratory rate in isolation of other data may not be cause for concern. But those same vitals, combined with all of the prior data on that patient, combined with years of data on other patients with similar risk factors, combined with unique characteristics of that patient's medical history, physical characteristics, gender, and age—all of that will eventually paint a far more detailed picture, with more predictive power.

Again, Boicey:

> For healthcare, we have never had the ability to do this. We have always taken the approach that we think we know what data elements are important. Now with all the data, we let the data determine what is important for predictive analysis. Yogi Berra might have said it like this: We are now able to capture the data that we know that we need as well as the data that someday we will know that we needed.

SOLUTIONS FOR RESEARCHERS

Researchers at the medical school will be using HDP for cohort discovery. For example, a biomedical researcher on prostate cancer may want to identify males between the ages of 45 and 55 who:

- Had prostate cancer at a certain stage,
- Underwent a prostatectomy, and
- Are taking a certain class of drugs.

Then researchers can easily present the anonymous sample cohort to their internal review board for approval, without ever having seen uniquely identifiable information. This speeds the process of preparing and approving a study while ensuring patient confidentiality.

FUTURE PLANS

UC Irvine Health has already benefited from integrating the Hortonworks Data Platform into its modern data architecture. Now UCIH is ready to tackle additional use cases.

UCIH plans to extend its research capabilities with data mining and data exploration. Now that the group has all of the data in one data lake, it can find previously undiscovered factors that are indicative of a certain outcome.

It also plans to include genomic data in the future.

New research made possible by this combined data will be shared with other practitioners and policy makers as they review publications that come out of the medical school.

For its biomedical device maintenance, the team wants to use geolocation and sensor data to better manage its medical equipment. The biomedical team needs to know where all the equipment is, so time is not wasted searching for an item.

Over time, the team can determine the usage of different devices. For example, the biomedical engineers will know how often a heart monitor is being used. They can use this information to make rational decisions about when to repair or replace the monitor.

ABOUT UCIH

UC Irvine Health (UCIH) is a team of nationally regarded physicians and nurses, researchers and clinicians, educators and students united by a single calling—to improve the lives of the people in Orange County, California, and beyond.

As the only university-based care provider in Orange County, UC Irvine Health's multifaceted organization is dedicated to the discovery of new medical frontiers, to the teaching of future healers, and to the delivery of the finest evidence-based care. The union of discovery, teaching, and healing gives them the expertise to diagnose and treat exceedingly rare conditions and diseases.

CASE STUDY

CASE STUDY 11: THE EXTENT OF SUBCLONAL VARIATION IS PREDICTED BY THE NUMBER OF DISTINCT DOMINANT CLONES

Diego Chowell, James Napier, Rohan Gupta, Karen S. Anderson, Carlo C. Maley, and Melissa A. Wilson Sayres

Genome sequencing has revolutionized our understanding of the process of somatic evolution in cancer. Increasing evidence shows that tumor clonal architectures

(*Continued*)

(*Continued*)

are often the consequence of a complex branched subclonal process. Yet little is known about the expected dynamics and the extent to which these divergent subclonal expansions occur. Here we study intratumor subclonal heterogeneity and its impact on treatment resistance by developing and implementing more than 88,000 realizations of a stochastic evolutionary model simulating the process. Under different combinations of the population genetic parameter values, including those that have been previously estimated for colorectal cancer and glioblastoma multiforme, our results show that the distribution of sizes of subclones carrying driver mutations has a heavy right tail at the time of tumor detection, with only one to four dominant clones present at ≥10% frequency, composing most of the tumor cell population. In contrast, our model also predicts that the vast majority of subclones will be present at <10% frequency. We find that these minor, and often undetectable, subclones can harbor treatment-resistant mutations. In our analysis, the number of dominant clones (≥10%) in a tumor has a strong correlation with the number of minor subclones. Model predictions are consistent with empirical data on the number of dominant clones at detectable levels across different cancer types. Our results contribute to explaining why tumors with greater numbers of detectable clonal populations are associated with poorer prognosis in multiple types of cancer.

Cancer, a subclonal evolutionary process, is governed by the dynamic interplay of mutation, stochastic drift, and selection [1, 2, 3, 4, 5]. Although most mutations that steadily accumulate in our cells are neutral or weakly deleterious, a fraction of these mutations in a gene or a regulatory element can confer a selective advantage to the cell by increasing its fitness [6, 7, 8, 9] and in cancers can result in increased survival of a clone [6, 10, 11]. In the field of cancer biology, the term "driver mutation" is used to refer to mutations that increase cell fitness (and thus are increased in frequency due to positive selection) [6, 12]. The term "passenger mutation" is used for mutations that are neutral or deleterious [6, 12, 13] and increase in frequency due to hitchhiking alongside driver mutations. A common model for the evolutionary process of tumor growth envisions driver mutations causing clonal expansions that sweep through the cancer cell population and reach fixation (100% frequency) [14, 15]. If such a driver mutation did reach fixation, it would appear as a "trunk" mutation, present in all the tumor cells. However, across multiple cancer types, tumor clonal architectures are often observed experimentally to be the consequence of a complex branched subclonal processes, with divergent subclones evolving simultaneously [16, 17, 18, 19, 20, 21, 22, 23, 24, 25, 26, 27].

While a few clones may dominate the composition of a tumor, minor and often undetectable subclones can dominate the clinical course of disease progression and recurrence [28, 29, 30, 31, 32, 33]. For example, in patients with chronic lymphocytic leukemia who received chemotherapy, the presence of detectable subclones harboring one or more cancer-driver genes in the primary leukemia adversely impacted clinical outcome [28, 33]. More recently, similar findings have shown that there is a clear association between a greater number of detectable subclonal populations and poorer clinical outcome in lower-grade glioma, prostate, clear cell kidney, head and neck, breast cancers, and localized lung adenocarcinomas [34, 35, 26, 37]. The generation of genetic variation and subclonal diversity may be an indicator of the potential of a tumor to adapt under different selective pressures and has important implications on disease progression and drug resistance. When studying cancers in patients who have relapsed, several studies have revealed that tumor cells in the relapsed clone were often present as an undetectable subclone in the primary tumor before the initiation of therapy. These revelations suggest that mutations contributing to recurrence are selected for during treatment [38, 39, 40, 41, 42, 43, 44, 45].

A "Big Bang" model of tumor evolution has been recently observed in an analysis of 349 samples from 15 independently derived colorectal tumors [46]. This model shows that colorectal tumors grow as a single expansion generating several intermixed subclones where both clonal and most detectable subclonal mutations occur early during transformation [46]. These subclones are defined from the founding clone and are established by the additional mutations they acquired, which may not be present in the bulk of the tumor. Many subclones carrying driver mutations can remain rare and undetectable because their abundance falls below the detection limit of standard genome or exome sequencing techniques [21, 29, 47, 48, 49, 50]. Current standard sequencing methods have low sensitivity and high false positive rates when detecting mutations below 10% frequency in the DNA extracted from the tumor sample [47]. Although the Big Bang model anticipates uniformly high levels of subclonal mutations throughout the neoplasm, a quantitative assessment of this subclonal diversity across cancers is needed.

We develop and implement a computational model to gain insight into the dynamics of the subclonal evolution of cancer and to assess the extent to which heterogeneous subclonal expansions occur. We simulate tumor growth via a birth-and-death branching process, where we keep track of all subclones that arise and die out or are maintained and grow during the evolutionary process. Under different combinations of the evolutionary parameter values, including those that have been previously estimated for two cancer types (glioblastoma multiforme and colorectal cancer), simulations lead to the conclusion that the distribution of sizes of subclones carrying driver mutations has a heavy right tail at the time of tumor detection, with only one to four dominant clones present at ≥10% frequency, composing most of the tumor cell population. Our model predicts that the vast majority of subclones will be present at <10% frequency. We find that most treatment-resistant subclones harboring driver mutations are present at low frequency, below the detection limit of standard sequencing techniques. Our results suggest that the number of minor subclones is strongly correlated with the number of numerically dominant clones in a tumor. Here we discuss empirical data that supports our simulation results, the implications of our model predictions, the strengths of the model, and its limitations.

(*Continued*)

(*Continued*)

RESULTS

Subclonal Evolutionary Model of Cancer Cell Populations

Previous dynamic models developed to study tumor evolution [15, 51, 52, 53] assume that each driver mutation affects the fitness of a tumor cell lineage equally (with the exception of ref. [52]). They also assume that the fitness effect of a driver mutation is independent of the other driver mutations carried by the cell. However, epistatic interactions are a central aspect of the dynamics of adaptation of asexual populations [54, 55] and should be relevant to asexual tumor populations as well [56]. Moreover, as it is a computationally prohibitive task, cancer evolution models have not studied the extent of heterogeneous subclonal expansions that can occur simultaneously during the neoplastic process. Clonal heterogeneity is particularly important because multiple subclones carrying favorable (and potentially even treatment-resistant) mutations can emerge and compete with each other, increasing variation in evolutionary outcomes, as shown previously in laboratory evolution experiments [54, 57, 58].

Our computational model is based on a branching evolutionary process [15, 59], where we model selection as an epistatic process [55, 60]. In the model, a subclone is defined as a subpopulation of cells that descended from another clone but then diverged by accumulating another driver mutation.

Similar to the framework presented in ref. [15], each simulation is initiated with a single cell carrying a single driver mutation (the potential founder of a primary tumor) that provides a selective growth advantage over normal neighboring cells. At each time step, a cell may either die or divide. If it divides, then it can further acquire an additional driver mutation in one of the daughter cells at a rate μ_d. For each driver mutation occurring during cell division, we randomly sample a selection coefficient from an exponential distribution of mean $\bar{s}$ [57, 61] and update the cell fitness f. We assume that each subsequent driver mutation increases the probability of cell division, defined as $b = \frac{1}{2}f = \frac{1}{2}\left[w_{wt} + d\left(1 - \prod_{i=1}^{n}(1 - s_i)\right)\right]$ [60, 62, 63 64]. The probability of cell death is $1 - b$. The fitness change in a cell produced by a driver is thus dependent on the other driver mutations and the temporal order at which they occur in the cell; consequently, each cell lineage has its own fitness trajectory during the neoplastic process. The parameter w_{wt} represents the fitness of the wild-type cell in which the first driver occurs, and without loss of generality it is assumed to be 1. The parameter d is a measure of the maximum possible fitness gain through adaptation; we assume $d = 1$ [62]. The parameters $s_1, s_2, \ldots, s_n$ characterize the fitness effects associated with each of n driver mutations that a cell lineage carries.

By employing an optimized algorithm on a Hadoop cluster (see the section titled "Materials and Methods" for details), we are able to keep track of all subclones that arise and die out or are maintained and grow during the evolutionary process. Because of the limited quantitative knowledge of parameter values across cancers, we test a range of values for μ_d and $\bar{s}$. The ranges we explored are centered on values obtained from the literature. The values selected for the driver mutation rate, μ_d, are: 1×10^{-8}, 1×10^{-7}, 1×10^{-6}, and 1×10^{-5} mutations per cell division [7, 8, 15, 46, 53, 65]. And the values chosen for the mean, $\bar{s}$, of the exponential distribution of fitness effects are: 0.1, 0.01, and 0.005 [15, 53, 65].

DRIFT DOMINATES EARLY NEOPLASTIC DYNAMICS

A necessary step in neoplastic initiation is that the first mutated cell lineage survives stochastic drift to result in a clone growing at the expense of its normal neighbors. The growth of the first clone is important in increasing the number of cells in which a second driver mutation could occur, and subsequently, another clone could emerge from the cell with the second driver and so on until a clinically apparent tumor is formed (Figure CS7.1) [66]. To quantify the effect of stochastic drift in neoplastic initiation, we ran our simulations until we generated at least 100 clinically detectable simulated tumors (defined as a tumor cell population reaching $\approx 10^9$ cells) for each combination of the chosen parameter values, for a total of 88,265 simulations of the process (Table CS7.1). Overall, we observe that out of the total number of realizations executed, only 1,432 became clinically detectable tumors, despite each simulation being initiated with a driver mutation. Thus, on average, ≈ 98% of all the initiating mutated cell lineages carrying a driver mutation die out early, which is in line with theoretical expectations [67]. This result highlights the importance of genetic drift affecting neoplastic initiation.

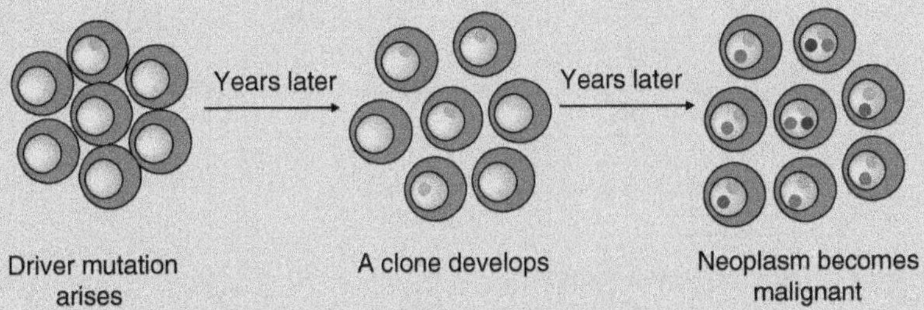

Figure CS7.1 Clone Mutation Development

To test how this model works with parameter values from a known cancer type, we use estimates from colorectal cancer. It has been experimentally estimated that colorectal cancer cells divide every four days [15, 68]. Assuming this cell division time in the simulations, we find that the average expected time from onset to clinical detection of the simulated tumors ranges from 1.64 years to 27.97 years, depending on the values for $\bar{s}$ and μ_d (Table CS7.1). Additionally, using the parameter values

(Continued)

(*Continued*)

$\bar{s} = 0.005$ and $\mu_d = 1 \times 10^{-5}$ per cell division, which have been estimated for colorectal cancer [15], our model predicts that it would take an average of 18.28 years for a colorectal tumor to develop after the first driver mutation appears (Table CS7.1). This estimate is concordant with previous estimates of tumor development in colorectal cancer [15, 68].

Table CS7.1 Number of Simulations Performed for Each Combination of Parameter Values ($\bar{s}$, μ_d).*

$\bar{s}$	μ_d	Number of Realizations	Number of Simulations That Reached 10^9 Cells	Percentage of Simulations That Reached 10^9 Cells	Mean Number of Generations to Detection	Mean Time to Detection (Years)
0.1	1×10^{-8}	10,155	162	1.6%	1,596.66	17.50
0.1	1×10^{-7}	1,948	112	5.7%	475.08	5.21
0.1	1×10^{-6}	748	134	17.9%	158.54	1.74
0.1	1×10^{-5}	748	111	14.8%	147.50	1.62
0.01	1×10^{-8}	6,867	125	1.8%	1,807.63	19.80
0.01	1×10^{-7}	6,866	113	1.6%	1,406.75	15.41
0.01	1×10^{-6}	6,866	120	1.7%	1,263.80	13.85
0.01	1×10^{-5}	6,865	115	1.7%	1,018.40	11.16
0.005	1×10^{-8}	11,951	102	0.9%	2,552.70	27.97
0.005	1×10^{-7}	11,751	112	1.0%	2,546.85	27.91
0.005	1×10^{-6}	11,750	126	1.1%	2,046.78	22.43
0.005	1×10^{-5}	11,750	100	0.9%	1,668.07	18.28
		88,265	1,432	1.6%		

*The mean time from initiation to clinical detection of a simulated tumor is shown. The generation time assigned in the simulations is $T = 4$ days. Extent of Intratumor Subclonal Variation at Detection.

By having generated a total of 1,432 clinically detectable simulated tumors under a wide range of parameter values, we can determine the general contribution of each of the parameters to initiation and neoplastic progression. We find, consistent with a previous report [53], that selection has a larger effect on neoplastic initiation than the driver mutation rate. Moreover, we find that the average expected time from initiation to detection of a tumor increases with decreasing the average fitness effect of driver mutations and with decreasing the driver mutation rate.

To gain insight into the extent of subclonal populations within a tumor at the time of detection and to determine how the different evolutionary parameters impact the subclonal composition, we analyzed all the 1,432 detectable tumors generated by our model. In most tumors, we find that the number of dominant clones, defined here as a subclone present at ≥10% frequency in a tumor, ranges from 1 to 4.

However, the average number of dominant clones in a tumor tends to increase with decreasing the average fitness effect of driver mutations and with increasing the driver mutation rate. Across all the 1,432 detectable simulated tumors, the average number of dominant clonal populations is 1.46. Of note, the predicted range by the model on the number of numerically dominant clones in a tumor is largely concordant with the findings reported in two recent pan-cancer analyses of intratumor heterogeneity, which found that there were typically from one to four dominant detectable clones in most cancer types analyzed [35, 36]. Importantly, we find that even though only a few dominant clones compose the majority of the cancer cell population in a simulated tumor (range 90.6%–99.5%), the number of minor subclones present at <10% frequency is substantial; this number increases with decreasing the average fitness effect of drivers and with increasing the driver mutation rate.

Given the parameter values $\overline{s} = 0.005$ and $\mu_d = 1 \times 10^{-5}$, which have been estimated for glioblastoma multiforme and colorectal cancer [15], the model predicts that, on average, 1.8 dominant clones and 2,705 minor subclonal populations carrying driver mutations compose a tumor. We also find that there is a strong, statistically significant correlation between the average number of dominant clones and the average number of minor subclones across all simulated tumors (Pearson $r = 0.91$, $P < 0.001$). This result suggests that the number of detectable clonal populations by standard sequencing techniques may serve as a proxy to reflect the extent of undetectable minor subclones in a tumor.

For each combination of parameter values, we computed the probability density function for the subclone sizes present in the simulated tumors. Overall, we find that the distribution of subclone sizes harboring driver mutations has a heavy right tail, with only a few clones present at ≥10% frequency in the tumor and with most subclones present at frequencies as low as 10^{-7}.

DIFFERENTIAL FITNESS BETWEEN DOMINANT AND MINOR SUBCLONES

A key aspect of our computational model is that simulates and tracks subclonal heterogeneity, where each clone evolving as a cellular lineage has its own fitness, which is dependent on the fitness effects conferred by the driver mutations and their epistatic interactions. For illustrative purposes, we show the subclonal composition and their corresponding fitness in two clinically detectable simulated tumors using the parameter values $\overline{s} = 0.01$ and $\mu_d = 1 \times 10^{-5}$; and $\overline{s} = 0.005$ and $\mu_d = 1 \times 10^{-5}$. The corresponding population dynamics of both simulated tumors are shown as well. We observe that the simulated tumor has three dominant clones present at 41%, 19%, and 10% frequency in the tumor, carrying one to two driver mutations. The simulated tumor, however, has only two dominant clones present at 80% and 17% frequency, harboring two and one driver mutations, respectively. Additionally, we also observe that, as would be expected, there is substantial intra- and

(*Continued*)

(*Continued*)
inter-subclonal variation in both cases. More important, we find that, on average, the relative fitness of some minor subclones is greater than the fitness of the dominant clonal populations. These results show that, even though cells acquire subsequent driver mutations with accompanying fitness advantages, they do not sweep through the population within the time scale of tumor growth. Consequently, a substantial number of minor—and often fitter—subclones harboring driver mutations remain in the tumor at very low frequency.

RESISTANT SUBCLONES CARRYING DRIVER MUTATIONS ARE PRESENT AT LOW FREQUENCY AT DETECTION

Populations can adapt to novel environments in two different ways: selection can act on preexisting genetic variants or on de novo mutations [69]. Adaptation from standing genetic variation is probably faster than from novel mutations, not only because beneficial mutations are immediately available in the new environment, but also because they may start at higher frequencies [69]. We thus tested whether subclones carrying driver mutations could also carry at least one resistance mutation in the clinically detectable simulated tumors. To test this, we assume that multiple different mutations can independently cause resistance and assume a resistance mutation rate of 1×10^{-8} [70, 71] in a cell that coincidentally acquires a driver mutation during cell division. Additionally, we assume that the resistance mutation does not affect fitness. Under these assumptions and parameter values, we find that the majority of resistant subclones carrying driver mutations are often present at low frequency, below the detection limit of standard DNA sequencing techniques. We then calculated the number of independent resistant subclones within each clinically detectable simulated tumor. We find that the maximum number of independent resistant subclones in a particular simulated tumor is 18, and the minimum is 0. Overall, we find that the number of independent resistant subclones in a simulated tumor increases with decreasing the average fitness effect of the drivers and with increasing the driver mutation rate. We finally "treated" all clinically detectable simulated tumors with a hypothetical targeted drug and calculated the average time from the moment when the drug is applied to the time at disease recurrence (cancer cell population reaching $\approx 10^9$ cells). Our analysis suggests that there is on average an eight-fold decrease in the time from the start of treatment to the time at recurrence relative to the average time from initiation to clinical detection of the simulated tumors. Therefore, these results, along with other studies [38, 39, 40, 41, 42, 43, 44, 45] suggest that the extent of standing subclonal variation in a tumor may be the most important factor for the evolution of acquired resistance to treatment.

DISCUSSION

In this study, we developed and implemented a stochastic evolutionary modeling framework to study the subclonal dynamics of cancer progression. First, we show that despite the selective advantage of the driver mutation, drift substantially affects neoplastic initiation. This result is expected from population genetics theory, as selection is less efficient in small populations [67]. That said, we find that the mean selective coefficient has a much larger effect on neoplastic initiation than the driver mutation rate. These results are in agreement with a report where the authors quantified the competitive benefit of *Apc* loss, *Kras* activation, and *P53* mutations in intestinal tumor initiation [65]. They showed that most mutated cells are lost and that clones in colitis-affected intestines carrying *P53* mutations are particularly favored in tumor initiation.

We show that the average expected time from the first driver mutation to clinical detection of a tumor increases with both decreasing the average fitness effect associated with the driver mutations and with decreasing the driver mutation rate. Based on this, we hypothesize that the fitness effects conferred by driver genetic alterations in certain sporadic childhood cancers, which arise within a few years, should be greater than those associated with drivers in sporadic adult cancers. For example, in childhood chronic myeloid leukemia, the fitness effect conferred by the chromosome translocation juxtaposing the *BCR* and *ABL* genes may be quite large, and consequently, this single genetic alteration may be all that is required for tumor initiation and rapid progression of this childhood sporadic cancer [72, 73].

A statistical strength of this study is that we simulated 88,265 tumor initiation events for a range of biologically realistic parameters, resulting in more than 1,400 clinically detectable tumors, from which we could analyze and gain important biological insights. Across all the combinations of the chosen evolutionary parameter values, our analysis shows that the distribution of sizes of subclones carrying driver mutations has a heavy right tail at the time of tumor detection. We find that the vast majority of subclones are predicted to be present at <10% frequency in the tumor and only one to four dominant clones present at ≥10% frequency, composing the majority of the tumor cell population. We also find that the number of the minor subclones present at <10% increases with decreasing the average fitness effect of drivers and with increasing the driver mutation rate. Additionally, we find that there is a strong, statistically significant correlation between the average number of numerically dominant clones and the average number of minor subclones across all simulated tumors.

The distribution of subclone sizes inferred by our model is qualitatively similar to that found in a recent empirical study where the authors used ultra-deep sequencing technology to detect mutations in specific known cancer genes in biopsies of sun-exposed eyelids from different individuals [74]. The authors found that aged sun-exposed skin has already thousands of subclones with driver mutations subjected to selection, with some clones as large as several square millimeters

(*Continued*)

(*Continued*)

in surface area [74]. Moreover, the predicted range by the model on the number of dominant clonal populations is largely concordant with a recent pan-cancer analysis of intratumor heterogeneity [35]. In this study, the authors analyzed over 3,300 tumors and integrated SNP array copy number and whole exome sequencing mutational data from TCGA to infer that 92% of all the tumors analyzed had between one and four clonal populations at detectable levels by standard sequencing methods [35].

Understanding the expected levels of subclonal variation is important for treating primary cancers and predicting recurrence. By employing ultra-deep sequencing technology to study intratumor subclonal diversity in patients with chronic lymphocytic leukemia, the presence of rare subclones at frequencies down to the limit of detection for depth of this specific sequencing method, 10^{-4}, has been shown [21]. Our model predicts that minor subclones carrying driver mutations can be present in a tumor at lower frequencies, 10^{-7}. Importantly, we find that these often-undetectable minor subclones can harbor treatment-resistant mutations. These results are in line with multiple previous reports showing that tumor cells corresponding to the relapsed clone were often present as a rare subclone in the diagnostic tumor before the initiation of treatment [38, 39, 40, 41, 42, 43, 44, 45, 75]. We also find that the number of independent resistant subclones in a simulated tumor depends on the population genetic parameter values—increasing with decreasing the average fitness effect of the driver mutations and with increasing the driver mutation rate.

Given that cancer is the result of a very complex process, our approach has some limitations. First, we have not taken spatial structure into consideration in our computational model, which may restrict the expansion of certain subclonal populations during the neoplastic process. Thus, our modeling framework may be more suitable for cancers that develop in the absence of spatial constraints. Second, the host immune system has not been taken into account, although it has been demonstrated to have an important role for both cancer suppression and promotion [76]. Third, future studies should extend this work and consider noncell autonomous interactions, as well as "common good" factors, which are likely to be a strong influence on subclonal dynamics [77]. Despite these caveats, our model captures some essential features of the dynamics of subclonal evolution of cancer progression. The subclonal dynamics predicted by our model are consistent with the Big Bang model [46], where clonal driver mutations and most detectable subclonal drivers occurred relatively early during tumor growth. This result is in contrast with the traditional clonal selection model, where sequential stepwise accumulation of drivers leads to fitter clones that sweep through the population [14, 15].

In conclusion, our modeling provides a theoretical framework for tumor growth, predicting that a substantial number of subclonal populations carrying driver mutations will remain rare and undetectable within a tumor because their abundance falls below the detection limit of standard genome sequencing methods.

Additionally, these minor and often undetectable subclones can harbor treatment-resistant mutations, which present a major challenge for personalized medicine and clinical management. These results suggest that driver mutations that have been identified in individual tumors through standard genome sequencing [78] are likely to constitute only the tip of the iceberg, with several mutations never rising above very low frequencies. However, these "low-frequency" mutations can expand post-treatment and are critical for the evolutionary dynamics of cancer progression and relapse. Altogether, our findings explain why tumors with greater numbers of detectable clonal populations are associated with poorer prognoses across multiple cancer types [28, 34, 35].

MATERIALS AND METHODS

Mathematical Modeling Framework

Software Required. The following open source platforms and programming languages were used for tumor simulation, monitoring, and analysis:

- Apache Hadoop (HortonWorks 2.6.0). Software framework written in Java for distributed storage and processing of very large data sets over commodity hardware clusters.
- Apache Hive (1.2.1 Spark HiveMetastoreConnection version 1.2.1, interactive hive-cli-0.14). External data warehousing stacked on Hadoop, provides simulation monitoring, data summarization, query, and analysis.
- Apache Scala (2.10.5). Functional programming language that utilizes the Java Virtual Machine for platform independency. Controls tumor simulation logic.
- Apache Spark (1.6.0 with a minimum of 1.4.0). Computing framework originally developed at UC Berkeley AMPLab, stacked on top of Scala and distributed over Hadoop. Tracks tumor array memory across multiple machines.
- Bash (Sun AMD64 Linux 2.6.32–504.el6.x86_64). Bash is a UNIX shell and command language. Various scripts used for monitoring, analysis, and data export to spreadsheets or other visualizations.
- Java/JDK (Oracle 1.7). Spark, Scala, and Hive are converted to run in the Java Virtual Machine for platform independence.
- Microsoft Excel (2013)—for aggregates and table visualizations. Module (3.2.10). Bash environment management scripting un/loader.
- Tableau (public 9.1 to 9.3). For visualization of subclonal composition of simulated tumors.
- YARN (2.2.4.2–2). Yet Another Resource Manager. Manages Hadoop data and hardware resources. We used a hierarchical data structure to store common attributes for all cells within the same subclonal population.

(*Continued*)

(*Continued*)

Run Environment. The computation- and data-intensive piece includes a 44-node HDP 2.3 cluster on Dell PowerEdge 720xd servers. Each of the 40 worker nodes has 128 GB RAM, 2x Intel E5–2640 6 core processors, and 22 TB of disk. The cluster backbone network consists of 10 Ge HA top of rack switching combined with Intel x520 10 Ge NICs in each server. Although the tumor simulator can run parallel jobs utilizing multiple resources, the demands on the Hadoop NameNode (worker, memory, disk resource management) are quite exhaustive; therefore, it is suggested to run sequential jobs on a single node for as many images as needed to emulate parallelization.

Statistical Analysis. We created scripts on RStudio (Version 0.99.891) to analyze the data sets and perform statistical analysis.

Code Accessibility. The computer code tumorsim.scala is available at: https://github.com/WilsonSayresLab/TumorHeterogeneity. For details on the steps necessary to run the tumorsim application, see SI Appendix and the readme on GitHub (https://github.com/WilsonSayresLab/TumorHeterogeneity /blob/master/README .md). All the R scripts are also available at https://github.com/WilsonSayresLab/TumorHeterogeneity.

ACKNOWLEDGMENTS

We thank Sergey Kryazhimskiy, Andriy Marusyk, and Jay Taylor for their helpful comments and insightful discussions. This research was partially supported through startup from the School of Life Sciences and the Biodesign Institute to MAWS, the Flinn Foundation to Melissa A. Wilson Sayres and C. Carlo Maley, and through computational resources provided by ASU Research Computing.

NOTES

1. Greaves M, Maley CC. Clonal evolution in cancer. *Nature.* 2012; 481(7381):306–13. Available from: http://www.ncbi.nlm.nih.gov/pmc/articles/PMC3367003/.
2. Marusyk A, Almendro V, Polyak K. Intra-tumour heterogeneity: A looking glass for cancer? *Nat Rev Cancer* [Internet]. Nature Publishing Group; 2012; 12(5):323–34. Available from: http://dx.doi.org/10.1038/nrc3261\nhttp://www.ncbi.nlm.nih.gov/pubmed/22513401.
3. Nowell PC. The clonal evolution of tumor cell populations. *Science* (80–). 1976; 194(4260):23–8.
4. Lipinski KA, Barber LJ, Davies MN, Ashenden M, Sottoriva A, Gerlinger M. Cancer evolution and the limits of predictability in precision cancer medicine. *Trends in Cancer* [Internet]. Elsevier; 2016; 2(1):49–63. Available from: http://linkinghub.elsevier.com/retrieve/pii/S2405803315000692.
5. Frank SA. *Dynamics of cancer: Incidence, inheritance, and evolution.* Princeton University Press, Princeton, NJ; 2007.
6. Martinocorena I, Campbell PJ. Somatic mutation in cancer and normal cells. *Science* (80–). 2015; 349(6255):1483–9.
7. Shendure J, Akey JM. The origins, determinants, and consequences of human mutations. *Science.* 2015; 349(6255):1478–83. Available from: C:\Users\kirsl_000\OneDrive\Documents\ReadCube\Shendure et al-2015-Science.pdf.

8. Lynch M. Mutation and human exceptionalism: Our future genetic load. *Genetics* [Internet]. 2016; 202(3):869–75. Available from: http://www.genetics.org/cgi/doi/10.1534/genetics.115.180471.

9. Hanahan D, Weinberg RA. Hallmarks of cancer: The next generation. *Cell*. Elsevier; 2011; 144(5): 646–74.

10. Genovese G, Kähler AK, Handsaker RE, Lindberg J, Rose SA, Bakhoum SF, et al. Clonal hematopoiesis and blood-cancer risk inferred from blood DNA sequence. *N Engl J Med* [Internet]. 2014; 371(26):2477–87. Available from: http://www.ncbi.nlm.nih.gov/pubmed/25426838\nhttp://www.nejm.org/doi/abs/10.1056/NEJMoa1409405.

11. Fisher JC. Multiple-mutation theory of carcinogenesis. *Nature*. 1958; 651–2.

12. Vogelstein B, Papadopoulos N, Velculescu VE, Zhou S, Diaz Jr. LA, Kinzler KW. Cancer genome landscapes. *Science* (80–) [Internet]. 2013; 339(6127):1546–58. Available from: http://science.sciencemag.org/content/sci/339/6127/1546.full.pdf.

13. McFarland CD, Korolev KS, Kryukov G V, Sunyaev SR, Mirny LA. Impact of deleterious passenger mutations on cancer progression. *Proc Natl Acad Sci* USA [Internet]. 2013; 110(8):2910–5. Available from: http://www.pubmedcentral.nih.gov/articlerender.fcgi?artid=3581883&tool=pmcentrez&rendertype=abstract.

14. Fearon EF, Vogelstein B. A genetic model for colorectal tumorigenesis. *Cell*. 1990; Jun 1;61(5):759–67. Available from: http://www.cell.com/cell/pdf/0092-8674(90)90186-I.pdf.

15. Bozic I, Antal T, Ohtsuki H, Carter H, Kim D, Chen S, et al. Accumulation of driver and passenger mutations during tumor progression. *Proc Natl Acad Sci* USA [Internet]. 2010; 107(43):18545–50. Available from: http://www.pubmedcentral.nih.gov/articlerender.fcgi?artid=2972991&tool=pmcentrez&rendertype=abstract.

16. Navin N, Krasnitz A, Rodgers L, Cook K, Meth J, Kendall J, et al. Inferring tumor progression from genomic heterogeneity. *Genome Res*. 2010; 20(1):68–80. Available from: https://www.researchgate.net/publication/38080487_Navin_N_et_al_Inferring_tumor_progression_from_genomic_heterogeneity_Genome_Res_20_68-80.

17. Campbell PJ, Yachida S, Mudie LJ, Stephens PJ, Pleasance ED, Stebbings LA, et al. The patterns and dynamics of genomic instability in metastatic pancreatic cancer. *Nature* [Internet]. Nature Publishing Group; 2010; 467(7319):1109–13. Available from: http://www.pubmedcentral.nih.gov/articlerender.fcgi?artid=3137369&tool=pmcentrez&rendertype=abstract.

18. Anderson K, Lutz C, van Delft FW, Bateman CM, Guo Y, Colman SM, et al. Genetic variegation of clonal architecture and propagating cells in leukaemia. *Nature* [Internet]. Nature Publishing Group; 2011; 469(7330):356–61. Available from: http://www.nature.com/doifinder/10.1038/nature09650\nhttp://www.ncbi.nlm.nih.gov/pubmed/21160474.

19. Notta F, Mullighan CG, Wang JC, Poeppl A, Doulatov S, Phillips LA, et al. Evolution of human BCR-ABL1 lymphoblastic leukaemia-initiating cells. *Nature* [Internet]. Nature Publishing Group; 2011; 469(7330):362–7. Available from: http://www.ncbi.nlm.nih.gov/pubmed/21248843.

20. Sottoriva A, Spiteri I, Piccirillo SGM, Touloumis A, Collins VP, Marioni JC, et al. Intratumor heterogeneity in human glioblastoma reflects cancer evolutionary dynamics. *Proc Natl Acad Sci* USA [Internet]. 2013; 110(10):4009–14. Available from: http://www.pubmedcentral.nih.gov/articlerender.fcgi?artid=3593922&tool=pmcentrez&rendertype=abstract.

21. Campbell PJ, Pleasance ED, Stephens PJ, Dicks E, Rance R, Goodhead I, et al. Subclonal phylogenetic structures in cancer revealed by ultra-deep sequencing. *Proc Natl Acad Sci* USA. 2008; 105(35): 13081–6. Available from: https://lifescience.roche.com/wcsstore/RASCatalogAssetStore/Articles/BIOCHEMICA_2_09_p4-7.pdf.

22. Gerlinger M, Rowan AJ, Horswell S, Larkin J, Endesfelder D, Gronroos E, et al. Intratumor heterogeneity and branched evolution revealed by multiregion sequencing. *N Engl J Med*. 2012; 366(10):883–92. Available from: http://www.nejm.org/doi/full/10.1056/NEJMoa1113205#t=article.

(*Continued*)

(*Continued*)

23. Nik-Zainal S, Van Loo P, Wedge DC, Alexandrov LB, Greenman CD, Lau KW, et al. The life history of 21 breast cancers. *Cell*. 2012; 149(5):994–1007. Available from: http://www.sciencedirect.com/science/article/pii/S0092867412005272.
24. Shain AH, Yeh I, Kovalyshyn I, Sriharan A, Talevich E, Gagnon A, et al. The genetic evolution of melanoma from precursor lesions. *N Engl J Med* [Internet]. 2015; 373(20):1926–36. Available from: http://www.nejm.org/doi/abs/10.1056/NEJMoa1502583.
25. Burrell RA, McGranahan N, Bartek J, Swanton C. The causes and consequences of genetic heterogeneity in cancer evolution. *Nature* [Internet]. 2013; 501(7467):338–45. Available from: http://www.ncbi.nlm.nih.gov/pubmed/24048066.
26. Burrell RA, Swanton C. Re-evaluating clonal dominance in cancer evolution. *Trends in Cancer* [Internet]. Elsevier; 2016; 64:1–14. Available from: http://dx.doi.org/10.1016/j.trecan.2016.04.002.
27. Zhao B, Hemann MT, Lauffenburger DA. Modeling tumor clonal evolution for drug combinations design. *Trends in Cancer* [Internet]. Elsevier; 2016; 2(3):144–58. Available from: http://dx.doi.org/10.1016/j.trecan.2016.02.001.
28. Landau DA, Carter SL, Stojanov P, McKenna A, Stevenson K, Lawrence MS, et al. Evolution and impact of subclonal mutations in chronic lymphocytic leukemia. *Cell*. Elsevier; 2013; 152(4):714–26. doi: http://dx.doi.org/10.1016/j.cell.2013.01.019.
29. Schmitt MW, Loeb LA, Salk JJ. The influence of subclonal resistance mutations on targeted cancer therapy. *Nat Rev Clin Oncol* [Internet]. Nature Publishing Group; 2015; Available from: http://www.nature.com/doifinder/10.1038/nrclinonc.2015.175\nhttp://www.ncbi.nlm.nih.gov/pubmed/26483300.
30. Maley CC, Galipeau PC, Finley JC, Wongsurawat VJ, Li X, Sanchez CA, et al. Genetic clonal diversity predicts progression to esophageal adenocarcinoma. *Nat Genet* [Internet]. 2006; 38(4):468–73. Available from: http://www.nature.com.libproxy1.nus.edu.sg/ng/journal/v38/n4/full/ng1768.html.
31. Chowell D, Boddy AM, Mallo D, Tollis M, Maley CC. When (distant) relatives stay too long: Implications for cancer medicine. *Genome Biol* [Internet]. 2016; 17(34):1–4. Available from: http://dx.doi.org/10.1186/s13059-016-0906-3.
32. Bozic I, Nowak MA. Timing and heterogeneity of mutations associated with drug resistance in metastatic cancers. *Proc Natl Acad Sci* USA [Internet]. 2014; 111(45):15964–8. Available from: http://www.pubmedcentral.nih.gov/articlerender.fcgi?artid=4234551&tool=pmcentrez&rendertype=abstract.
33. Landau DA, Tausch E, Taylor-Weiner AN, Stewart C, Reiter JG, Bahlo J, et al. Mutations driving CLL and their evolution in progression and relapse. *Nature* [Internet]. 2015; 526(7574):525–30. Available from: http://www.nature.com/doifinder/10.1038/nature15395\nhttp://www.ncbi.nlm.nih.gov/pubmed/26466571.
34. Zhang J, Fujimoto J, Zhang J, Wedge DC, Song X, Zhang J, et al. Intratumor heterogeneity in localized lung adenocarcinomas delineated by multiregion sequencing. *Science* [Internet]. 2014; 346(6206):256–9. Available from: http://www.ncbi.nlm.nih.gov/pubmed/25301631.
35. Morris LGT, Riaz N, Desrichard A, Şenbabaoğlu Y. Pan-cancer analysis of intratumor heterogeneity as a prognostic determinant of survival. *Oncotarget*. 2016 Mar 1; 7(9):10051-63. doi: 10.18632/oncotarget.7067.
36. Andor N, Graham TA, Jansen M, Xia LC, Aktipis CA, Petritsch C, et al. Pan-cancer analysis of the extent and consequences of intratumor heterogeneity. *Nat Med* [Internet]. 2015; 22(1):105–13. Available from: http://dx.doi.org/10.1038/nm.3984.
37. Pereira B, Chin S-F, Rueda OM, Vollan H-KM, Provenzano E, Bardwell HA, et al. The somatic mutation profiles of 2,433 breast cancers refines their genomic and transcriptomic landscapes. *Nat Commun* [Internet]. 2016; 7(May):11479. Available from: http://www.nature.com/doifinder/10.1038/ncomms11479.
38. Mullighan CG, Phillips LA, Su X, Ma J, Miller CB, Shurtleff SA, et al. Genomic analysis of the clonal origins of relapsed acute lymphoblastic leukemia. *Science* (80–). 2008; 322(5906):1377–80.

39. Bhang HC, Ruddy DA, Krishnamurthy Radhakrishna V, Caushi JX, Zhao R, Hims MM, et al. Studying clonal dynamics in response to cancer therapy using high-complexity barcoding. *Nat Med* [Internet]. 2015; 21(5):440–8. Available from: http://www.ncbi.nlm.nih.gov/pubmed/25849130.

40. Roche-Lestienne C, Lai JL, Darre S, Facon T, Preudhomme C. A mutation conferring resistance to imatinib at the time of diagnosis of chronic myelogenous leukemia. *N Engl J Med.* 2003; 348(22):2265–6. doi: 10.1056/NEJMc0350895.

41. Morrissy AS, Garzia L, Shih DJH, Zuyderduyn S, Huang X, Skowron P, et al. Divergent clonal selection dominates medulloblastoma at recurrence. *Nature* [Internet]. 2016. Available from: http://www.nature.com/nature/journal/vaop/ncurrent/full/nature16478.html?WT.ec_id=NATURE-20160114&spMailingID=50459781&spUserID=NzE3MzA2NzYwNAS2&spJobID=841825502&spReportId=ODQxODI1NTAyS0.

42. Diaz LA Jr, Williams RT, Wu J, Kinde I, Hecht JR, Berlin J, et al. The molecular evolution of acquired resistance to targeted EGFR blockade in colorectal cancers. *Nature* [Internet]. Nature Publishing Group; 2012; 4–7. Available from: http://www.nature.com/nature/journal/v486/n7404/pdf/nature11219.pdf.

43. Ding L, Ley TJ, Larson DE, Miller CA, Koboldt DC, Welch JS, et al. Clonal evolution in relapsed acute myeloid leukaemia revealed by whole-genome sequencing. *Nature* [Internet]. Nature Publishing Group; 2012; 481(7382):506–10. Available from: http://www.pubmedcentral.nih.gov/articlerender.fcgi?artid=3267864&tool=pmcentrez&rendertype=abstract.

44. Roche-Lestienne C, Soenen-Cornu V, Grardel-Duflos N, Laï JL, Philippe N, Facon T, et al. Several types of mutations of the Abl gene can be found in chronic myeloid leukemia patients resistant to STI571, and they can pre-exist to the onset of treatment. *Blood.* 2002; 100(3):1014–8. Available from: http://www.bloodjournal.org/content/bloodjournal/100/3/1014.full.pdf?sso-checked=true.

45. Roehe-Lestienne C, Deluche L, Corm S, Tigaud I, Joha S, Philippe N, et al. RUNX1 DNA-binding mutations and RUNX1-PRDM16 cryptic fusions in BCR-ABL + leukemias are frequently associated with secondary trisomy 21 and may contribute to clonal evolution and imatinib resistance. *Blood.* 2008; 111(7):3735–41. Available from: http://www.bloodjournal.org/content/111/7/3735.

46. Sottoriva A, Kang H, Ma Z, Graham TA, Salomon MP, Zhao J, et al. A Big Bang model of human colorectal tumor growth. *Nat Genet* [Internet]. Nature Publishing Group; 2015; 47(3):209–16. http://dx.doi.org/10.1038/ng.3214.

47. Barber LJ, Davies MN, Gerlinger M. Dissecting cancer evolution at the macro-heterogeneity and micro-heterogeneity scale. *Curr Opin Genet Dev.* Elsevier; 2015; 30:1–6. Available from: http://www.sciencedirect.com/science/article/pii/S0959437X14001464.

48. Tirosh I, Izar B, Prakadan SM, Ii MHW, Treacy D, Trombetta JJ, et al. Dissecting the multicellular ecosystem of metastatic melanoma by single-cell RNA-seq. *Science* (80–). 2016; 352(6282):189–96. Available from: http://science.sciencemag.org/content/352/6282/189.

49. Wang Y, Waters J, Leung ML, Unruh A, Roh W, Shi X, et al. Clonal evolution in breast cancer revealed by single nucleus genome sequencing. *Nature* [Internet]. Nature Publishing Group; 2014; 512(7513):1–15. Available from: http://dx.doi.org/10.1038/nature13600\npapers2://publication/doi/10.1038/nature13600.

50. Gerstung M, Beisel C, Rechsteiner M, Wild P, Schraml P, Moch H, et al. Reliable detection of subclonal single-nucleotide variants in tumour cell populations. *Nat Commun* [Internet]. Nature Publishing Group; 2012; 3(May):811. Available from: http://www.ncbi.nlm.nih.gov/pubmed/22549840\nhttp://www.nature.com/ncomms/journal/v3/n5/pdf/ncomms1814.pdf.

51. Waclaw B, Bozic I, Pittman ME, Hruban RH, Vogelstein B, Nowak M. Spatial model predicts dispersal and cell turnover cause reduced intra-tumor heterogeneity. *Nature.* 2015; 525:261–7. doi: 10.1038/nature14971.

52. Durrett R, Foo J, Leder K, Mayberry J, Michor F. Intratumor heterogeneity in evolutionary models of tumor progression. *Genetics.* 2011; 188(2):461–77. doi: 10.1534/genetics.110.125724.

53. Beerenwinkel N, Antal T, Dingli D, Traulsen A, Kinzler KW, Velculescu VE, et al. Genetic progression and the waiting time to cancer. *PLoS Comput Biol.* 2007; 3(11):2239–46. Available from: http://journals.plos.org/ploscompbiol/article/asset?id=10.1371%2Fjournal.pcbi.0030225.PDF.

(*Continued*)

(*Continued*)

54. Lang GI, Rice DP, Hickman MJ, Sodergren E, Weinstock GM, Botstein D, et al. Pervasive genetic hitchhiking and clonal interference in forty evolving yeast populations. *Nature* [Internet]. Nature Publishing Group; 2013; 500(7464):571–4. Available from: http://www.pubmedcentral.nih.gov/articlerender.fcgi?artid=3758440&tool=pmcentrez&rendertype=abstract.
55. Breen MS, Kemena C, Vlasov PK, Notredame C, Kondrashov FA. Epistasis as the primary factor in molecular evolution. *Nature* [Internet]. Nature Publishing Group; 2012; 490(7421):535–8. Available from: http://dx.doi.org/10.1038/nature11510.
56. Sprouffske K, Merlo LMF, Gerrish PJ, Maley CC, Sniegowski PD. Cancer in light of experimental evolution. *Curr Biol* [Internet]. Elsevier; 2012; 22(17):R762–71. Available from: http://dx.doi.org/10.1016/j.cub.2012.06.065.
57. Hegreness M, Shoresh N, Hartl D, Kishony R. An equivalence principle for the incorporation of favorable mutations in asexual populations. *Science*. 2006; 311(5767):1615–7. Available from: http://kishony.med.harvard.edu/pdf/Hegreness_2006.pdf.
58. Levy SF, Blundell JR, Venkataram S, Petrov DA, Fisher DS, Sherlock G. Quantitative evolutionary dynamics using high-resolution lineage tracking. *Nature* [Internet]. 2015; 519(7542):181–6. Available from: http://dx.doi.org/10.1038/nature14279.
59. Haccou P, Jagers P, Vatutin VA, Dieckmann U. Branching processes: Variation, growth, and extinction of populations (Cambridge Studies in Adaptive Dynamics). 2005; 82(106). Available from: http://www.langtoninfo.com/web_content/9780521832205_frontmatter.pdf.
60. Kryazhimskiy S, Draghi JA, Plotkin JB. In evolution, the sum is less than its parts. *Science* [Internet]. 2011; 332(6034):1160–1. Available from: http://www.ncbi.nlm.nih.gov/pubmed/21636764.
61. Orr HA. The distribution of fitness effects among beneficial mutations. *Genetics* [Internet]. 2003; 163(4):1519–26. Available from: http://dx.doi.org/10.1016/j.jtbi.2005.05.001.
62. Nagel AC, Joyce P, Wichman HA, Miller CR. Stickbreaking: A novel fitness landscape model that harbors epistasis and is consistent with commonly observed patterns of adaptive evolution. *Genetics*. 2012; 190(2):655–67. doi: 10.1534/genetics.111.132134.
63. Kryazhimskiy S, Rice DP, Jerison E, Desai MM. Global epistasis makes adaptation predictable despite sequence-level stochasticity. 2014; 344(6191). Available from: http://biorxiv.org/lookup/doi/10.1101/001784
64. Wiser MJ, Ribeck N, Lenski RE, Littell JS, Muller CJ, Dunne KA, et al. Long-term dynamics of adaptation in asexual populations. *Science*. 2013; 342(December):1364–7.
65. Vermeulen L, Morrissey E, Heijden M van der, Nicholson AM, Sottoriva A, Buczacki S, et al. Defining stem cell dynamics in models of intestinal tumor initiation. *Science* (80–) [Internet]. 2013; 342(6161):995–8. Available from: http://www.damtp.cam.ac.uk/user/st321/CV_&_Publications_files/STpapers-pdf/Vermeulen13.pdf.
66. Vogelstein B, Kinzler KW. The path to cancer—three strikes and you're out. *N Engl J Med* [Internet]. 2015; 373(20):1895–8. Available from: http://www.ncbi.nlm.nih.gov/pubmed/26559568.
67. Charlesworth B. Effective population size and patterns of molecular evolution and variation. *Nat Rev Genet* [Internet]. 2009; 10(3):195–205. Available from: http://www.nature.com/nrg/journal/v10/n3/abs/nrg2526.html\nhttp://www.nature.com/nrg/journal/v10/n3/pdf/nrg2526.pdf.
68. Jones S, Chen W-D, Parmigiani G, Diehl F, Beerenwinkel N, Antal T, et al. Comparative lesion sequencing provides insights into tumor evolution. *Proc Natl Acad Sci* USA [Internet]. 2008; 105(11):4283–8. Available from: http://www.pubmedcentral.nih.gov/articlerender.fcgi?artid=2393770&tool=pmcentrez&rendertype=abstract.
69. Barrett RDH, Schluter D. Adaptation from standing genetic variation. *Trends Ecol Evol*. 2008; 23(1):38–44.

70. Komarova NL, Burger JA, Wodarz D. Evolution of ibrutinib resistance in chronic lymphocytic leukemia (CLL). *Proc Natl Acad Sci* USA [Internet]. 2014; 111(38):13906–11. Available from: http://www.pnas.org/content/111/38/13906.full.

71. Komarova NL, Wodarz D. Drug resistance in cancer: Principles of emergence and prevention. *Proc Natl Acad Sci* USA [Internet]. 2005; 102(27):9714–9. Available from: http://www.pubmedcentral.nih.gov/articlerender.fcgi?artid=1172248&tool=pmcentrez&rendertype=abstract.

72. Michor F, Iwasa Y, Nowak MA. The age incidence of chronic myeloid leukemia can be explained by a one-mutation model. *Proc Natl Acad Sci* USA [Internet]. 2006; 103(40):14931–4. Available from: http://www.pubmedcentral.nih.gov/articlerender.fcgi?artid=1595453&tool=pmcentrez&rendertype=abstract.

73. Tomasetti C, Marchionni L, Nowak MA, Parmigiani G, Vogelstein B. Only three driver gene mutations are required for the development of lung and colorectal cancers. *Proc Natl Acad Sci* USA [Internet]. 2015; 112(1):118–23. Available from: http://www.pubmedcentral.nih.gov/articlerender.fcgi?artid=4291633&tool=pmcentrez&rendertype=abstract.

74. Martincorena I, Roshan A, Gerstung M, Ellis P, Van Loo P, McLaren S, et al. High burden and pervasive positive selection of somatic mutations in normal human skin. *Science* [Internet]. 2015; 348(6237):880–6. Available from: http://www.ncbi.nlm.nih.gov/pubmed/25999502.

75. Siravegna G, Mussolin B, Buscarino M, Corti G, Cassingena A, Crisafulli G, et al. Clonal evolution and resistance to EGFR blockade in the blood of colorectal cancer patients. *Nat Med* [Internet]. 2015; 21(7):795–801. Available from: http://www.nature.com/nm/journal/v21/n7/full/nm.3870.html?WT.ec_id=NM-201507&spMailingID=49045495&spUserID=MTEwMjUwNjE0MzgxS0&spJobID=720844904&spReportId=NzIwODQ0OTA0S0.

76. Schreiber RD, Old LJ, Smyth MJ. Cancer immunoediting: Integrating immunity's roles in cancer suppression and promotion. *Science* (80–) [Internet]. 2011; 331(6024):1565–70. Available from: http://www.sciencemag.org/content/331/6024/1565.abstract.

77. Marusyk A, Tabassum DP, Altrock PM, Almendro V, Michor F, Polyak K. Non-cell-autonomous driving of tumour growth supports sub-clonal heterogeneity. *Nature* [Internet]. Nature Publishing Group; 2015; 514(7520):54–8. Available from: http://dx.doi.org/10.1038/nature13556\npapers3://publication/doi/10.1038/nature13556.

78. Lawrence MS, Stojanov P, Polak P, Kryukov G V, Cibulskis K, Sivachenko A, et al. Mutational heterogeneity in cancer and the search for new cancer-associated genes. *Nature* [Internet]. 2013; 499(7457):214–8. Available from: http://dx.doi.org/10.1038/nature12213.

Appendix: A Brief Statistics Primer

Content Contributed by Daniel Peñaherrera, July 13, 2016

This section will cover the conceptual framework of statistics and probability in hopes of familiarizing you with the statistical thinking process. Some at least minimal prior exposure to statistics is assumed. After reviewing the basics, this chapter will conclude with a section on regression analysis and model fitting. While many statistical tools offer shortcuts and built-in analytical capabilities, it is worth being familiar with the underlying math.

FOUNDATIONS

Scientific determinism postulates that we may predict how a system will develop over time if only we knew (i) the laws governing that system and (ii) the initial state of the system. Unfortunately, we live in an extraordinarily complex and uncertain world. Because of our imprecise knowledge and measurement errors, our reductionist attempts to describe reality will at best give us only approximations. As George Box once said, "All models are wrong, but some are useful."

For these reasons, we must deal with uncertainty, and statistical inference is of great help with this. Statistics offers a methodology for developing theorems and procedures that allow us to extract meaning from data that has been generated by stochastic processes.

POPULATION AND SAMPLE

In statistical inference, we are concerned with deducing the underlying distribution of the data which will provide the foundation of our statistical models. This entails inferring properties about a **population** through **sampling**. The population is assumed to be larger than the data set, which is our sample. There are different ways one might go about attaining this subset of the population and one ought to be aware of this sampling mechanism. Sampling mechanisms can introduce ***biases*** into the data.

It is also important to note that today, with the advent of greater computational abilities and big data, one may be able record every observation of interest. At this point, is sampling even necessary? Should we just focus on preforming statistical analyses on entire populations? Well, not exactly.

Sampling still solves some engineering problems and the amount of data you might need largely depends on what your goals are. For instance, sampling may be more convenient and computationally efficient as we do not have to store all the data all the time. Additionally, even if we were working with all the data, one may still think of it as a subset of an even larger data set not yet observed. One should also be wary of the hidden bias of big data; that is to say, although we may be working with the entire data set, that does not necessarily mean that the data is objective. There may still be potential errors and biases that occur during the data collection process.

RANDOM VARIABLES

When conducting an experiment or developing a model, we deal with characteristics of interest that take on random values during the experimental phase. The exact numerical values obtained during the experimental phase will depend on many factors that account for the measurement's randomness and the size and complexity of the sample space as well as the experimentalists' resources. Sometimes, it may not be possible to directly observe the outcome. Thus, what one might typically do is measure some quantity X that reveals some information about the outcome. Being that the value of X depends on the outcome of the experiment, which is stochastic, we say that X is a **random variable**.

Because the measured value of the random variable must be numeric, we are often restricted to some domain of possible values. The two types of random variables one will encounter are either *discrete* or *continuous*. A discrete random variable is one whose domain of possible values will be finite or countably infinite. Countably infinite just means one can count all the elements in a set in such a way that you will get to any particular element in a finite amount of time. Typically, discrete random variables are usually the result of count data. Examples of discrete random variables include the result from a die roll, the number of coin tosses till the first heads, the number of matching bases when comparing two strands of DNA of the same length, or the number of alleles in generation t+1.

A continuous random variable is one whose domain of possible values is uncountably infinite; that is, it takes values in the set of all real numbers $\mathbb{R}$. Continuous random variables are often measures of times, lengths, weights, and percentages. Examples include the time until a certain cellular molecule degrades or the molecular weight of a randomly selected RNA molecule.

Discrete Random Variables

Mathematically, we say that a real-valued variable X is said to be discrete if there is a countable set of values $E = \{x_1, x_2, \ldots\} \subset \mathbb{R}$ such that $\mathbb{P}(X \in E) = 1$. In this case, the ***probability mass function*** (PMF) of X is the function $p_x : E \rightarrow [0, 1]$ defined by $p_x(x) = P(X = x)$.

To illustrate how the PMF of a discrete random variable relates to the probability distribution of that variable, suppose $A \subset E$. Then

$$\mathbb{P}(X \in A) = \sum_{x \in A} p_X(x),$$

that is, the probability that X belongs to A is equal to the sum of the PMF evaluated at all of the elements of A. For a probability distribution to be valid it must satisfy two properties:

(i)

$$\sum_{x \in A} \mathbb{P}(X = x) = 1$$

(ii)

$$\mathbb{P}(X = x) \geq 0$$

$$\forall x \in A$$

The first property states that the probabilities assigned to each value in the domain of X must sum to 1. The second simply states that the probabilities must be non-negative numbers.

Another special function of the discrete random variable is the ***cumulative distribution function*** (CDF). This function is defined for any real valued number x as the probability that the random variable will be less than or equal to x. By this definition, we express it mathematically as

$$F_X(x) = \mathbb{P}(X \leq x),$$

If p_x is the PMF of a discrete random variable X with range $\{x_1, x_2, \ldots\}$ and F_x is its CDF, then

$$F_X(x) = \sum_{x_i \leq x} p_X(x_i).$$

Although both the PMF and CDF convey the same information and one can always be derived from the other, one should be able to acknowledge their difference.

Example: Suppose we want to estimate the genetic drift in a population of interest that has been maintained at 100 diploid individuals through 5 generations. In population genetics, the neutral theory of evolution claims that genetic mutations insert genetic variation into populations and are countered by the process of genetic drift which eliminates genetic variation from populations.

In mating, an allele either does or does not get passed on to the next generation. Thus, random mating produces discrete binary observations and we can simulate the amount of genetic drift with a Monte Carlo simulation. We will create 1,000 random walks through 5 generations and take a random sample from a **binomial distribution** of size 200 (because 100 diploids implies 200 genomes).

A discrete random variable X is said to be a ***Binomial random variable*** *with parameters n and p* $\in$ *[0, 1] if X takes values in the set {0, 1, . . . , n} and the PMF of X is equal to*

$$p_X(k) \equiv \mathbb{P}(X = k) = \binom{n}{k} p^k (1 - p)^{n-k}.$$

The name of this distribution come from the relationship between the probabilities $p_x(k)$ and the coefficients in a binomial expansion:

$$\sum_{k=0}^{n} p_X(k) = \sum_{k=0}^{n} \binom{n}{k} p^k (1 - p)^{n-k} = (p + 1 - p)^n = 1$$

It's worth noting that a *Bernoulli* random variable is also a binomial random variable with parameters n=1 and p.

Theorem: *Let* $X_1, \ldots, X_n$ *be independent Bernoulli random variables, each with the same parameter p. Then the sum* $X = X_1 + \ldots + X_2$ *is a binomial random variable with parameters n and p.*

In our exercise, the random sampling process always starts with a probability of sampling our allele at 50% in the first generation. In each subsequent generation the probability is updated to reflect the realized frequency from the previous generation. Once we get to the final generation, the simulated allele frequency will typically drift away from the initial 50%. Below, I have included the R code to run the simulation.

```
##code for sampling
x = 0.5 #initial allele frq
sz = 100*2
k = matrix(-999, nr=100m nc=4) #matrix to store results

for(i in 1:1000){
    xf = x #initial frq of 0.5, will also store updated allele frq
    for(j in 1:4){ #5 generations require 4 mating rounds
        xf = rbinom(1,size=200, xf) / 200 #random sample
        k[i,j] = xf #updates matrix
    }
}

k = cbind(rep(0.5,1000),k) #add first gen

##code for plotting
#plotting 1000 random walks
plot(1,1,xlim=c(1,5),ylimc(0,1),ty='n',
    xlab='generation',ylab='allele frq')

for(i in 1:1000){
```

```
    lines(1:5,k[i,],lwd=.1) #draw 1000 random walks as lines
    points(5.1,k[i,5],pch='-',col=adjustcolor(2,alpha.f=0.1))
}

##Monte Carlo results in final gen
MC_final = sort(k[,5])
hist(MC_final) #histogram

mean(MC_final)
[1] 0.49883

#lower and upper 95% confidence intervals
c(MC_final[25], MC_final[975])
[1] 0.355 0.640
```

The resulting computations have yielded a mean of about 0.5, implying no net directional change in allele frequencies. We can also expect the starting allele frequency of 50% to fall between 36% and 64% in the fifth generation 95% of the time given our population size. However, it is important to keep in mind that these are just approximations and that we could do a larger number of simulations to improve accuracy.

Continuous Random Variables

A real-valued random variable X is said to be continuous if there is a function $f_x : \mathbb{R} \rightarrow [0, \infty]$, called the ***probability density function*** (PDF or density), such that

$$\mathbb{P}(a \leq X \leq b) = \int_a^b f_x(x)dx = F(b) - F(a)$$

for every $-\infty \leq a \leq b \leq \infty$.

The density of a continuous random variable X is different than the PMF of a discrete random variable. A PDF is defined for all real numbers in the range of the random variable. It is a continuous function that can be derived by taking the derivative of CDF of X. The choice of such a function to use for a certain random variable has everything to do with how we want to model probabilities of various sets of values occurring. The way we use the PDF for interpretation is that the area under the PDF curve between points a and b is equivalent to the probability that the random variable will have a particular value between a and b. It is important to note that if we evaluated the integral at a single point then the resulting value will be zero. That does not necessarily mean that it is improbable for the continuous random variable X to take on that value.

There are also certain restrictions to the PDF we should bear in mind in order for us to interpret the area within its curve as a probability. The first being that the function should be non-negative for all x and the second restriction is that the function should integrate to one when we integrate from $-\infty$ to ∞.

While these restrictions are important they actually don't completely limit our choices for the PDF *f(x)* as there are an infinite number of possible functions that meet these requirements.

The CDF of a continuous random variable is thus a continuous function defined as $F_X(x) = \mathbb{P}(X \leq x) \ \forall \ x \in \mathbb{R}$. From the definition provided at the beginning of the section one should be able to see how the PDF and CDF are related. As previously mentioned, if we know the density of a random variable, then we can find its CDF by integration. Similarly, if we know the CDF, then we can find the density through differentiation.

Example: From the earlier example, we used a Monte Carlo simulation to model genetic drift in a population. We can also approximate the amount of genetic drift using the **beta distribution**. The beta distribution is a fairly flexible generalization of the standard uniform distribution that is often used to model distributions of frequencies.

A continuous random variable X is said to have the ***beta distribution*** *with parameters a,b > 0 if its density is*

$$f_X(x) = \begin{cases} \frac{1}{\beta(a,b)} x^{a-1}(1-x)^{b-1} & \text{if } x \in (0,1) \\ 0 & \text{otherwise,} \end{cases}$$

where the ***beta function*** *β(a,b) is defined (for a,b > 0) by the formula*

$$\beta(a,b) = \int_0^1 x^{a-1}(1-x)^{b-1} dx.$$

It should be noted that the beta function can be expressed in terms of a ratio of **gamma functions**

$$\beta(a,b) = \frac{\Gamma(a)\Gamma(b)}{\Gamma(a+b)} = \frac{(a-1)!(b-1)!}{(a+b-1)!}$$

Notice also that if a = b = 1, then X is simply the standard uniform random variable.

As mentioned before, random mating produces discrete binary observations and we can use the beta distribution to model allele frequencies given a characterization of the random matings we expect in our population of 100 individuals. In order to do this we'll have to solve for our two "shape" parameters a and b. If we compute the expected value or mean (μ) and sample variance (σ^2) of our allele frequencies then we may use them to solve for a and b. For this exercise, suppose that the initial generation t_0 has an allele at a frequency of 0.5 and we expect the final frequency to also be 0.5 at generation t_4, so μ = 0.5. To find the variance in this context, we will rely on the following formula from Falconer and Mackay [1]

$$\sigma^2 = p_0 q_0 (1 - (1 - \frac{1}{2N})^t)$$

where t is the number of generations it takes to go from the initial population to the final while maintaining N diploid individuals. In our case t = 4, since it takes 4 mating rounds to arrive at our fifth generation and N = 100. The starting and ending allele frequencies, which we stated were both 0.5, are p_0 and q_0, respectively. Thus after a simple plug-n-chug we get $\sigma^2 = 0.00496$.

Now that we have our expected value of allele frequencies and the sample variance we may begin to estimate our shape parameters. The *method of moments* estimates of the parameters are the following formulas:

$$a = \mu(\frac{\mu(1-\mu)}{\sigma^2} - 1).$$

$$b = (1-\mu)(\frac{\mu(1-\mu)}{\sigma^2} - 1)$$

The result is that a = b = 24.688. We can now specify our beta distribution and get our estimate of the genetic drift. Below is some simple R code to run the estimation at the 95% confidence intervals:

```
n = 100
p = 0.5
q = 1-p
u = p
t = 4
v = p*q*(1-(1-(1/(2*n)))**t) #Falconer and Mackay eqn
a = u*((u*(1-u))/v-1)
b = (1-u)*((u*(1-u))/v-1)

#estimated lower and upper conf. intervals
qbeta(0.025, shape1=a, shape2=b) #lower
 [1] 0.3625435
qbeta(1-0.025, shape1=a, shape2=b) #upper
 [1] 0.6374565
```

The R code tells us that the estimated 95% confidence intervals for our beta distribution estimation of allele frequency drift are about 36.3% and 63.7%. Very close to our original results from the Monte Carlo estimates! We can extend the R code to conduct a direct comparison between the beta distribution model and the Monte Carlo simulation.

```
##return the original results from the M.C. and fit our beta est.
x = 0.5
sz = 200
k = matrix(-999, nr=100m nc=4) #matrix to store results

for(i in 1:100000){
    xf = x
    for(j in 1:4){
        xf = rbinom(1,size=200, xf) / 200 #random sample
        k[i,j] = xf
    }
```

```
}

##plot M.C. result as histogram
hist(k[,4], br=100, freq=F, main=''Monte Carlo (bars)
      vs. Beta (red line)'', xlab='allele freq')

##add beta as red line
lines(seq(0,1,0.01), dbeta(seq(0,1,0.01),
      shape1=a, shape2=b), ty='l', col=2)
```

As you can see from the figures, the beta estimates are pretty close! Despite the results, we need to address some caveats. Namely, the fact that we are using a continuous distribution to model a discrete process means that the beta distribution will be a better estimator of drift if the population size is really large. This is the case because there will be so many discrete possibilities that they are virtually continuous. If we had chosen increasingly smaller population sizes then the beta distribution's performance would suffer.

EXPECTED VALUE AND VARIANCE

The previous example illustrated the use of the expected value and variance in statistical modeling with the beta distribution. In other scenarios we also use the expected values and variance to summarize the distribution of random variables more concisely. In addition to parameter estimation, it provides a measure of comparison between random variables. This section covers how to derive these values from discrete and continuous distributions.

Suppose that X is a real-valued random variable which is either discrete with probability mass function $p_x(x)$ or continuous with probability density function $f_x(x)$. Then, the expected value of X is the weighted average of the values of X given by

$$\mathbb{E}[X] = \begin{cases} \sum_{x_i} p_X(x_i)x_i & \text{if } x \text{ is discrete} \\ \int_{-\infty}^{\infty} f_X(x)x\,dx & \text{if } x \text{ is continuous,} \end{cases}$$

provided that the sum or the integral exists.

Expectations also grant us the convenience of finding the expected value of a function of a random variable through what is commonly known as ***the Law of the Unconscious Statistician***.

Suppose that X is a real-valued random variable which is either discrete with probability mass function $p_x(x)$ or continuous with probability density function $f_x(x)$. Then, for any real-valued function $g : \mathbb{R} \to \mathbb{R}$

$$\mathbb{E}[X] = \begin{cases} \sum_{x_i} p_X(x_i)g(x_i) & \text{if } x \text{ is discrete} \\ \int_{-\infty}^{\infty} f_X(x)g(x)\,dx & \text{if } x \text{ is continuous,} \end{cases}$$

provided that the sum or the integral exists.

An important property of the law of the unconscious statistician is that expectations are linear.

Corollary: *If a and b are constants, then*

$$\mathbb{E}[aX + b] = a\mathbb{E}[X] + b$$

This same property will prove useful in the following section on regression. For now, we will utilize this property in solving for the variance.

*The nth **moment** of a real-valued random variable X is the quantity*

$$\mu_n' = \mathbb{E}[X^n] = \begin{cases} \sum_{x_i} p_X(x_i) x_i^n & \text{if } x \text{ is discrete} \\ \int_{-\infty}^{\infty} f_X(x) x^n dx & \text{if } x \text{ is continuous,} \end{cases}$$

*provided that the sum or the integral exists. Similarly, if $\mu = \mathbb{E}[X]$ is finite, then the nth **central moment** of X is the quantity*

$$\mu_n = \mathbb{E}[(X - \mu)^n] = \begin{cases} \sum_{x_i} p_X(x_i)(x_i - \mu)^n & \text{if } x \text{ is discrete} \\ \int_{-\infty}^{\infty} f_X(x)(x - \mu)^n dx & \text{if } x \text{ is continuous,} \end{cases}$$

provided that the sum or the integral exists.

Notice that the first central moment vanishes, since the linearity of expectations implies that

$$\mu_1 = \mathbb{E}[X - \mu] = \mu - \mu = 0.$$

The second, third, and fourth central moments are important in statistics and applied probability. In fact, the second central moment is the variance of the random variable.

$$\begin{aligned} \sigma^2 &= \mathbb{E}[(X - \mu)^2] \\ &= \mathbb{E}[X^2 - 2\mu X + \mu^2] \\ &= \mathbb{E}[X^2] - 2\mu^2 + \mu^2 \\ &= \mathbb{E}[X^2] - \mu^2. \end{aligned}$$

The square root of the variance is the standard deviation, denoted as σ. The standard deviation will have the same units as the random variable X, whereas the variance has the units of X^2. This means that if the units of X are cm, then the units of σ are also cm, whereas the units of σ^2 are cm^2.

REGRESSION ANALYSIS

In this section, we will start by covering *linear regression* and finish the chapter by reviewing *logistic regression*. Linear regression is a very simple approach for what is called supervised learning in machine learning and generally an all-around useful tool for predicting a quantitative response. Here, we begin by reviewing its key ideas as well as the ordinary least squares approach.

In *simple linear regression,* we are predicting a quantitative response for our dependent variable Y on the basis of a single independent variable X, assuming there is approximately a linear relationship between the two. Mathematically, we express this relationship as

$$Y \approx \beta_0 + \beta_1 X + \epsilon,$$

where ϵ is the mean-zero error term; meaning the expected value of the error term is zero.

In this equation, our population parameters β_0 and β_1 are unknown constants that represent the *intercept* and *slope* of the linear model. Because they are unknown we must use our sample or training data to compute our estimators $\hat{\beta}_0$ and $\hat{\beta}_1$. Once we have done that, we can use the model for forecasting by computing

$$\hat{y} = \hat{\beta}_0 + \hat{\beta}_1 x + \epsilon,$$

where $\hat{y}$ indicates a prediction of Y on the basis of X = x.

Ordinary Least Squares (OLS)

If we observe a random sample of size (n) from the population then for each ith observation we have $Y_i = \beta_0 + \beta_1 x_i + \epsilon_i$, where $\epsilon_i = y_i - \hat{y}_i$ is the ith residual—the difference between the ith observed y value and the ith predicted y value. Furthermore, we define the *residual sum of squares* (RSS) as

$$RSS = \epsilon_1^2 + \epsilon_2^2 + \ldots + \epsilon_n^2,$$

or equivalently as

$$RSS = \left(y_1 - \hat{\beta}_0 - \hat{\beta}_1 x_1\right)^2 + \left(y_2 - \hat{\beta}_0 - \hat{\beta}_1 x_2\right)^2 + \ldots + \left(y_n - \hat{\beta}_0 - \hat{\beta}_1 x_n\right)^2.$$

In the OLS method, we choose our estimators to minimize the residual sum of squares. To derive estimators for the model we must rely on the following assumptions:

$$\mathbb{E}[\epsilon] = 0$$
$$\mathbb{E}[\epsilon \mid x] = 0.$$

The expectation of ϵ given x is known as the *zero conditional mean* assumption and it implies that the error term and x are statistically independent. From these two expectations and the sample means $\bar{y} = \frac{1}{n}\sum_{i=1}^{n} y_i$ and $\bar{x} = \frac{1}{n}\sum_{i=1}^{n} x_i$, one can show that the minimizers are

$$\hat{\beta}_0 = \bar{y} - \hat{\beta}_1 \bar{x},$$
$$\hat{\beta}_1 = \frac{\sum_{i=1}^{n}(x_i - \bar{x})(y_i - \bar{y})}{\sum_{i=1}^{n}(x_i - \bar{x})^2}.$$

These equations define the least squares coefficient estimates for the simple linear regression. Notice that for $\hat{\beta}_1$ the numerator is the *covariance* between (x) and (y), while the denominator is the variance of x.

Estimator Accuracy

After deriving our OLS estimators, we turn our attention to assessing their accuracy. Recall that the OLS estimators are different from the population parameters. Even though these coefficients are different, we can expect that in general the OLS coefficients will act as good estimates of the population parameters. If it is indeed the case that, on average, we expect $\hat{\beta}_0$ and $\hat{\beta}_0$ to estimate β_0 and β_1 then we say that the OLS estimators are *unbiased*. Thus, an unbiased estimator does not systematically over- or underestimate the true parameter. The following are the four conditions that must be satisfied for the OLS estimators to be unbiased:

The true population regression must be linear in its parameters

Data are a random sample of size (n) from the population $\{(x_i, y_i) : i = 1, .., n\}$

Sample contains variation in $\{x_i : i = 1, .., n\}$

Zero Conditional Mean : $\mathbb{E}[\epsilon \mid x] = 0$

Homoskedasticity: The error term ϵ has the same variance given any value of x: $\mathrm{Var}(\epsilon \mid x) = \sigma^2$

Having established that the average of the OLS estimators will be very close to β_0 and β_1, we may still encounter substantial under- or overestimation in a single estimator. We can measure how off a single estimator is from a population parameter by computing the *standard error*.

$$SE\left(\hat{\beta}_0\right)^2 = \sigma^2\left[\frac{1}{n} + \frac{\overline{x}^2}{\sum_{i=1}^{n}(x_i - \overline{x})^2}\right],$$

$$SE\left(\hat{\beta}_1\right)^2 = \frac{\sigma^2}{\sum_{i=1}^{n}(x_i - \overline{x})^2},$$

where $\sigma^2 = \mathrm{Var}(\epsilon)$. Generally, σ^2 is unknown and must be estimated from the data. This estimate is known as the *residual standard error* and is given by the formula $\mathrm{RSE} = \sqrt{RSS/(n-2)}$. Observe that we rely on the *zero conditional mean* assumption here in order for these formulas to be strictly valid; however, it is unrealistic for this to actually be true. Nonetheless, the formulas still turn out to be a good approximation.

Interpreting these formulas reveals useful properties of the estimators. Notice that $\mathrm{SE}(\hat{\beta}_1)$ is smaller when x_i is more spread out, meaning that we have more flexibility to estimate a slope when this is the case. We also use standard error to compute confidence intervals as follows:

$$\hat{\beta}_0 \pm 2 * SE(\hat{\beta}_0),$$
$$\hat{\beta}_1 \pm 2 * SE(\hat{\beta}_1).$$

Standard errors are also used to perform *hypothesis testing* on the OLS estimators, the most common of which is testing the *null hypothesis* of H_0 : *There is no relationship between X and Y* versus the *alternative hypothesis* of H_1 : *There is some relationship between X and Y*. Mathematically, we represent this as

$$H_0 : \beta_1 = 0$$

versus

$$H_1 : \beta_1 \neq 0.$$

If β_1 were indeed 0 then the model reduces to $Y = \beta_0 + \epsilon$, indicating that X and Y have no association. To test the null, we must determine whether β_1 is sufficiently far from zero that we can conclude that β_1 is non-zero. This will depend on the $SE(\hat{\beta}_1)$, for if it is small then even relatively small values of $\hat{\beta}_1$ may provide strong evidence that $\beta_1 \neq 0$. Conversely, if the $SE(\hat{\beta}_1)$ is large, then $\hat{\beta}_1$ must be large in absolute value in order to reject the null hypothesis. This brings us to the *t-statistic,* defined as

$$t = \frac{\hat{\beta}_1 - 0}{SE(\hat{\beta}_1)}.$$

The t-statistic measures the number of standard deviations that $\hat{\beta}_1$ is away from zero. The t-distribution is bell shaped and for large enough values of n it becomes similar to the normal distribution. If we find that the relationship between X and Y is nonexistent then we expect that the above equation will have a t-distribution with n-2 degrees of freedom. To draw a conclusion on the strength of the relationship between X and Y, we simply compute the *p-value*.

The p-value is the probability of observing a t-statistic as extreme or greater, assuming the null hypothesis is true. This means that if we observe a small p-value, then we can infer that there is an association between the dependent and explanatory variables. Thus, we *reject the null hypothesis*. Conversely, if we observe large enough p-values, then we have evidence to conclude that there is hardly any association between X and Y—in doing so we *fail to reject the null hypothesis*. Our conclusions will of course depend on the p-value cutoffs that we set. Typically cutoffs for rejecting the null are 5% or 1%.

Goodness of Fit

Having rejected the null hypothesis in favor of the alternative, it is appropriate to next measure the accuracy of the model. We typically assess the overall quality of the simple linear regression residual standard error (RSE) and the R^2 statistics.

Due to the presence of error terms, even if the true regression parameter were known, it would still not be possible to perfectly predict Y from X. Thus we need a way to measure the average amount that the predicted value of the dependent variable ($\hat{y}$) will deviate from the true regression line. The RSE does just that; it is an estimate of the standard deviation of ϵ given by the formula

$$RSE = \sqrt{\frac{1}{n-2} RSS} = \sqrt{\frac{1}{n-2} \sum_{i=1}^{n} (y_i - \hat{y}_i)^2}.$$

The RSE may also be interpreted as a measure of the lack of fit of the model to the data. A model with a predictive value that closely matches the true outcome values is a model that fits the data very well. However, beware of *overfitting* the model to closely match the sample data. In that scenario, the model will be incredibly accurate with regard to the sample or training data used, but once new data is introduced it performs poorly.

Despite its usefulness, RSE is measured in units of Y, makes it not always clear what constitutes a good RSE value. For that reason, we also rely on the R^2 statistics to provide an alternative measure of fit that is independent of the scale of Y. The R^2 is the proportion, bounded between 0 and 1, of variance calculated as

$$R^2 = \frac{TSS - RSS}{TSS} = 1 - \frac{RSS}{TSS} = 1 - \frac{\sum_{i=1}^{n} (y_i - \hat{y}_i)^2}{\sum_{i=1}^{n} (y_i - \bar{y})^2},$$

where TSS = $\sum_{i=1}^{n}(y_i - \bar{y})^2$ is the *total sum of squares*. TSS is a measurement of the total variance in the dependent variable Y. In contrast, recall that the RSS is a measure of the amount of variability that is left unexplained after the regression is performed. So then one can interpret TSS – RSS as the amount of variability in Y that is explained by performing the regression. From the formula above, the R^2 measures the *proportion of variability in Y that can be explained by X*.

In interpreting the R^2, a value close to 1 indicates that a large proportion of the variability in Y is explained by the model. Because the R^2 is bounded between 0 and 1, it has an interpretative advantage over the RSE. However, determining what is a good R^2 may still pose a challenge and will largely be dependent on the model's application. In many cases, such as in biology, linear models will at best provide a rough approximation. Under those circumstances, observing only a very small proportion of the variance in Y explained by X is not unexpected. Thus, a low R^2 might be more realistic.

MULTIVARIATE LINEAR REGRESSION

In practice, when analyzing large data sets, we often have more than one explanatory variable included in the regression model. In general, a multiple linear regression takes the form

$$Y = \beta_0 + \beta_1 X_1 + \beta_2 X_2 + \ldots + \beta_k X_k + \epsilon,$$

for X_j is the jth predictor and β_j quantifies the relationship between that variable and Y. We interpret β_j as the *average* impact on Y from a *marginal* increase in X_j while holding all else constant.

OLS Estimators

We again use the least squares method to choose our parameter estimates that minimize the sum of square residuals. In this case, the model predictions take the form

$$\hat{y} = \hat{\beta}_0 + \hat{\beta}_1 X_1 + \hat{\beta}_2 X_2 + \ldots + \hat{\beta}_k X_k + \epsilon,$$

and the RSS is represented as

$$RSS = \sum_{i=1}^{n} (y_i - \hat{y}_i)^2 = \sum_{i=1}^{n} \left(y_i - \hat{\beta}_0 - \hat{\beta}_1 x_{i1} - \hat{\beta}_2 x_{i2} - \ldots - \hat{\beta}_k x_{ik}\right)^2.$$

Relationship Strength

For conciseness, I will only go over hypothesis testing and deciding on which important variables to include in the model as much of the simple linear regression material already covered overlaps with the multivariate case.

In multiple regression with k predictors, we need to determine whether $\beta_1 = \beta_2 = \ldots = \beta_k = 0$. We use this as our null hypothesis and test it against the alternative of at least one β_k being non-zero. This hypothesis test is conducted by computing the *F-statistic,*

$$F = \frac{(TSS - RSS) / k}{RSS / (n - k - 1)},$$

where TSS and RSS are the same from the simple linear regression. When there is no relationship between the Y and the $X_j's$ then the F-statistic will take a value close to 1. An F-statistic ≈ 1 occurs because the numerator and denominator will both take on the value σ^2, provided that H_0 is true. If H_1 is true, the numerator will take on a value greater than σ^2, so we expect F to be greater than 1.

Suppose we compute the F-statistic and examine its associated p-value to conclude that at least one of the explanatory variables is related to Y. Naturally, we would like to know which of our estimators best explains the variance seen in Y. We could examine the individual p-values for each of the predictors; however, if the number of explanatory variables is large then we are likely to make some false discoveries. In a process called *forward selection*, we start with a model containing nothing but the intercept term called the *null model*. Then we fit k simple linear regressions and add to the null model the variable that results in the lowest RSS. This procedure is continued until we arrive at a model that can no longer have its RSS lowered. Unfortunately, for models with many explanatory variables this is infeasible as there are a total of 2^k models that contain subsets of k variables. Under such constraints one must rely on automated processes that are beyond the scope of the material covered in this section.

LOGISTIC REGRESSION

We now turn to the problem of *classification*. Where before we were concerned with making quantitative predictions, with *logistic regression* we can make qualitative predictions. A suitable application could be medical diagnosis or classifying DNA mutations to a given disease.

Once again we begin with a sample or training data set, but the response now falls into one of two categories. Logistic regression accomplishes this by modeling the probability that Y belongs to a particular category. This means that our prediction will be a value bounded between 0 and 1 for all values of X. There are indeed infinitely many functions that satisfy this requirement. Here, we will use the *logistic function* represented as,

$$p(X) = \frac{e^{\beta_0 + \beta_1 X}}{1 + e^{\beta_0 + \beta_1 X}}.$$

As can be seen, the logistic regression model produces a sigmoidal curve. With a fair bit of manipulation, we observe,

$$\frac{p(X)}{1 - p(X)} = e^{\beta_0 + \beta_1 X}.$$

The quantity on the left hand side is called the *odds*, which may take a value anywhere between 0 and ∞. Values close to 0 or ∞ indicate a very low or very high probability of the data. By taking the log of both sides, we get

$$\log\left(\frac{p(X)}{1 - p(X)}\right) = \beta_0 + \beta_1 X.$$

The left hand side of this equation is called *log-odds* or *logit*. Recall from the previous section that β_1 gives the average change in Y from a marginal increase in X. Here, a marginal increase in X corresponds to a change in the log-odds by β_1.

This is also equivalent to multiplying the odds by e^{β_1}. In contrast, because the relationship between p(X) and X is nonlinear, a marginal increase in X does not correspond to a change of β_1 in p(X). The rate of change in p(X) actually depends on the current value of X. Furthermore, if β_1 is positive, a marginal increase in X will be associated with increasing p(X), and if β_1 is negative, a marginal increase in X is associated with decreasing p(X).

Estimating Parameters

Again we are faced with unknown parameters β_0 and β_1 that must be estimated, and we do so using the method of *maximum likelihood*. The intuition behind this procedure is that we seek estimates for β_0 and β_1 such that the predicted probability $\hat{p}(x_i)$ corresponds closely to the data's observed classification. We express this intuition mathematically as the *likelihood function*

$$l(\beta_0, \beta_1) = \prod_{i:y_i=1} p(x_i) \prod_{i':y_{i'}=0} (1 - p(x_{i'})).$$

Maximum likelihood is a very general approach for choosing $\hat{\beta}_0$ and $\hat{\beta}_1$ that maximize this likelihood function. In fact, the least squares method covered in the previous sections is a special case of the maximum likelihood method. With the use of statistical programming languages like R, we need not concern ourselves with the details of the maximum likelihood fitting procedure.

In determining the accuracy of our estimators, the process is largely the same. The exception is that here we use the *z-statistic* in place of the t-statistic.

So Why Logistic Regression?

When it comes to problems of classification, linear regression is not suitable when our model's output is a qualitative response. Consider the problem where, given a data set of DNA samples, we seek to identify which DNA mutations are deleterious and which are not. Potentially, there is the option of utilizing the dummy variable approach, where the independent variable Y is 0 if the DNA mutation is nondeleterious or 1 if it is. In special cases, it has been proven that this approach fitted with a linear regression can in fact estimate $\mathbb{P}(Y \mid X)$. However, by using linear regression, it's possible that some of our estimates may take values beyond the [0,1] interval. This is where logistic regression becomes appropriate and it is the data analyst's responsibility to identify whether a particular problem is a classification problem or not. So in summary, simple linear regression and multiple linear regression models are appropriate when core assumptions hold, chief among them being that there is a clear linear relationship between the independent and dependent variables. Last, logistic regression is suitable when trying to classify your data into two distinct categories.

This ends our brief primer on statistics. Hopefully when you are analyzing data you will keep in mind the foundational concepts covered here. For additional details on the techniques discussed, you can refer to:

- Flagel, Lex. "A Hopeful Monster." Modeling Genetic Drift Part 2. Blogger, December 4, 2013. Web: January 7, 2016. http://ahopefulmonster.blogspot.com/2013/12/modeling-genetic-drift-part-2.html.
- James, Gareth, Daniela Witten, Trevor Hastie, and Robert Tibshirani. "Linear Regression, Classification." In *Introduction to Statistical Learning: With Applications in R*. New York: Springer, 2013, pp. 59–72, 127–134.
- Maiste, Paul. "Probability and Statistics for Bioinformatics and Genetics." Course Notes, pp. 28–37. Johns Hopkins University, May 2, 2006. http://www.ams.jhu.edu/~dan/550.435/notes/COURSENOTES435.pdf.

REFERENCES

1. Falconer, D. S. "Small Populations I." In *Introduction to Quantitative Genetics*. New York: Ronald, 1960.

CHAPTER 8

Next-Generation Cyberinfrastructures

So far in this book we have covered many components of biomedical data management and analysis. Of course, as you have already certainly realized, the neat separation of topics into chapters doesn't hold in real life. In research, clinical, and administrative settings, they overlap and interrelate in ways that are at once messy and fascinating. There are countless such scenarios—far, far more than we can cover in this book. But in this last chapter we share one example that we hope is rich and compelling.

Larger research institutions, in particular, find themselves dealing with many, if not all, of the issues covered in this book: genomic analysis, data management, data storage, networking, infrastructure, and data science. As a way of synthesizing the various strands and themes of this book and providing a specific example, we share the story of Arizona State University (ASU). We detail how we have chosen to meet our community's data and compute needs in ways that we hope will continue to put us on good footing and foster first-rate research. ASU offers a valuable example because it is a very large research institution, with over 90,000 enrolled students and over 3,000 faculty. And to sing our own praises, we were honored in the 2016 university ratings by *U.S. News & World Report*, where we ranked No. 1 among the Most Innovative Schools in America. It is also, of course, best to write about what you know.

In 2014 I accepted the appointment to director of research computing at ASU. In this role I have been intimately involved and often directly responsible for many of ASU's large-scale computing initiatives. A final note before we begin: I am certainly not holding out ASU as the only or even the best way of meeting these challenges. But I do suspect that most successful institutional approaches use some of the strategies we are using at ASU, including: hybrid cloud, a mix of standing and on-demand resources; full-time staff bolstered by short-term contractors as needed; and the adoption of ubiquitous compute, to extend research computing capacity to all who require access.

NEXT-GENERATION CYBER CAPABILITY*

The biomedical research community faces major challenges in addressing the integration and analysis of the rapidly growing volumes of highly diverse data and their application to discovery, translation, and support for improved patient care. The challenge presented by this revolution is the need to develop and implement hardware and software that can store, retrieve, and analyze mountains of complex data and transform it into knowledge to improve our understanding of the human condition. These factors have impacted not only research sciences but also inter- and intrauniversity collaboration. Addressing

* Some material taken from Jay Etchings, "New Models for Research Computing, Part I," HPCwire, March 9, 2015, https://www.hpcwire.com/2015/03/09/new-models-for-research-computing-part-i/.

the current challenges required a novel resolution path, disruptive to the traditional university high-performance computing model: a sustainable, collaborative, elastic, distributed model that promises to overcome legacy barriers and open new avenues into research sciences.

Arizona State University charged the Research Computing and Complex Adaptive Systems Network (CASN) teams with articulating the cyberinfrastructure necessary to successfully execute 21st-century research projects. It is the assessment of the team that what we have termed a Next Generation Cyber Capability (NGCC) is required to meet the unique needs of research projects and major collaborations. Conceptually, the NGCC is composed of standing capabilities and dynamic, on-demand, virtual resources that grow and contract as efforts require. The NGCC is a synergistic system that uniquely synthesizes physical and logical infrastructure that is fulfilled through dedicated resources working in unison.

The NGCC is the concept of Dr. Kenneth Buetow. As the director of the Computational Science and Informatics Core Program and the Complex Adaptive Systems Initiative, Ken serves as a professor in ASU's School of Life Sciences. He is regarded as an expert in addressing the major challenges facing the biomedical research community in the integration and analysis of the rapidly growing volumes of highly diverse data and their application to improved patient care. ASU is emerging as a leader in this revolution.

While components of the NGCC reside in various isolated niches throughout many research university communities, successfully meeting the needs of large-scale holistic projects requires a dedicated enterprise. Mirroring the dynamic nature of the complex adaptive systems life cycle, the NGCC is executed through a construct that utilizes local, virtual, and "cloud-based" resources. Central to the project is the ability to leverage a portfolio of virtual capabilities on demand for short-term engagements. The ASU NGCC has adopted a novel approach that extends the norms of traditional high-performance computing (HPC). The rich collection of assets represents a first-generation data science research instrument through the choreography of a diverse collection of physical and logical capabilities that perform as an integrated whole.

The physical infrastructure integrates differing hardware platforms configured to support transactional computing, HPC, and big data problems. Each of these elements utilizes alternative hardware configurations optimized to support the unique characteristics of the computational problems it addresses. The transactional component supports day-to-day utility computing and is composed of a cluster of cost-efficient commodity hardware. Its unique characteristic is a very large data storage reservoir. An HPC component supports computationally intensive efforts in three alternative configurations, all with high-speed connectivity to the transactional storage reservoir. The first configuration is composed of a large cluster of fast processors with modest memory. The second configuration is a smaller cluster of fast processors that access a common, shared large memory resource. The third configuration, which supports big data problems, is composed of a cluster of fast processor nodes interconnected with high-speed links, with each node having large memory and large data storage. This cluster similarly is interconnected at high speed to the transactional data storage reservoir via a unified high-speed, low-latency fabric. To support access to outside virtual capacity, all components are connected to the research network over Internet2 and the Research Education Network by high-speed connections at speeds of 40 gigabit and 100 gigabit Ethernet.

The NGCC embraces the following foundational components:

- Research centers without walls that are not only National Institute of Standards and Technology compliant but are collaboration-centric
- Open big data frameworks that support global metadata management for digital curation of omics data
- Dedicated bandwidth, free of policy or capacity restrictions, supporting research collaboration
- OpenFlow-based software-defined networking, dedicated bandwidth supporting research collaboration
- Programmable, pluggable architectures for the next generation of research computing
- Efficient and effective touchless network management free from the bottlenecks of legacy hardware–defined networking in a secure computing environment
- Research as a Service workload-based provisioning for holistically defined scientific challenges.

The rest of this chapter explores in greater detail the organization and functioning of the NGCC. We also offer valuable information about funding and implementation, sharing lessons about both deployment (implementation) and architectural design (sustainability) that we have already learned from our experiences.

NGCC DESIGN AND INFRASTRUCTURE

The NGCC is now well into year three of a five-year proposal and has contributed to a significant uptick in bioinformatics proposals submitted to the National Institutes of Health and the National Science Foundation. The typical gestation period for these proposals is 12–18 months before an award is processed and funding becomes available. Therefore, this year is the target year to refresh many of the components now ripe for upgrade.

The unwritten policy at most organizations, public or private, is to award seed monies in an amount, such as $10 million over five years, and then dispense a percentage, in this case $4 million up front, with the remainder available in subsequent years. Keep in mind, in private industry, it is common when an initiative fails to meet an intended milestone to freeze further funding in order to recoup the remainder for new seed projects. This could happen in the public realm as well, but due to the extended period by which success is measured in public awards, this is less likely, although not entirely unheard of.

The NGCC is based on an open source ideology and is thus a bit different from most enterprise and research systems. Think of the NGCC as a collaborative, where resources are utilized and payment, at least in the immediate term, comes in the way of code development and contribution back to the cluster in the form of software enhancements, much the way the open source Apache project functions.

One of the most significant accomplishments of this effort is the Precision Medicine Consortium to Explore Next Generation Genomics Open Source Platform. Harnessing the full potential of precision medicine demands a platform to store a massive volume of genomic information, an analytic interface, and real-time querying at scale, among other requirements. The consortium will further define these requirements and address the limitations of current technologies through an open and collaborative approach using Design Thinking. It will also leverage knowledge across multiple domains, including medical genetics, programming, HPC, and big data to ensure that organizations of any size have the opportunity to store and analyze genomics in a single platform. At the 2016 Hadoop Summit in San Jose, California, the consortium members launched the collaborative effort to define an open source platform for genomics.

The logical infrastructure makes the NGCC a whole more than the sum of its parts and includes the software products that support NGCC research projects. This software is executed against combinations of the physical infrastructure components and can be subdivided into transactional, analytic, and big data capabilities. Cross-cutting these are semantic capabilities that permit data to move between individual components. A core collection of operations tools interconnects logical components and is used to support and develop software. The transactional component represents the software infrastructure necessary to capture, manage, and share data. The analytic infrastructure is composed of tools that transform and interpret data. The big data infrastructure supports the management, processing, and mining of data of large volume, varying structure, and diverse content. The semantic component supports data use/reuse and provides context for converting data to information. As a whole, the components create the Transdisciplinary Common Ontologic Representation (TransCORE) framework. TransCORE enables data liquidity and facilitates discovery. TransCORE underpins a universal knowledge engine. Figure 8.1 shows the TransCORE Framework.

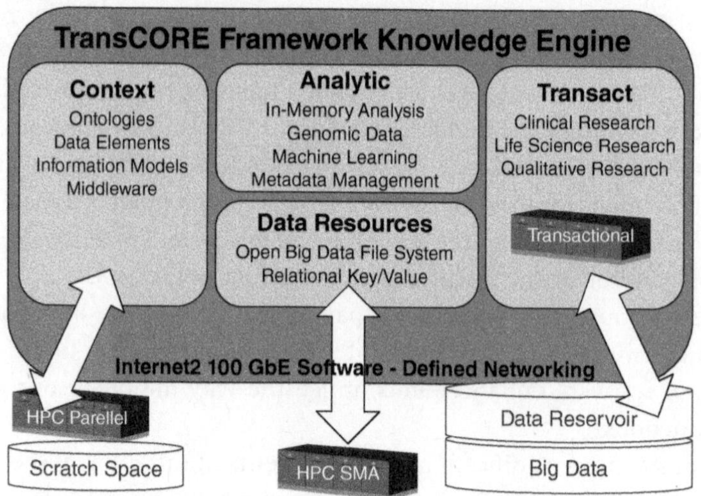

Figure 8.1 TransCORE Framework of ASU's NGCC
TransCORE Framework ASU NGCC 2012 Ken Buetow—Jay Etchings.

Staff resources are required to design, manage, and execute the capabilities represented in the infrastructure and to manage the enterprise. The composition of the NGCC staff mirrors the subcomponents described above and shown in Figure 8.1. The dynamic capabilities proposed for the NGCC dictate that staff is the most critical component. The success of the enterprise depends on staff with expertise that can bridge the gaps, especially in coordinating standing and on-demand resources.

Space is also required to support the NGCC. Two broad categories describe the space requirements: space supporting physical infrastructure and space to house staff. The physical infrastructure requires specialized power, cooling, network access, and security. Staff space requires high-speed Internet connectivity and team space.

The current ASU computational environment has some NGCC components in place. However, where they exist, these resources are committed to other activities, cannot be seamlessly connected to other resources, or are not cost-effectively priced to make them competitive with *de novo* generating new components or utilization of outside resources. Moreover, there are significant gaps in existing capabilities. Nowhere within the current ASU enterprise are the resources assembled in a manner that makes them consumable in the systems manner required to address current and future projects. Therefore, the NGCC is being created *de novo* using a phased approach that utilizes on-demand contract resources in parallel with the development of the complex core structure.

Systems Architecture

The NGCC addresses large-scale, multistakeholder, transdisciplinary research initiatives. It is supported by a dynamic, evolving, multidimensional system of physical, logical, and staff resources. The capabilities include extensive and mixed computational capacity, state-of-the-art networks, large and heterogeneous storage resources, diverse software and data services, and personnel who can administer and support complex environments and analytic tooling. To describe the composition of the NGCC, it is useful to project the system's architecture along alternative views derived from the Reference Model of Open Distributed Processing systems architecture (ISO/IEC 10746). The following paragraphs provide an elaboration of the NGCC based on five key system points of view:

1. **Enterprise.** The purpose, scope, and policies for the system (i.e., business requirements)
2. **Physical infrastructure.** The hardware components necessary to support the system
3. **Logical infrastructure.** The software, data management, and data resources that comprise the system
4. **Staff resources.** The staff necessary to develop, execute, and maintain the system
5. **Space.** Characteristics associated with space to house components of the system within a high-availability enterprise data center

Enterprise

The research project life cycle is a key consideration from the enterprise point of view. This project life cycle requires the NGCC to evolve consistent with the maturation of each specific project. First, there is a design phase where proof-of-concept work is performed to assess feasibility and establish credibility. In a second build phase, the lessons from the first phase are used to establish the working project, expanding the NGCC's resources as needed to meet specific project needs. The final launch phase draws on the NGCC resources identified previously. Each phase has unique characteristics. Figure 8.2 shows the NGCC's enterprise model.

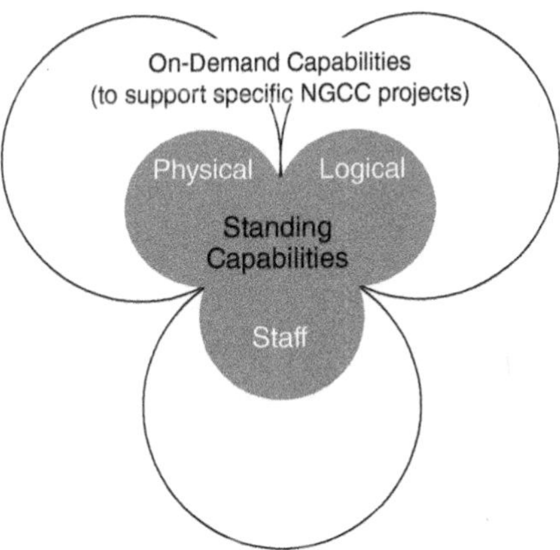

Figure 8.2 NGCC Enterprise Model

During the design phase, the NGCC leverages standing capabilities. These capabilities represent a collection of core competencies that permit continuity of operations, economies of scale (components that are reused across projects), exploratory capacity, and ASU ownership of innovation. In the build phase, these capabilities are expanded on demand, as determined by the specifics of the project. The build phase leverages standing capacity for program and project management. Project-specific actions leverage a portfolio of vendors in specific areas that can be utilized for short-term engagements to deliver desired components. In the final launch phase, decisions are made regarding the permanence of project-specific resources and capabilities. Multiple options exist for sustainability. If it is felt the component will enhance future projects and has a clear line of support, it may be added to the portfolio of standing NGCC capabilities. Alternatively, the on-demand resource may be used as a means of maintaining long-term continuity of the effort, minimizing longer-term commitments and risk. Similarly, the capability may be packaged and licensed to a third-party group not associated with the original build, again minimizing commitments and risk.

To meet project commitments in the short term, it will be necessary to bootstrap the NGCC as standing capabilities are ramped up to redress the lead time of recruiting staff, procuring infrastructure, and identifying space. Immediate capabilities will be delivered through contracted services of limited duration utilizing known entities. Such entities may represent groups that will later provide on-demand capacity and/or provide sustainable postlaunch support for activities outside the core NGCC. The services will be procured with an explicit commitment to perform knowledge transfer to establish the standing capabilities. These contracted services therefore may incur a cost premium associated with expediency versus the longer-term investment in stable capacity. The magnitude of this bootstrap resource will depend on the rate at which NGCC projects are identified and mature. Regardless, this component will be of limited duration.

It is neither practical nor desirable to procure equipment, import software, or hire all staff at once. Therefore, complementing the bootstrap phase is a buildup sequence. The buildup sequence will complete by the end of year 2. Within this buildup sequence, key leadership staff are brought on board first, permitting these staff to tailor hiring to emerging specific NGCC project needs and to have ownership in the recruitment of their personnel. A similar buildup will be used for acquiring equipment. Computer equipment rapidly grows obsolete. As such, it is not desirable to procure equipment before its full-time use is required. Also, the portfolio will evolve as specific projects come on board and computer technology evolves. As such, the equipment will be procured over a two-year period. Following this build, a capability refreshment fund will support replacing equipment or substituting it with on-demand services.

The evolution of the NGCC Enterprise is summarized in Figure 8.3.

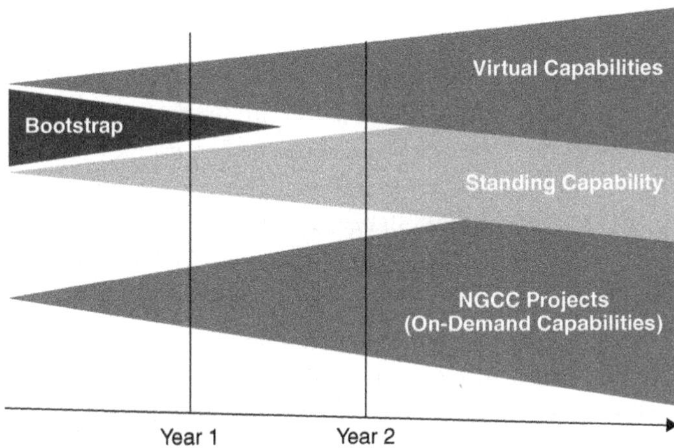

Figure 8.3 Next-Generation Cyber Capability Evolution

Physical Infrastructure

The physical infrastructure supporting an NGCC is a composite of computational capacity, storage, and networking. These components are intimately intertwined in the physical infrastructure and not easily segregated. Of equal importance is the recognition that there is not a single one-size-fits-all physical infrastructure that will accommodate the diversity of NGCC activities. Different physical configurations are needed to optimally address different cyber needs. These capabilities can be broken into three general categories: transactional, high performance, and big data. However, a given project may need multiple capabilities so it is important that projects can seamlessly transition among the different types of infrastructure. The NGCC physical infrastructure is summarized in Figure 8.4.

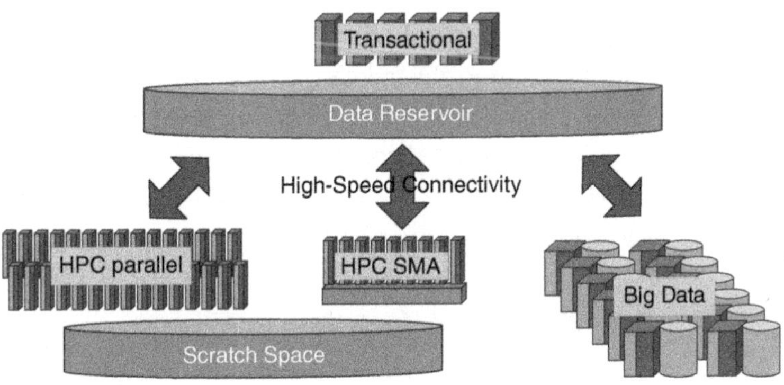

Figure 8.4 NGCC Physical Infrastructure

Transactional

Transactional systems are the central component of the NGCC. They represent the general day-to-day utility platforms and are used for tasks such as routine computing, ad hoc computational capacity, and presentation layer services, such as hosting services (including web servers, database servers, and applications), hosting data, and supporting middleware.

Within the transactional componentry, common computation tasks such as data ingestion, denormalization, extract-transform-load operations, and raw computational tasks with templated virtual nodes takes place in both commodity server hardware and specialized compute-intensive graphics processing units.

The standing physical infrastructure to support utility computing would be comprised of a server cluster composed of 64 commodity x86 servers, each with latest-generation Intel 14nm Broadwell processors (Intel Xeon E5–2699 v4). The servers are outfitted with dual-socket 22 core @ 2.20 gigaHertz (GHz) and 256 gigabyte DDR4 Memory @ 2133. Transactional systems would have access to directly connected 10 gigabit Ethernet (10 GbE) Internet Small Computer System Interface (iSCSI) Network all-flash storage to support data-intensive computation (400 terabytes [TB]). The 409 TB all-flash array stands as a scratch space that replicates data to the larger file storage research computing capacity storage array of 4 petabytes. This component requires access to high-speed Internet (Internet2) as well as access to high-performance data transfer nodes (DTNs).

Purpose-built, high-availability, networked computer server systems used for wide area large-scale data transfers over Internet2 are referred to as DTNs. Their function is to serve as endpoints where large data sets can be shared, ingested, and moved to HPC clusters or, more appropriately, data-intensive computing clusters. Modern-day, efficient DTNs typically have large memory footprints, fast disk subsystems comprised of solid-state disks, and high-bandwidth, redundant interfaces at speeds of 10, 40, or even 100 gigabits per second (Gbps).

The server itself has been commoditized and/or converted to an appliance and serves no other general-purpose computing tasks. Furthermore, the server has interfaces that sit on the unprotected side of a firewall where potentially "stateless" checking can occur via access control lists; however, no "stateful" inspection or further security exists in this zone. The server zone is described as friction free. This configuration offers the most efficient transfer of data across the wide area network.

High-Performance Computing

High-performance systems are necessary to address computationally intensive tasks. These tasks can be broken into two subclasses: tasks that require a large number of computations and those that require large memory stores. Each requires a different physical infrastructure.

The first configuration supports embarrassingly parallel tasks that are either naturally parallel or have specialized code to utilize parallel computing. This configuration needs a large collection of compute node/cores connected via high-speed internal connections with fast-access storage space to read/write information and to store intermediate information.

The standing infrastructure to support this need would be a 100-node Intel Xeon E5–2667 v4 Processors @ 3.20 GHz 1,600 core cluster with 128 Gb DDR4 2133 memory /node connected via 14 data-rate InfiniBand FDRinterconnects. The cluster has an additional 500 TB of fast scratch storage space in a Lustre file system. High-speed 40 Gbps network connections to the transactional infrastructure are configured for optimal file transfer.

The second high-performance configuration requires large shared memory. This environment processes jobs with high complexity/interdependencies requiring processing of a common data space or code that isn't or can't be straightforwardly parallelized. This environmental component supports jobs run in Apache Spark (in memory).

The infrastructure to support this component is composed of 16-node Intel Xeon Phi (Knights Landing) Cluster with 128 Gb DDR4/node and Omni-Path fabric integration.

Big Data

New models of computing intimately combine processing, large data stores, and data transfer through a unique file system (Hadoop/MapReduce) that provides novel computational strategies. The in-memory computational model still leverages the underpinnings and robustness of the Hadoop Distributed File System.

Standing big data capacity consists of two 44-node commodity clusters interconnected with a mixture of 40 gigabit Ethernet (GbE) and 10 GbE. Nodes are optimized to have larger memory pools and facilitate multiple disk configurations for maximum disk density. To facilitate potential expansion, the servers would be configured over multiple racks, with an appropriate mixture of 100–40–10 GbE switches added as growth might dictate. High-speed L2/L3 connections make these elements highly available to one another.

Mixed Capacity

The standing capacity described would be augmented with virtual capacity obtained via partnership and/or procurement. The models for provisioning physical infrastructure are in the midst of radical transformation. More specifically, Infrastructure as a Service (IaaS), Platform as a Service (PaaS), and

Big Data as a Service (BDaaS) business models are rapidly transforming the economics of local versus cloud-based capabilities. The base framework for all of the hybridized components and the Research as a Service platform (RaaS) is built on OpenStack.

While initially used for "on-demand" expansion during project build phases, ongoing analysis will assess what fraction of standing capacity can be addressed though virtualization. The analysis of what fraction of infrastructure should be local versus virtually provisioned is based on calculations of capital versus operations expenditure priorities; true assessment of total cost of ownership (comparing apples to apples); assumptions about actual use versus projected use; assessment of the cost of rapid hardware obsolescence (the need for recurring capital investment); and the need for physical and logical control of environments not always possible through virtualized environments.

The most mature virtualized capabilities support transactional computing. Internal resources, large-scale providers (e.g., Penguin Computing, Amazon, Microsoft, and Google), and small business all offer capabilities at various price points that can complement local infrastructure and incrementally replace local capacity. For example, Amazon is providing increasingly competitive pricing for large-scale storage and computing. Amazon's compute services, such as Elastic Compute Cloud, provide pay-as-you go utility computing. Amazon's increasingly diverse offerings of storage services (Simple Storage Service, Elastic Block Storage, and Glacier) provide competitive pricing for short-term, intermediate-term, and archival storage. Finally, Amazon's Virtual Private Cloud, Elastic Load Balancing, and Direct Connect can be directly connected to local standing capabilities. The HPC capacity of Penguin Computing (Penguin on Demand; POD) offers elastic capacity in the form of ready-to-launch HPC nodes for capacity spikes.

Access to virtual HPC capabilities currently is more limited but includes many of the same options just mentioned (POD, Amazon, and small business). Internet2 continues to build the innovation platform partnership among academic and private-sector companies to provide on-demand HPC. Emerging opportunities are also arising from groups that are marketing their own HPC resources (e.g., Intel, Dell, Amazon, Rackspace, and Reliable Site), packaging resources provided by others, or combining their resources with large HPC vendors.

Big data virtual resources are currently even more limited (Amazon and small business). However, the physical infrastructure offered by many of the groups just mentioned can be configured on demand to support big data tasks. Amazon currently offers limited but useful (Elastic MapReduce) cloud-based Big Data as a Service (BDaaS) resources. Interestingly, one of the most dynamic small business growth areas is in the provisioning of BDaaS.

Logical Infrastructure

NGCC's logical infrastructure is what creates the functionality and represents the software tooling that is used to solve problems. The logical infrastructure is what makes data accessible, usable, and reusable. It facilitates the conversion of data to information and positions it so that it is actionable knowledge. The NGCC's logical infrastructure provides the analytic tools that generate discovery and itis the substrate that connects the transdisciplinary ecosystem. The logical infrastructure ensures that the NGCC operates as a cohesive system. It blends the different physical infrastructure capabilities into a logical whole. When coupled with the underlying physical infrastructure, the logical infrastructure generates a unique knowledge engine.

The software architecture used to create the logical infrastructure is modular and layered. This permits components to be used as needed for individual projects, ensuring that activities are not overburdened by complex cyberinfrastructure. However, conformance to a common information architecture permits appropriate capabilities to be choreographed to create solutions to complex projects. Moreover, this adherence breaks down silos and facilitates data liquidity.

Like the physical infrastructure, the logical infrastructure comes in multiple, interconnected categories. It supports the transactional collection, processing, management, and preservation of data and supports analysis of data. A new generation of tooling intimately blends the transactional and analytic components, enabling big data use cases. Logical infrastructure supports semantic capabilities that maintain data about data (metadata) and the "context" of the data. Finally, a broad category contains the logical infrastructure necessary to conduct operations ranging from logically connecting infrastructure to software development environments. Seamless user access and a unique knowledge engine are an emergent property of the system. The logical infrastructure is summarized in Figure 8.5.

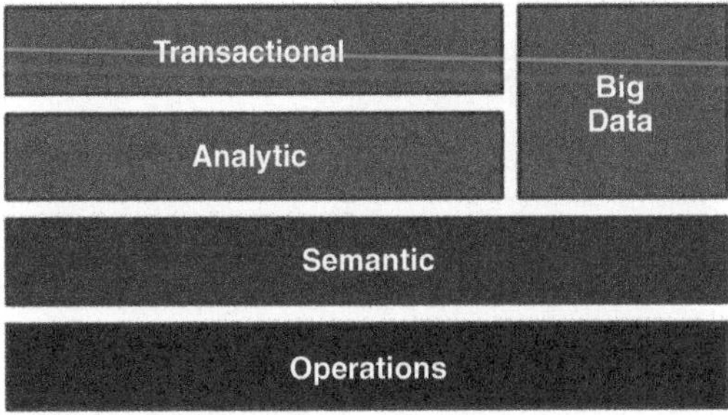

Figure 8.5 NGCC Logical Infrastructure

Transactional

The transaction capabilities represent the utility computing capabilities of the NGCC (i.e., the infrastructure necessary to capture, manage, and share data). They may be coupled with analytic capabilities in workflows. The NGCC will use open source software where it exists in robust, production-ready form. Open source software provides the capability to customize software to reflect the research problems being solved and the capacity to redistribute software in on-demand settings with partners. Standards-compliant software will also be used preferentially as it amplifies the utility of the data managed and reduces the barriers to creating automated pipelines.

A diverse portfolio of applications is necessary to support the anticipated NGCC portfolio. Software already identified as key components of NGCC projects includes:

- Clinical research—clinical trial management (CCTS), adaptive trials management (TRANSCEND), in vivo image management (NBIA suite), clinical investigator credential registry (National Cancer Institute [NCI] online credential repository), and regulatory submissions management (CTR); and
- Life science research—biospecimen management (caTissue), molecular characterization (caArray), pathology image management (caMicroscope), laboratory information management system (caLIMS), and molecular analysis output visualization (CGWB).

The applications are complemented by data services. These services package data from numerous, distributed sources, making it available through well-described computer interfaces. Early attention will be paid to life and clinical science data resources.

In addition to specialized data services already described, data is also persisted in relational database tools. The logical infrastructure will support Oracle, Postgres, and MySQL database applications. These transactional databases are complemented by data marts and data warehouses. The infrastructure will support a biomolecular data mart (NCI's caIntegrator) and a clinical research data warehouse that utilizes semantic web technology (caCIS).

Analytic

Analytic capabilities transform and interpret data. In the life science space, a vast collection of such tools exists, especially for the processing of large-scale genomic data. Individual analytic tools and tool suites that support analysis of diverse molecular data will be deployed (e.g., Bowtie, Tophat, Cufflinks, bioConductor, GenePattern, and geWorkbench). Specialized tools that analyze networks will also be deployed. Commonly, molecular analytic tools are executed in pipelines that sequentially process combinations of raw and derived data. Existing pipelines developed by the NCI and pipelines that are part of the Galaxy consortium will be instantiated. The workflow engine Taverna, permits custom generation of pipelines will be deployed.

General-purpose analytic tools complement the set of capabilities already described. These applications or collections of tools support analysis of diverse data types and represent general analytic utilities and agent-based analysis. A portfolio of tools is required, including R, SAS, MatLab, NVivo, and MAXQDA.

Big Data

A next generation of logical infrastructure has recently emerged that is designed from first principles to efficiently handle data of large volume of diverse constitution. These tools assume access to high-capacity, high-performance physical infrastructure. Underpinning many of these tools is a unique software system that utilizes this hardware: Hadoop. A central component of this capability is Hadoop MapReduce, which is software for distributed processing of large data sets. Apache has generated an open source collection of capabilities that sits on top of this system, including a distributed database that supports structured data storage for large tables (HBase), a data warehouse infrastructure that provides data summarization and ad hoc querying (Hive), a machine learning and data mining library (Mahout), and a high-level data-flow language (Pig). Two other components round out the NGCC big data portfolio: CouchDB and Culvert. Apache CouchDB is a NoSQL database that complements HBase through its use of JavaScript Object Notation and JavaScript. Culvert is a big data utility that permits the use of semantic relationships in a big data framework.

The NGCC will implement big data genomics tools that populate an HBase database to integrate mutation, copy number, gene expression, and epigenetic data to create a holistic genetic view with gene-to-network, gene-to-disease, disease outcome, and gene-to-drug information. A web-based, ultra-flexible data collection framework utilizing CouchDB (caCURE) has been created. It leverages the semantics of data elements where they exist and creates a standards-based, reusable question library. This tool is complemented by a report generator that uses the same CouchDB data persistence, permitting ad hoc schema on-demand reporting.

Semantic

A key component of the NGCC is its use/reuse of data and its capacity to convert data to information. Both require the establishment of data context through the use of metadata. The NGCC provides a collection of integrated semantic components to support the establishment of context and use of metadata. Ontologies are managed through the lexEVS tool set. This tool set can be populated through the NCI's lexEVI application programming interface, which hosts the NCI Thesaurus, metaThesaurus, and the National Library of Medicine's Unified Medical Language System. The next tool manages common data elements (CDEs). CDEs represent atomic units of data collection and represent data using ontologies and are themselves described using ontologies. OpenMDR will be used to support CDE development and curation. OpenMDR leverages the NCI Center for Biomedical Informatics and Information Technology's ISO21090 Data Type Common Library for the construction of elements. OpenMDR also houses information models. These models represent aggregations of CDEs where the relationship between elements is captured through ontologies. The infrastructure uses UML to represent these models. The NCI caCORE SDK can utilize these models to create data services with a variety of application programming interfaces, including SOAP, REST, Java, and grid.

Operations

The logical infrastructure has multiple layers of capabilities to support operations. At the top level are capabilities that support the NGCC's service-oriented architecture. This services framework requires a connecting middleware infrastructure. The most mature middleware is the Globus toolkit with support for virtualization of both physical and logical resources. This resource has been extended to support extended security models, definitions of virtual organizations, and the provisioning of data and analytic services by NCI's caGrid. The caGrid utilizes both NCI Integration Hub and Mirth Connect as an enterprise service bus. These capabilities expose a diverse collection of granular life science services constructed by the NCI (NCI Enterprise Services) that facilitate the construction of complex applications through the choreography of composite components. The National Science Foundation's Integrated Rule-Oriented Data System (iRODS) will be used as a complementary means of exposing Data as a Service by facilitating data file access control and description through metadata.

Consistent with the diversity of tools it will encounter and projects it needs to support, the NGCC hosts a number of development tools. The Java EE platform and related build and deploy infrastructure (Ant, AnthillPro, and Maven) will represent the primary development platform. (The majority of the transactional, analysis, big data, and semantic capabilities are programmed in Java.) Java-supporting frameworks such as Hibernate, Spring, and Struts will be utilized. For high-performance applications, C will be available. Scripting capabilities will include Perl, Python, and PHP.

A variety of container technologies are necessary to operate the NGCC. The Apache Web server will host web services. Tomcat will be used as a lightweight servlet container and JBoss as a full-fledged application server to support Java EE.

Best practice in software development dictates the creation of multiple tiers. A development tier gives programmers complete latitude in altering software. When a new capability is stable, it graduates to a staging tier, where it can be tested by independent staff and evaluated for its compatibility with existing systems software. After passing these tests it is moved into a production tier with other software that is in day-to-day use.

Success of a complex enterprise is mediated through communication. Beyond traditional coordination activities (meetings, project plans, etc.), this is accomplished with a combination of public-facing and internal electronic resources. Consistent with the complexity of the tasks to be managed, these electronic tools include software release tools (JIRA for internal use, Apache Subversion for public use), websites (maintained using Drupal), wikis (using Confluence or Media Wiki depending on needs for security), and web conferencing tools (Adobe Connect).

The NGCC will combine two types of operating systems. The vast majority of infrastructure will utilize the Linux operating system (Red Hat). Windows Server (2008 R2) will be used as necessary.

The lowest layers of the logical infrastructure are related to network operations and access control. The logical infrastructure will require common network name space that can be managed by the NGCC staff, accessing ASU intra- and Internet connections. Similarly there is a need for common user/directory space that can be coordinated by NGCC staff but connects to ASU directories.

TransCORE Framework

The preceding capabilities can be à la carte. However, a key feature of the NGCC is the capacity to utilize the components as a system—the Transdisciplinary Common Ontologic Representation (TransCORE) framework. Briefly, in addition to persisting data in traditional stores, the transactional applications can also present data to big data resources. Similarly, data services can also be used to report their content into the big data reservoir. Finally, the analytic tools, running on HPC or big data physical infrastructure, can report in traditional form and to the big data capabilities. As the big data capability has semantic infrastructure components, it can connect data through information models and translate semantics. The TransCORE Framework Knowledge Engine was shown in Figure 8.1.

This system has two important emergent properties: data liquidity and discovery. Complementing traditional business intelligence tools, big data tools will be able to connect interrelated data not connected through existing formal models and without the need to construct complex supporting data warehouse infrastructure. Also, while it can utilize structure, it is not constrained by it. Using high-performance machine learning and data mining tools, it can discover patterns not previously described.

Mixed Capacity

As with physical capabilities, the capacity to use virtual logical capabilities is rapidly evolving. In the biomedical space, applications provided via Software as a Service (SaaS) are emerging. Clinical trials application providers are shifting to hosted models. Unfortunately, these SaaS offerings do not permit choreography with other clinical or life science capabilities unless they are offered by the vendor. A subset of the portfolio of tools generated by the NCI's caBIG program is available from third-party vendors for on-demand use.

Genomic analysis tools are also emerging in SaaS modes. A collaboration between Penn State and Emory University provides a complete collection of tools and workflows for genomic analysis. The Beijing Genomics Institute has launched the cloud service EasyGenomic that hosts complete genomic analysis pipelines. A collection of genome analysis tool generators have placed their capabilities in the Amazon Cloud (including Galaxy) to facilitate their virtual use (Genome Space). All of these services are candidates for on-demand capacity.

A limited number of groups have created virtual data services. The NCI Center for Biomedical Informatics currently hosts the most diverse set of resources, including clinical research, imaging, molecular, and biospecimen. Other groups are using Amazon to host data sets for download, including the 1,000 genome data set and Ensembl's annotated human genome. More specialized resources include the Cancer Genomics Hub. Data as a Service has yet to be systematically addressed within the biomedical community.

At a lower layer within the logical capability stack, an increasing number of vendors are offering PaaS. These vendors provide the basic operating system and programming environment on which one can deploy transactional and analytic capabilities. Amazon offers literally hundreds of virtual machine images that create diverse software environments in its cloud. Given complexities with network name space and access restrictions, it is often difficult to choreograph these capabilities in workflows, which in part limits their overall utility.

Staff Resources

The dynamic systems nature of the NGCC creates novel staffing approaches. Each of the components of the system requires staff expertise to ensure that they are state of the art and operate at high performance. As a system, each component has critical dependencies outside the realm of normal expertise, thereby requiring close coordination among diverse staff. Given the dynamic environment proposed for the NGCC, staff is the most critical component. This is true for two main reasons. First, it is only through staff that the system's component edges are bridged. This bridging is particularly important when mixing standing and on-demand capabilities. Second, given the enterprise strategy of using on-demand capabilities, staff is the reservoir of continuity of knowledge necessary to evaluate and maintain diverse, evolving operations.

Similar to the previously described capabilities, staff needs can be broken into categories corresponding to the major systems points of view: enterprise, physical infrastructure, and logical infrastructure. Each of these categories has subclasses related to the breakdowns within each point of view.

Enterprise

In order to provide overall coordination and administration of the on-demand components of the NGCC, program and project management staff will be required. This staff will be composed of a program manager who will oversee cross-cutting activities and a project manager responsible for the day-to-day aspects of individual NGCC projects. These individuals will be complemented by a business manager who is responsible for generating and tracking budgets, personnel, and so on, and an administrative assistant who will coordinate scheduling and NGCC staff communications. To support outward communications the enterprise team will have a dedicated writer to assist with documentation, generation of tutorials and educational material, and a communications staff member to provide and organize content for websites and wikis.

Physical Infrastructure

To support the standing physical infrastructure and connect it with on-demand capabilities, the NGCC will require systems personnel (a systems architect and a systems engineer). It will also need staff to develop and maintain the networking of the systems (senior network engineer and network engineer). Finally, an individual with cloud and big data experience will be required (big data systems engineer). These staff will be responsible for the installation and maintenance of many of the components in the operations software stack (web servers, databases, programming environment, etc.) and the maintenance of the development tiers.

Logical Infrastructure

The logical infrastructure component has the largest and most diverse staffing needs. In many instances staff in this component will have overlapping responsibilities with the other systems' points of view.

To support the transactional and big data component, software engineers will be required. These individuals will install, modify, integrate, and choreograph application software. A senior engineer, midrange engineer, and junior engineer will support and develop software, assist in software evaluation from on-demand developers and providers, bridge between environments, and provide Tier 3 support. In partnership with the systems staff, a quality assurance specialist will oversee the validation of software as it moves from development to production environments. A database administrator will provide configuration, programming, and support for relational database management system and NoSQL databases. A web developer will support the programming of websites and wikis and act as webmaster. A help desk staff member will provide Tier 1 and Tier 2 support for both physical and logical infrastructure.

Support for the analytic components of the program will come from analysts/programmers. Two senior analysts/programmers will execute analysis. They will be supported by a more junior data analyst with expertise in executing analytic/application software. This data analyst will also serve as data steward, curating the data resources that are part of the NGCC standing infrastructure and connecting outside data services. Analytic efforts will be supported by two postdoctoral fellows and two graduate students. The former are to guarantee a pipeline to rapidly developing advances, the latter to support training and to prevent burnout of permanent staff.

Staff will be required to create the overarching TransCORE framework and to support the capture of semantic information. A knowledge architect will design and implement the systems architecture. A knowledge engineer will create and manage metadata, ontologies, CDEs, and information models.

Mixed Capacity

It is critical that a core staff of senior individuals be available to create the systems point of view for NGCC. These individuals are also critical to provide review and oversight of contracted services and personnel. Many of the roles described can be accommodated through contracted personnel. The flexibility in terms of service is balanced by the additional costs associated with contracted labor.

Resource Management (Space Allocation)

The space required to support the NGCC reflects the alternative points of view of the systems architecture. Two broad categories describe the space requirements: space supporting physical infrastructure and space to support staff.

The nature of the physical infrastructure requires specialized space. The most critical components are power and cooling. Modern computing equipment has significant power and cooling demands. Electrical demands are measured in megawatts. Ideally, power is provided by independent electrical grid feeds. Cooling requires high-capacity circulating air supported by robust, redundant air conditioning. Emergency generating capacity to maintain key systems is required. Backup batteries should be available to support orderly system shutdown. Redundant, high-speed access to the Internet is essential, ideally at 100 Gb rate.

The physical infrastructure requires a collection of security components. Multiple rooms within the server space are required to provide physical barriers for servers requiring secure access. The space should have security cameras and restricted card key access. The space requires a fire suppression system.

Ideally, all NGCC staff will be housed in approximately contiguous space. The primary physical requirement is a high-speed network connecting staff space with server space. Staff require fiber to the desktop and redundant Ethernet drops in their individual space. A mix of differing types of space is required. Senior staff require modest-size private offices to support their supervisory needs. Midrange and junior staff can reside in cubicles. Additional cubicles are required to support visiting staff who are part of on-demand work teams. Team rooms are essential to support the transdisciplinary components of the NGCC. Team rooms are equipped with digital projection equipment and telepresence capabilities to support connections with on-demand team players. All staff require access to personal computers, ideally laptops to support access regardless of their physical location. Common, high-performance printers are required in this space.

CONCLUSION

The first three years of the NGCC have been very successful. We have migrated multiple workloads from traditional HPC and benefited from many improvements. As one use case found, for a tumor simulation project, simulating the life span of 100 tumors, for 12 types, we estimate it would have taken us 120,000 days, whereas it took about 20 minutes for the same simulation on Apache Spark. Additional lessons learned are divided into design and deployment.

Design

Research and technology is a rapidly evolving field, and to discuss it is much like taking aim at a moving target. Design for the future is a good strategy, although the reality in execution is far more challenging. How can infrastructure components keep pace with a field that changes almost daily? An integrator in the field of research computing can be key in the process to create a sustainable cluster with a life span that allows the asset to reach the projected return on investment mark specified in the proposal.

Big-box vendors struggle to meet this objective, as much of their focus is around delivery of enterprise-ready solutions that are easily supported from the perspective of technical support. Big-box vendors complete this through validated design components that they have tested with specific software components.

These are known as reference architectures in the field. However, it is important to state that reference architectures typically are created through partnerships with hardware suppliers/makers and software developers/distributors and at times take as long as a year to propose, design, develop, and distribute. What this means to the researcher is that the hardware architecture underneath the software overlay is no less than a year behind whatever is considered current generation.

Remember Moore's Law: "The number of transistors incorporated in a chip will approximately double every 24 months." Following the Tick–Tock model, we have watched Intel release E5 processor units starting with version 1, code-named Sandy Bridge, and then within the same 24-month period release E5 version 2, code-named Ivy Bridge, and then again with Haswell and Broadwell, the E5 versions 3 and 4. Each release has greater core density, memory capacity, and capabilities.

Therefore, the most significant challenge is choosing the next-generation processor during the current generation and ensuring that your desired applications will run. It is fairly likely that, in your research organization, there are applications that will require recompile to run or to optimize their capacity to utilize or, in some cases, ignore some features. The lesson learned in this section can be applied to not only central processor units but to memory, network speeds (adapters, route-switch gear), and disks as well. Reference architectures are for well-known applications in the enterprise, such as Oracle databases, Microsoft Exchange Server, Microsoft SharePoint, and others. None of these applications has a place in research other than as an external tool managed by an operations team whose primary responsibility is uptime and availability. In speaking to groups for whom this concept is foreign, I employ the following scenario: "If you come into your place of work and the e-mail service was slow or unresponsive, you would open a ticket and wait for help, you would not go about the task to build your own private e-mail server under your desk." In the research realm: "If you were to come into your place of work and the computational simulations you were running were slow or unresponsive (in research, 'slow' and 'unresponsive' are synonymous and equal 'broken'), you would take your research dollars, buy your own cluster, and create yet another silo in your institution's environment." Availability and performance are still critical, but there is a distinct difference between the methodologies for meeting those objectives between enterprise operations and research computing.

Design for the farthest future you can conceive and support. There is no such thing as "future proofing," but there is a way to become future resistant, and the shortest path to that objective is through obtaining funding before your asset is no longer competitive. This adds the element of relativity to the equation. If you have a great science objective that can be achieved in a single year, then your cluster asset needs to be competitive only for a single year. As a rule of thumb, I architect systems to last for no longer than three years, at which point I hope to repurpose the asset through virtualization within OpenStack, thus increasing the usefulness in a non–top-tier performance role. The best example I would cite would be the deprecation of an HPC cluster to create a classroom learning cluster on the same hardware.

Deployment

Deployment should be regarded as a straightforward exercise with little complexity prior to the go-live and application transition. There are scenarios where you may choose to contract or enter a service agreement that provides installation. You may lack the expertise or, in most cases, the time in terms of downtime and time away from operational support to undertake the installation with your own team. Most research institutions function on tight budgets and have small, highly focused teams that are not best suited to the task of rack and stack. A vendor that provides this service as a bundle is preferable. One word of caution and lesson learned in the NGCC is to be very circumspect in the evaluation and selection of a full-services package that includes hardware, software, installation, postinstallation configuration, and ongoing support through resident services.

In our experiences a full-services package proved to be less desirable. The analogy we use in sharing this experience is one where a prospective home buyer goes to a master planned community. Upon arrival, the sign book doubles as a soft agreement or lock out of a seller's agent, leaving the buyer to be dual represented by a single agent acting as both the buyer's and the seller's agent. Additionally, in these types of agreements, the buyer is offered a low interest rate or additional incentives (upgrades) by selecting the seller's finance company and/or lending institution. The master planned community has successfully captured all available revenue and profit from the deal, allowing for maximal margin. This is the plan behind large-scale service organizations, such as IBM Global Services, Hewlett Packard Enterprise, and Dell Enterprise Services. Unfortunately, in many cases, the greatest benefit goes to the seller. The buyer is convinced there are deeper discounts due to the bundling, but in reality there are costs buried in margin-rich items elsewhere. Once the check is tendered, it becomes difficult to hold the vendor accountable.

Methods for avoiding this type of risk are straightforward and account for lesson learned number two in deployment planning. Ensure that the vendor proposing the work not only deeply understands the product and industry best practices but also has the individuals on staff to handle the proposed work. Do not be hesitant to ask to interview the people being positioned. Many companies do not have those expensive resources on staff and go to external contracted firms that cannot guarantee availability at your desired deployment date or even within months of your desired date. Remember, the resources you are seeking are top-notch, highly compensated individuals who are in high demand. We once engaged a provider that supplied resources that were contracted through a global statement of work and then supplied by three separate contract handlers, each taking a pound of flesh on the hand-off. When this occurs, the customer receives a $50 per hour resource who is compensated at a rate of $200 per hour. There is little wonder why such organizations cannot complete the proposed work. In most cases there is no discount deep enough to accept bundled offers. In 20 years in a high-technology market, I have witnessed bundling fail more times than it succeeds. As discussed by Phil Simon:

> More than three in five new system implementations fail. Many miss their deadlines. Others exceed their initial budgets, often by ghastly amounts. Even systems deployed on time and under budget often fail to produce their expected results. Many experience major problems almost immediately. While the statistics are grim, there is at least some good news: These failures can be averted. [1]

Check out Simon's book for additional insight.

Our sense that the future will be highly collaborative, largely open source, and reliant on the hybrid cloud has been confirmed by our initial experiences with ASU's NGCC initiative. You can read about one of the NGCC's first projects, the National Biomarker Development Alliance, in the case study that follows. We are looking forward to many more terrific years of the NGCC, which will certainly evolve and change as needs and technologies change.

NOTE

1. Phil Simon. 2009. *Why New Systems Fail: Theory and Practice Collide* (Bloomington, IN: AuthorHouse).

CASE STUDY

CASE STUDY 12: THE NATIONAL BIOMARKER DEVELOPMENT ALLIANCE

Ken Buetow

Professor, Arizona State University; Director, Computational Science and Informatics Core Program; Director, Complex Adaptive Systems Initiative

The National Biomarker Development Alliance (NBDA) is one project that relies on ASU's Next Generation Cyber Capability (NGCC). The NBDA offers a good example of how a research initiative might use and benefit from the NGCC's resources.

The NBDA's mission is to create and support an efficient and effective pathway for biomarker (re)discovery, development, and regulatory approval. The NGCC is the mortar that makes the NBDA component bricks a whole. Conversely, the NBDA uses nearly all the diverse resources that constitute the NGCC.

The NBDA is a quintessential NGCC project. NBDA is organizationally composed of multiple institutions, each with unique, synergistic roles (ASU, Critical Path Institute (C-path), and the International Genetics Consortium (IGC)). It plans to provide service to multiple, transnational communities including academic institutions, biotechnology companies, and the pharmaceutical industry. The NBDA needs to support multidimensional data that is processed through diverse workflows. Important products of the NBDA are regulatory standards and regularized processes for the development and approval of biomarkers. The standards and processes will reflect regulatory bodies' differing evidentiary requirements for approving different classes of biomarkers.

To credibly attract customers, the NBDA will need to have demonstrable proof-of-concept capabilities. These capabilities will be expanded to address the production needs of the client. The capabilities will also likely require customization to meet specific project needs. As a client base accrues, the NBDA's capacity will need to expand accordingly.

The NGCC's enterprise architecture supports the dynamic nature of the NBDA. The NGCC's standing capacity will be used to demonstrate the proof-of-concept capabilities of the NBDA during the design phase. The NGCC program manager will work with the NBDA project manager to allocate appropriate capacity. As the NBDA is likely to be one of the earliest NGCC projects, this capacity will utilize emerging local capabilities and short-term contract bootstrap resources. During the build phase, the dynamic, on-demand capacity will be exercised. The project manager will identify novel capacity required to support the project and work with the business manager to contract for specific resources. As successive clients are engaged, strategic decisions will be made regarding internalizing expanded capabilities or continuing to provide them through virtual, contract partners. The program manager will work with the business manager and NGCC staff to perform the appropriate cost-benefit analysis.

The transactional infrastructure supports the diverse data management requirements of the NBDA. Within this infrastructure the workflows necessary to regularize the various biomarker qualification processes will be instantiated. These workflows will translate the processes described in the standards development efforts into software that supports the process and enforces the standards. The workflows will choreograph existing software components through custom software bridges. Data flow through the workflow is guaranteed by standards compliance of the data enforced through software and managed through the semantic infrastructure. Using the tooling of the operations infrastructure, the software engineers will

(*Continued*)

(*Continued*)

be responsible for the development and validation of the appropriate workflow infrastructure. As regulatory submission is a goal of the workflow, software will be developed in compliance with Title 21 Code of Federal Regulations (CFR) 11 guidelines.

The NBDA will require multiple interconnected management environments. To support biomarker (re)discovery, tools that support management of multidimensional molecular data will be used. These include tools that store and manipulate the various types of molecular data (e.g., Cancer Genome Workbench (CGWB) and tools for genome-wide association studies such as caArray, caLIMS) and the biospecimens (e.g., caTissue, caMicroscope) from which they have been derived. This infrastructure will need to interoperate with the International Genetic Consortium's (IGC) biospecimen management capabilities. Biomarker development will extend this capacity to include the management of reference data sets using tools such as caIntegrator. These data sets will allow validation of findings obtained from the discovery processes. Clinical qualification studies are critical to the success of the NBDA. This component will leverage the clinical research suite of tools (e.g., CCTS, TRANSCEND, NBIA) and the regulatory submission tools that manage investigator credentials and CDISC-compliant submissions.

The NBDA workflows will include analytic pipelines that support biomarker (re) discovery. These analytic pipelines will choreograph the processing of data stored and managed in the transactional data reservoir with the HPC resources necessary to conduct analysis. Utilities in the transactional environment will perform data transformations, formatting, and simple analytic tasks using traditional tools (e.g., Bioconductor, GenePattern). More compute-intensive tasks that require large shared memory (next-generation sequence assembly and analysis) or large-scale parallel processing (pathway analysis) will utilize the alternative HPC configurations. The data analysts/programmers will be responsible for the execution of the analytic pipelines and the interpretation of their outputs.

Critical to the execution of the NBDA workflow is the standards-based representation of data and information models that define the interfaces between components and exchange of information between them. These standards are instantiated in the NGCC semantic infrastructure (lexEVS, OpenMDR). These repositories also act as electronically accessible repositories to support the dissemination of the standards developed by the NBDA. The knowledge engineer will be responsible for instantiating the NBDA-developed standards and for facilitating the use of these and other data standards and information models.

In addition to providing support for the discovery and development of biomarkers, the NBDA intends to provide assistance in the interpretation of the clinical outcomes associated with their use. This component will leverage the big data capacity of the

NGCC. The big data infrastructure is populated from the input of the transactional and output of the analytic infrastructures via the data reservoir. The network engineer will assist with this piping. Additionally, the big data infrastructure will be populated with semistructured and unstructured information from the scientific literature, lay literature, Food and Drug Administration guidance, and physician insights. Data analysts, fellows, and students will assist in representing this information utilizing the qualitative research tools. The big data resource will support *in silico* validation of biomarker findings and assist in interpreting outcomes. Novel tools will be developed by the engineers and utilized by the analysts to support this effort.

A goal of the NBDA is to not only manage data but also to provide context for that data-generating information and making that information actionable. The NBDA will leverage the NGCC's TransCORE to make this possible. TransCORE will provide the knowledge engine underpinning efforts to support *in silico* medicine. The knowledge engineer and software engineers will assist in with this.

The NBDA leverages the transactional and operations infrastructure to create a web presence in the community. This includes the generation of an NBDA portal with appropriate access controls. The portal will host the NBDA's virtual communities and provide controlled access to the workflows.

Conclusion

Congratulations on reaching the end of *Strategies in Biomedical Data Science.* (And if you've skipped ahead and are sneaking a peek at the ending, that's fine too. You can read this book in whatever order you choose!)

When you finish your first pass through the book, you should have gained a deeper understanding of biomedical data challenges and strategies, tools, and opportunities. I hope you are better prepared to help the organization you work for and ultimately the individual patients who receive medical care and benefit from medical research. Certainly, this book is not exhaustive in its scope. Your reading may well have pointed you to other topics, applications, and resources. We wish you all the luck in your continued education and development.

Strategies in Biomedical Data Science has set out to survey some very rapidly changing fields, namely data-intensive research analytics, research data management, genomics-genetics, and high-performance computing. There is every reason to believe that these fields will continue to change rapidly. So this book's specific technical recommendations probably will not have a very long shelf life. For this I apologize, but the alternative approach, given the rapid pace of change, was simply to leave out these specifics entirely. The broader concepts and strategies presented in this book should have longer-lasting utility. And it is my sincere hope that these concepts and strategies offer more durable tools for meeting ever-changing data challenges. I hope this book has been of use to you and your organization.

The primary goals of this book are translational. My experiences working in healthcare and academic computing have convinced me that information technology (IT) professionals work more effectively when they know more about biomedicine. Biomedical researchers, in turn, are often better able to collaborate and manage large technical initiatives if they know a good bit about pertinent IT issues. Much translational work remains, especially with both fields changing so rapidly. But it is very encouraging to see biomedicine and IT become ever more tightly intertwined. We all stand to reap the benefits of this close relationship.

It is tremendously exciting to be part of such a dynamic and innovative field, and the experience of writing this book, while not always easy, has been tremendously rewarding. At moments of frustration or seeming stasis in the process of putting this book together, I was continually energized by the human stakes of biomedicine. We all benefit from remembering that ultimately we are working hard so that people have better health outcomes. My proceeds from this book go to the ASU Research Foundation to support the efforts of Joshua LaBaer's lab in researching effective targeted treatments for pediatric brain cancer.

Biomedical data management and data science are rapidly changing fields. I lack the foresight or the self-importance to make any bold proclamations. Instead I will share just a bit about what I hope the future is like. I sincerely hope that the future of these fields is marked by great collaboration and creativity. I hope the future is increasingly open source so that all will stand to benefit.

Finally, I would very much welcome any feedback or suggestions for improvement. Hopefully there will be a second edition that can benefit from your collective insight. We are always better off when we work together, and this work is no exception.

APPENDIX A

The Research Data Management Survey

From Concepts to Practice

Brandon Mikkelsen and Jay Etchings

Libraries have been managing data for 4,000 years and will continue to be critical facilitators in the sharing and preservation of data for the research process. Therefore, it is important to coordinate the development of research data management with the needs and characteristics of end users. During the spring semester of 2015, a large university in collaboration with the Research Data Governance Committee conducted a research data management survey to determine the data management strategic requirements and curation needs of the digital research community. The survey engaged faculty, researchers, graduate students, postdoctoral fellows, and selected staff at five research institutions. We have agreed to keep the sources of the surveys anonymous. The institutions all admitted to just recently tackling the problem of data management as it pertains to research and emerging models for research compliance.

The purpose was to discover how research data is being managed across various units at the university, determine what the demand is for existing services, and identify new services that university researchers require. For many institutions, this is the best starting point toward the adoption of a research data management plan as it aligns with the baselining principle of the National Institute of Standards and Technology.

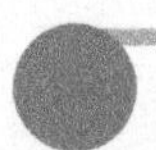

SOME QUICK DEFINITIONS

Research data Refers to any recorded, retrievable information necessary for the reconstruction and evaluation of reported results created in connection with the design, conduct, or reporting of research performed or conducted at or under the auspices of the university and the events and processes leading to those results, regardless of the form or the media on which they may be recorded. Research data can include both tangible and intangible data, such as statistics, findings, formulas, conclusions, and so on, and tangible/physical data including physical storage mediums to include removable media, mass storage devices, notebooks, and printed materials; and data stored on remote workstations, mobile devices, and public/private cloud storage.

Data curation According to the University of Illinois' Graduate School of Library and Information Science, "Data curation is the active and on-going management of data through its lifecycle of interest and usefulness to scholarship, science, and education; curation activities enable data discovery and retrieval, maintain quality, add value, and provide for re-use over time" [1].

Data archive Describes the practice where data that is no longer in an "active" state is migrated/moved to another storage device or medium. Data archival processes differ greatly from data backup processes as data backup focuses on the saving and restoration of active data for operational stability of production workloads. Data archival processes aim to maintain a single instance or a complete collection of historical records distinctly identified for long-term retention and future reference and in many cases candidates for data curation processes. The archival process is one that has evolved to meet the guidelines of regulatory compliance. Archival data process and enablement of long-term "available" cold storage, including search of deduplicated and/or encrypted storage that leverages indexing and object storage, is now a possibility, replacing the sequential tape-powered solutions of the past. Tjomsland, in 1980, declared: "The penalties for storing obsolete data are less than are the penalties for discarding potentially useful data" [2].

Data management policy The practice of creating a structured set of rules for enforcing the tracking of individual authors, curators, programmers, and contributors as they contribute to a shared data environment. The end goal is to provide accountability of who wrote, curated, approved, or managed other features of keeping data structure intact and up-to-date.

To better understand research data management within the research university in a pragmatic sense, we have compiled survey data from multiple institutions to gain insight as to current data management practices, storage techniques, sharing for collaboration, and methods by which access policies are applied. The discovery results and best practices analysis throughout the remainder of this appendix are directly from faculty, researchers, graduate students, postdoctoral fellows, contracted resources, and staff as well as internally created data management committees launched to work in unison with university research computing centers and their respective data management teams. The survey focus is on general opinions for the primary consumers/stakeholders regarding data creation, governance, sharing, archival preservation, and compliance. Included in the survey pool are questions related to the participants' demographics, data storage, data management, data sharing, and data reuse.

Demographics

One thousand participants in the survey, with 78% completing the survey (780). Figure A.1 represents the demographics of the participants. (Note: Approximately 240 participants did not provide demographic information.)

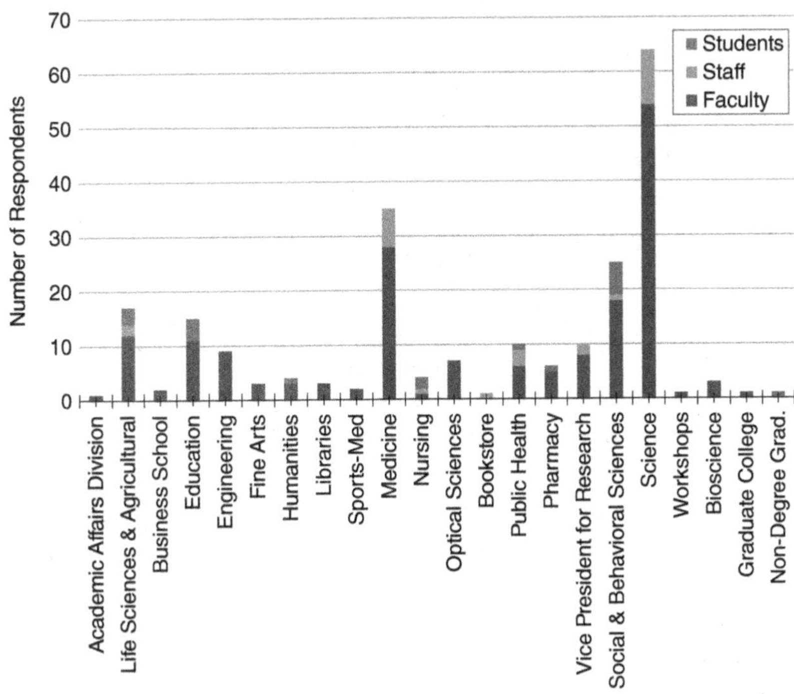

Figure A.1 Demographics: Faculty (398), Staff (125), Students (257) = Total Participants (780)

Research Data Characteristics

The majority of survey participants, 34%, indicated that the characteristics of the data they produce or utilize is observational, and 31% indicated that their data is experimental. Other data characteristics included reference, derived, simulated, or not applicable. The types of data most of the participants produce or use is automatically computer-generated data, sensor data, instruments output, application-created data, text files, ASCII data, and image data. There was insufficient data at the time of the survey to measure Internet of Things data. Figure A.2 summarizes the reported characteristics of research data.

Data Management Plans

With the continual evolution of compliance models, we can predict with a degree of certainty that a majority of federal funding agencies will require data management plans to be included with proposal submissions. Within the

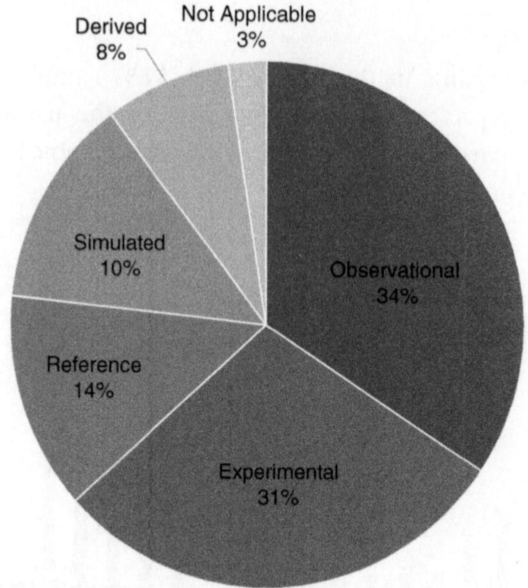

Figure A.2 Research Data Characteristics

survey are questions not only in regard to federal funding opportunities; journals and publications were also included. Figure A.3 summarizes the results from these questions. The majority of respondents (86%) indicated that data management plans were indeed required in proposals to funding agencies they currently were engaged with. Approximately 33.5% indicated that journals/publications to which they submit currently require them to submit related research data. Twenty percent were not certain.

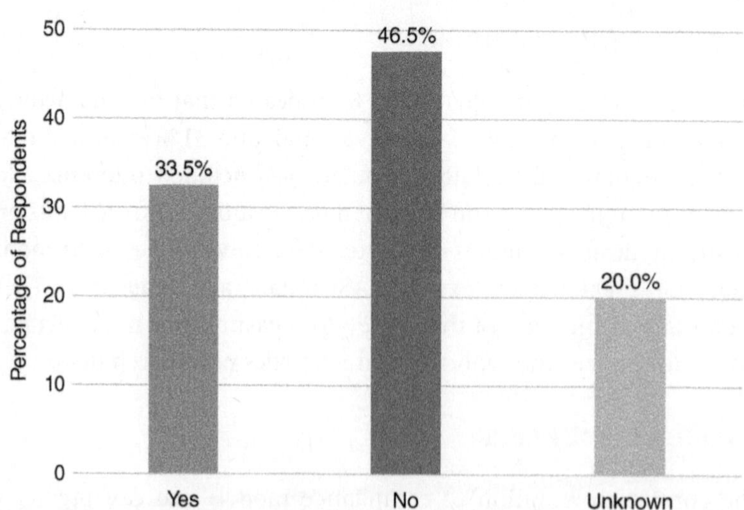

Figure A.3 Data Management Plan or Research Data Required with Submission to Journal or Publication

University Data Management Services

Many universities and institutions provide a wide range of data management services through either the libraries or the central technology offices. The respondents were asked which services were of interest and which services would add significant value to warrant paying for the service or including it as a budgeted item within a research proposal. Figure A.4 summarizes desired university research services.

Participants indicated the highest level of interest in the following services:

- Storage and preservation
- Preparation of data management plans
- Storage and collaboration tools
- "Best practices" for data management
- Unified campus data repository
- Data management workshops
- Documentation
- Data management requirements compliance
- Compliance, confidentiality, and legal issues

Participants indicated that they are willing to pay for these services:

- Storage, curation, and archive: 32%
- Personalized consultation: 20%
- Data management compliance assistance: 28%
- Unified campus data repository: 34%
- Data collaboration tools (sharing): 38%

Data Storage

The survey also contained a series of questions designed to assist with identification of data infrastructure components required on campus to support research data. The questions addressed the following categories:

Questions

- Data retention period
- Archival data access requirements
- Current data volume
- Data curation requirements
- Current storage infrastructure components

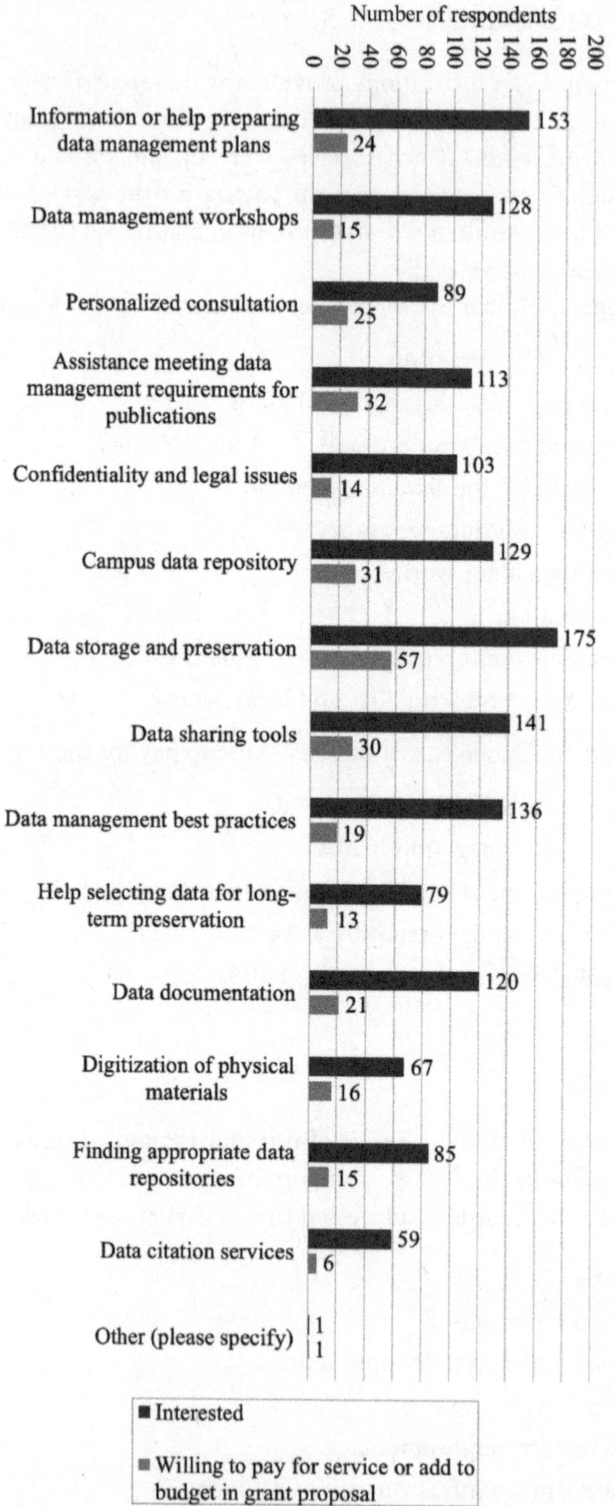

Figure A.4 Data Management Services

Responses

- Require five years of data storage following the close of their project: 75%
- Require one to four years of data storage following the close of their project: 23%
- Need daily 24/7 access during their funded research period: 85%
- Require weekly access to their data during the funded research period: 22%
- Require intermittent access (weekly) after project closure: 64%
- Require weekly or monthly data access following project closure: 22%

Note: In cases where data from federally funded human studies retain personally identifiable information (PII), there may be as much as a seven-year retention requirement. Agencies involved include the Food and Drug Administration, the Centers for Disease Control, and so on.

Desired Infrastructure Elements

The data storage infrastructure elements and physical components were not ranked, although the data was collected and is listed in Table A.1.

Table A.1 Desired Infrastructure Elements

Cloud storage features: Which infrastructure elements are desired?	Description: What is expected from each infrastructure element?
Network Attached Storage (NAS), Network File System (NFS)/ Server Message Block (SMB), Common Internet File System (CIFS)	Can provide NAS NFS/SMB (CIFS) support. Native support for network file systems ranks higher than NAS gateways.
Object-based storage support	Can provide object-based storage support. Native support ranks higher over the use of gateways.
40 GbE front-end connectivity	Supports 40 GbE and/or 10 GbE front-end connectivity.
Native block support fiber channel	Provides native block connectivity and detailed data for supported protocols for connectivity and performance.
Unified storage management	Minimal management interfaces for NAS support. Single pane of glass solutions are preferred, regardless of gateway usage.
Array efficiencies (dedupe/ compression/thin)	Ability to provide storage thin-provisioning, compression, and/or deduplication.
Native array encryption	Ability to provide data-at-rest storage encryption.
User-definable storage tiering	Ability to provide both automate and manual user-defined storage tiering.
Sub-LUN tiering	Ability to support sub-LUN tiering.

(*Continued*)

Table A.1 *(Continued)*

Cloud storage features: Which infrastructure elements are desired?	Description: What is expected from each infrastructure element?
Off-site replication	Ability to replicate to off-site/second site via synchronous and asynchronous methods.
Snapshots and local copy	Ability to perform read-only snapshots across storage tiers.
AD/LDAP integration	LDAP Integration in roles within the storage management interface as well as on share or export permissions.
Charge-back/Show-back functionality	Ability to provide charge-back or show-back storage utilization.
Monitoring and historical reporting	Ability to provide real-time as well as historical storage monitoring, alerting, and reporting.
OpenStack integration	Documented integration to Cinder and/or Swift API functionality.
Array partitioning/Multitenant	Ability to provide secure administrative segregation of users, hosts, and applications.

Current Data Volume

Data storage requirements among respondents ranged from megabytes (15%), to gigabytes (41%), terabytes (38%), and petabytes (3%). Participants indicated that the current method of data storage and backup as network-attached storage servers, desktop storage and external hard drives, departmental servers and Internet-based cloud storage were least popular and considered cost prohibitive to select groups. Figure A.5 shows current data storage volume.

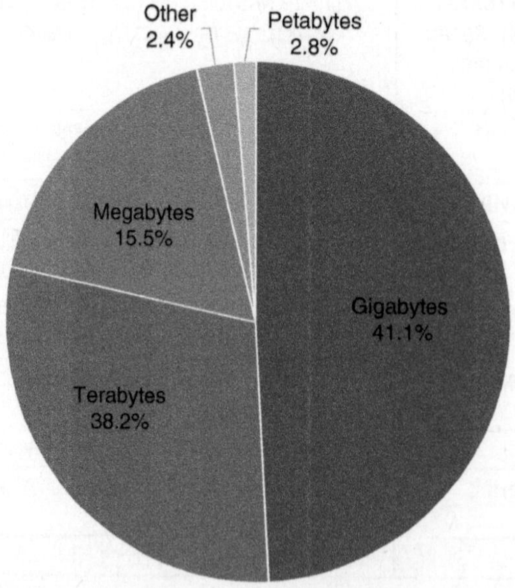

Figure A.5 Current Data Storage Volume

Forecasting Future Data Storage Volumes

As a metric to estimate future data storage volumes, respondents were asked to forecast data growth with projected research initiatives. More than 50% could not forecast the expected data volumes, although in comments they indicated an expected growth in volume. The largest group of responses (40%) indicated growth measured in terabytes; not surprisingly, the category of data volume growth in the petabyte scale was estimated at 4% and was aligned most with health informatics, genomic analysis, and large-scale epidemiology studies. The 2% margin for error included volumes less than gigabytes. Forecasted data growth is shown in Figure A.6.

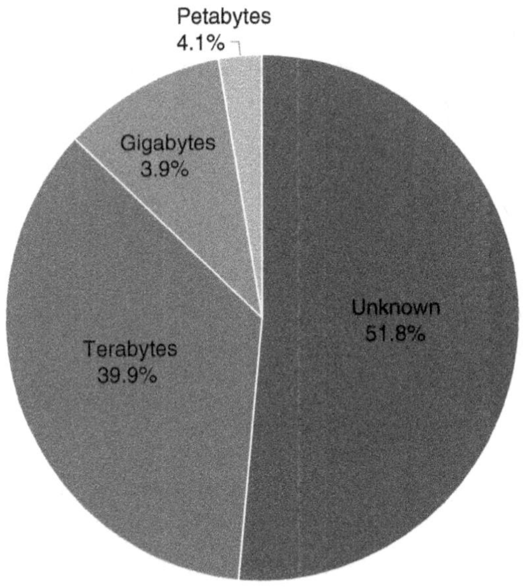

Figure A.6 Data Storage Volume Forecast

Data Management

About 75% of respondents indicated that they or their collaborators manage the data in their lab. Fewer than 10% indicated that data in their lab was managed by central technology offices, collaborators, postdoctoral fellows, graduate students, and/or student workers. No respondents outsourced the management of data to a third-party or contracted resource.

Collaborative Challenges

The great majority of participants (75%) conducted their research as a member of a research team or as part of a center. Numerous challenges to collaborative efforts were identified, as illustrated in Figure A.7.

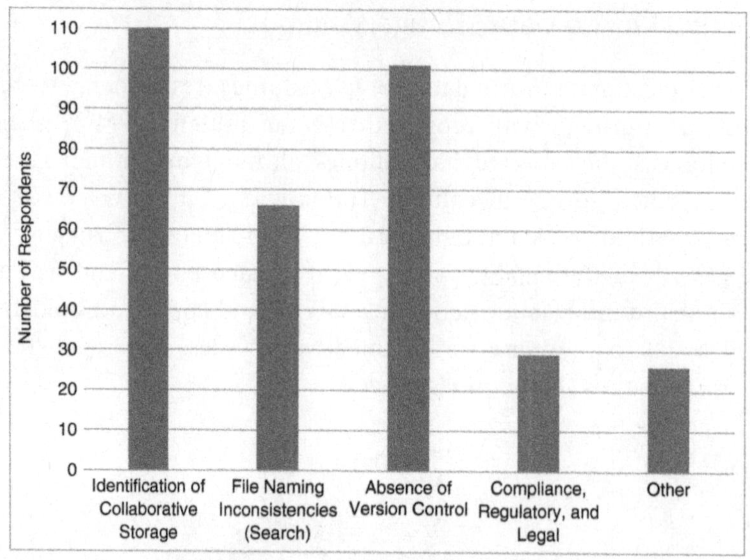

Figure A.7 Challenges to Collaborative Processes

(Note: The "Other" category included costs related to cloud options, robust availability, privacy, inadequate bandwidth, space limitations and backup, university account requirements for access, and management of provenance/history and adherence to change management policy.)

Research Data Sharing

There was a rough split as to whether respondents shared their data outside their research group. About 42% were willing to share their data during the project, 39% were willing to do so after the project is complete, and 19% indicated other—that they would share both during and after the project, depending on who was requesting access or depending on the research.

The majority of respondents (57%) were willing to share their data during the project with researchers outside the project; 68% were willing to share with funders. About equal numbers—21 to 25%—were willing to share their data with instructors, the public, and others, such as collaborators and selected stakeholders. After the project is complete, more were willing to share their data—91% with researchers outside the project, 81% with funders, 74% with the public, 64% with publishers, 57% with instructors, and 14% indicated other (i.e., some data cannot be shared with the public, data sharing varies by project and institutional review board restrictions, and some data can be shared with commercial entities for a fee).

To get a sense of how often a particular data set would be accessed and possibly downloaded, the survey asked how many people the researcher thinks would be interested in using their data per year. About 71% estimated that 1 to 50 people would be interested, 14% thought 51 to 100 people would be interested, and 9% indicated more than 200, in the thousands, or unknown.

Resistance to Data Sharing

History

Previous federal legislation governing data from funded research focused on privacy and security. Examples include the national security requirements surrounding data for Departments of Defense and Energy (DOD/DOE) grants. The Health Insurance Portability and Accountability Act (HIPAA) Privacy Rule of 1996 sought to regulate and protect health information and most specifically PII and the related personal health information (PHI). The regulations imposed significantly limited the accessibility of health data for research. Burdens on time and serious financial impacts became roadblocks to research institutions. Still under way are new techniques to reliably provide "deidentified" health information and in itself could lead to HIPAA reform. On October 1, 2003, the National Institutes of Health (NIH) took a step forward by releasing a memo to research institutions. Investigators submitting an NIH application seeking $500,000 or more in direct costs in any single year were expected to include a plan for data sharing or state why data sharing is not feasible. This significant compliance change systemically moved through government offices. Beginning January 18, 2011, the National Science Foundation required that all grant applicants submit a two-page research data management plan. Sharing for the purpose of advancing science is now a mandate and requirement toward funding [3].

Even with the knowledge of the trend within federal funding agencies, many researchers still resist sharing research data. Additional concerns around sharing data are summarized in Figure A.8.

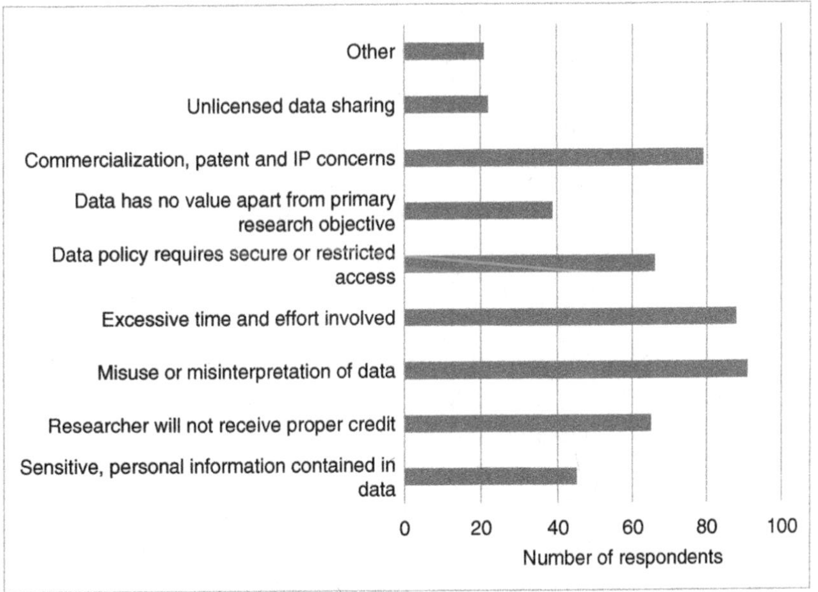

Figure A.8 Concerns with Sharing of Research Data

Grant or Legal Requirements

Grant and legal requirements have always varied widely by discipline and agency. The emerging trends in sharing tend to be more common with expensive-to-gather data, such as astronomy and meteorology, or certain kinds of earth science data.

GenBank is a well-established model for how data sharing models could prevail. The National Center for Biotechnology Information (NCBI) has employed this model for large-scale genome studies for years with success. Researchers are permitted to delay public access to submitted sequences in GenBank for a reasonable amount of time in order to publish their findings. GenBank currently holds more than 150 billion bases. It is theorized that this sharing facilitated the speed at which the Human Genome Project was first completed and has provided extensive medical benefits, such as the 2005 identification of an isolated case of polio in the United States.

In our study, approximately 30% of respondents indicated that researchers' ability to update policies related to research data was inhibited by grant or legal requirements related to data retention and specific contracts with external agencies or tribes, or an existing data management plan still in force.

The research community is expecting the number of federal granting agencies requiring data management plans to increase as the agencies release their responses to the Office of Science and Technology Policy memorandum. The memorandum, titled "Public Access to Federally Supported Research and Development Data and Publications" and dated February 22, 2013, directs federal agencies with more than $100 million in research and development expenditures to develop plans to make the published results of federally funded research freely available to the public within one year of publication and requires researchers to better account for and manage the digital data resulting from federally funded scientific research [4].

Updated policy information became available from the DOE Office of Science on Digital Data Management on July 28, 2014, and the NIH released the NIH genomic data sharing policy on August 27, 2014.

Methods for Data Sharing

The majority of respondents indicated that they use a public cloud service to share data, and the results were spread across a handful of public providers. While other departments, centers, and research groups utilize Microsoft SharePoint or another type of collaborative portal such as a university or department website that offers secure file transfer protocol (FTP), a fair number of researchers still utilize e-mail and sneakernet (aka portable drives sent via snailmail) to share data. At the time of the study, Microsoft Lync and

Slack were not in widespread use for file sharing in the universities polled and were grouped into the other category. Figure A.9 summarizes data sharing methods.

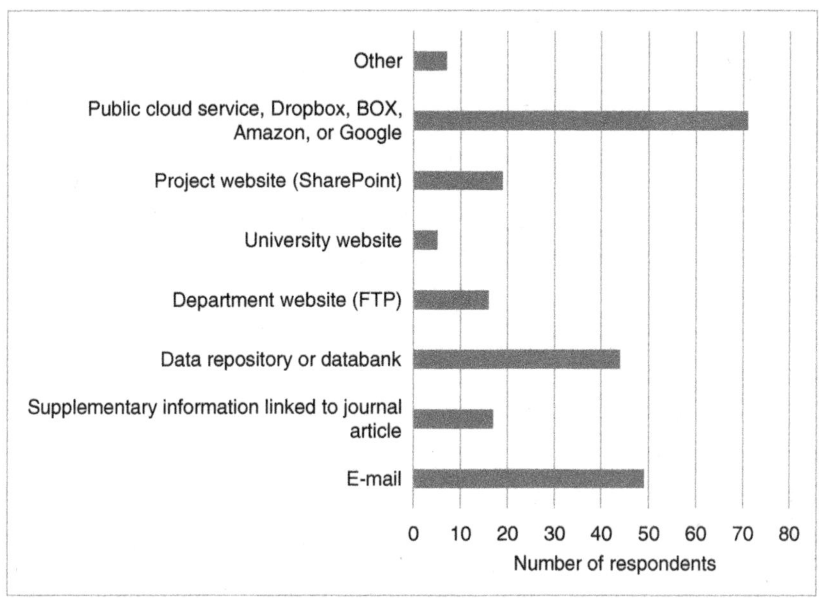

Figure A.9 Methods of Sharing Data

Proprietary Formats

Proprietary data formats were also identified as a barrier to sharing as specific applications are not cloud or sharing friendly or enabled, and shared data cannot be read without a licensed version of the application, which imposes an unforeseen expense.

Data Repository Interest (Metadata Indexed)

Greater than 80% of respondents were either very interested or somewhat interested in the potential of a university-supported data repository. Two of the four universities polled had an initiative under way led either by a committee assigned to data management or by the library. As many as 60% indicated that they were either very familiar or somewhat familiar with the concept of metadata and metadata management to manage, index, and search large data repositories.

At Scale Research Data Repositories

Multiple science disciplines have data repositories that are managed by universities, professional societies, nonprofit organizations, government agencies, publishers, or others. Some funding agencies, such as the NIH, require researchers to deposit their data in specific data repositories. Even if a funding agency does not require researchers to do so, researchers may prefer to make their data available in a repository that archives data similar to their own. A few examples of disciplinary repositories are listed next.

DataONE Data Observation Network for Earth (DataONE) is the foundation of an innovative environmental science through a distributed framework and sustainable cyberinfrastructure that meets the needs of science and society for open, persistent, robust, and secure access to well-described and easily discovered Earth observational data. Supported by the U.S. National Science Foundation (Phase 1 Grant #ACI-0830944, Phase 2 Grant #ACI-1430508) as one of the initial DataNets, DataONE will ensure the preservation, access, use, and reuse of multiscale, multidiscipline, and multinational science data via three primary cyberinfrastructure elements and a broad education and outreach program. (From https://www.dataone.org.)

Dataverse Network The Dataverse is an open source web application to share, preserve, cite, explore, and analyze research data. It facilitates making data available to others, and allows you to replicate others' work. Researchers, data authors, publishers, data distributors, and affiliated institutions all receive appropriate credit. A Dataverse repository hosts multiple Dataverses. Each Dataverse contains data sets or other Dataverses, and each data set contains descriptive metadata and data files (including documentation and code that accompany the data). (From http://dataverse.org/.)

DRYAD The Dryad Digital Repository is a curated resource that makes the data underlying scientific publications discoverable, freely reusable, and citable. Dryad provides a general-purpose home for a wide diversity of data types. (From http://datadryad.org/.)

GenBank GenBank is the NIH genetic sequence database, an annotated collection of all publicly available DNA sequences. GenBank is part of the International Nucleotide Sequence Database Collaboration, which comprises the DNA Databanks of Japan (DDBJ), the European Molecular Biology Laboratory (EMBL), and GenBank at NCBI. These three organizations exchange data on a daily basis. (From http://www.ncbi.nlm.nih.gov/genbank/.)

GEON GEON is an open collaborative project developing cyberinfrastructure for integration of three- and four-dimensional earth science data. The National Science Foundation has recently awarded a grant to researchers at the San Diego Supercomputer Center to explore new ways to manage extremely large data sets hosted on massive clusters, which have become known as computing clouds. The project will study dynamic strategies for provisioning such applications by doing a performance evaluation of alternative strategies for serving very large data sets. The cloud platforms that will be used in the project will be the Google-IBM CluE cluster and the HP-Intel-Yahoo cluster, both of which have been assembled in collaboration with the National Science Foundation for cloud computing research. The LiDAR processing application hosted at the Open Topography portal has been selected as the representative application for this study. The project will study alternative implementations for each step using database technology as well as Hadoop (http://www.hadoop.org) and run a series of performance evaluation experiments. Cloud platforms with thousands of processors and access to hundreds of terabytes of storage provide a natural environment for implementing Open Topography processing routines, which are highly data-parallel in nature. (From http://www.geongrid.org/.)

NCBI The National Center for Biotechnology Information (NCBI) provides the user community with a variety of educational resources including courses, workshops, webinars, training materials on research data downloads, tools, and documentation. (From http://www.ncbi.nlm.nih.gov/.)

NCEI The National Center for Environmental Information (NCEI; formerly National Climatic Data Center [NCDC]) is responsible for hosting and providing access to one of the most significant archives on Earth, with comprehensive oceanic, atmospheric, and geophysical data. From the depths of the ocean to the surface of the sun and from million-year-old sediment records to near real-time satellite images, NCEI is the nation's leading authority for environmental information. (From https://www.ngdc.noaa.gov/ngdcinfo/aboutngdc.html.)

NSSDCA The NASA Space Science Data Coordinated Archive (NSSDCA) serves as the permanent archive for NASA space science mission data. "Space science" means astronomy and astrophysics, solar and space plasma physics, and planetary and lunar science. As permanent archive, NSSDCA teams with NASA's discipline-specific space science "active archives," which provide access to data to researchers and, in some cases, to the general public. (From http://nssdc.gsfc.nasa.gov/about/about_nssdc.html.)

SLDR/ORTOLANG Speech and Language Data Repository (SLDR) is now engaged with the Centre National de Ressources Textuelles et Lexicales (CNRTL) and Nanterre Orléans Centre in building Open Resources and Tools for Language (ORTOLANG). SLDR continues its work of gathering and sharing language data. All services currently offered will remain part of the new platform. Thus, SLDR/ORTOLANG allows you to browse data already collected in the area of speech/multimodal linguistics. Resources are grouped into four main types of items: primary data, secondary data, tools, and collections. Downloading is possible on the basis of various provisions of archival law and intellectual property rights. (From http://sldr.org/.)

TCGA The Cancer Genome Atlas (TCGA) is a comprehensive and coordinated effort to accelerate our understanding of the molecular basis of cancer through the application of genome analysis technologies, including large-scale genome sequencing. TCGA is a joint effort of the National Cancer Institute (NCI) and the National Human Genome Research Institute (NHGRI), two of the 27 institutes and centers of the National Institutes of Health, U.S. Department of Health and Human Services. (From http://cancergenome.nih.gov/.)

tDAR The Digital Archaeological Record (tDAR) is an international digital repository for the digital records of archaeological investigations. tDAR's use, development, and maintenance are governed by Digital Antiquity, an organization dedicated to ensuring the long-term preservation of irreplaceable archaeological data and to broadening the access to these data. (From https://www.tdar.org.)

This listing only includes a small sampling of the many discipline-specific cloud data repositories. There are really three large-scale DNA databases—EMBL European Bioinformatics Institute, GenBank, and the DNA Bank of Japan. However, there are far more DNA repositories specific to aligning domains such as entomology, marine biology, and so on. Many of these data sources have limitations on file formats, file sizes, and types of data they will accept, which complicates the potential for large-scale interdisciplinary studies. With so many sources for research data, researchers often question the long-term viability of emerging data repositories.

See a bio-specific list assembled by Weill Cornell Medical College at http://med.cornell.libguides.com/content.php?pid=401060&sid=3966477.

NOTES

1. Council on Library and Information Resources, https://www.clir.org/initiatives-partnerships/data-curation.
2. Gil Press. 2013. "A Very Short History of Big Data." *Forbes*, May 9. http://www.forbes.com/sites/gilpress/2013/05/09/a-very-short-history-of-big-data/#591a0a2555da.
3. Abigail Goben and Dorothy Salo. 2013. "Federal Research Data Requirements Set to Change." *College & Research Libraries News* 74, no. 8: 421–425. http://crln.acrl.org/content/74/8/421.full.
4. Michael Stebbins. 2013. "Expanding Public Access to the Results of Federally Funded Research." The White House, February 22. https://www.whitehouse.gov/blog/2013/02/22/expanding-public-.access-results-federally-funded-research.

APPENDIX B

Central IT and Research Support*

Gregory D. Palmer

* Much of this chapter is reprinted from Central IT and Research Support. EUNIS Congress, April 22, 2016, http://www.eunis.org/eunis2016/wp-content/uploads/sites/8/2016/02/EUNIS2016_paper_5.pdf. Used with permission.
The author acknowledges funding and collaborative support from Temple University, May 2015.

In 2012, the Educause Center for Applied Research (ECAR) surveyed 675 institutions about their role in enabling research computing. The report indicated that the need for advanced infrastructure and computing capacity was on the rise but that the central information technology (IT) organization was not keeping up with the demand. This report asked many of the same questions that were put forward in the ECAR survey but differed in its focus in that only universities that are considered research intensive were approached. Four public and four private institutions responded to the request for an interview and were in various stages of developing a strategic plan to improve their support of the on-campus research initiatives.

In 2014, the total National Science Foundation (NSF) budget allocation in all categories decreased from the 2010 level of $147 million to $134 million. Other federal agencies have experienced similar decreases, and the emphasis on cross-institutional collaborations has become the standard criterion for successful awards. While this may stretch the available funding among multiple institutions, it reduces the total dollar volume per institution. This forces the university researcher to look for greater economies within the university at the same time that IT budgets are being scrutinized for potential reductions.

As the funding has either decreased or become more difficult to attain, university presidents and provosts are actively investing in the recruitment of big-name scientists while simultaneously expanding research initiatives as a requirement at the undergraduate level. All this has increased the pressure on the chief information officer (CIO) to enhance services to investigators without necessarily receiving more funding.

Some IT organizations are taking measures to improve their service levels in areas such as campus network infrastructure, data centers, shared computing, and the addition of specialized staff members. While the effect these modifications have had on overall grant funding appears to be making a difference, many of the universities interviewed are still in the early stages, with the full impact not to be realized for another three to five years.

In most cases where there is a decentralized IT environment, participants noted that the lack of communication and discovery of synergies was a major roadblock to taking what the NSF calls a "collaborative science" approach. Individualized IT budgets and ownership issues create an environment that is far from conducive for finding economies of scale and shared technologies across fields of study.

The ECAR report also pointed to the rapid growth of big data projects. Data collection, computing, and storage requirements are no longer limited to physics and bioinformatics. Research in the humanities and the growth of digital collections are presenting an additional strain on the campus infrastructure. This report looks at eight research-intensive universities and presents an overview of how they are dealing with the rapid growth of data management and communications.

The next five sections of this appendix provide an overview of the institutions, discuss the nature of the central IT organization, cover the campus infrastructure, explain offered services, and discuss the mechanisms in place that provide the funding for IT initiatives. The final summary and conclusions section is my subjective interpretation of the data in conjunction with personal experience.

INSTITUTIONAL DEMOGRAPHICS (BACKGROUND)

This section is intended to provide general demographics of the institutions surveyed. Of the eight universities, four are considered private and four are considered public. In the search for correlations, faculty populations become relevant only when compared to the number of IT staff available to support them.

Population statistics were requested in the following categories:

- Undergraduate: Full-time registered students
- Graduate: Full- and part-time registered students
- Faculty: Full-time faculty

Total Student Population

Participating institutions range from 7,910 to 37,619 enrolled undergraduate and graduate students for the 2014–2015 academic year. Figure B.1 reports combined enrollment for surveyed institutions.

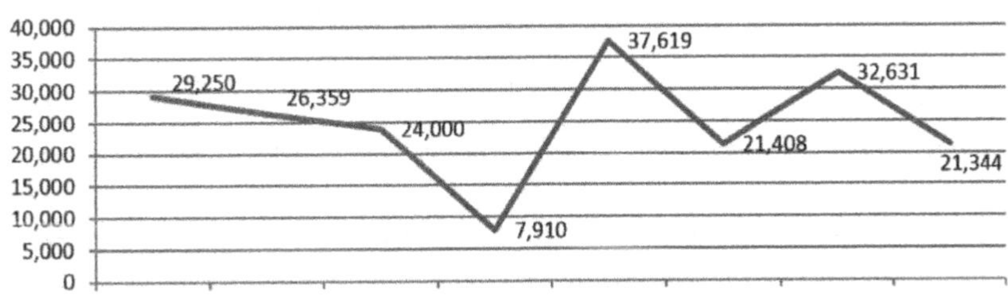

Figure B.1 Combined Student Population for Surveyed Institutions

Undergraduate, Graduate, and Faculty Populations

In Figure B.2 we see the comparative breakdown in student and faculty populations. No correlation is made at this time; however, in three cases, graduate students enrolled in private universities outnumbered undergraduates. While this does not seem to have any relevance to research expenditures, history reveals that the greater the number of graduate students at an institution, the higher the likelihood that research initiatives will not draw on the resources of central IT since they are fulfilling the technology functions.

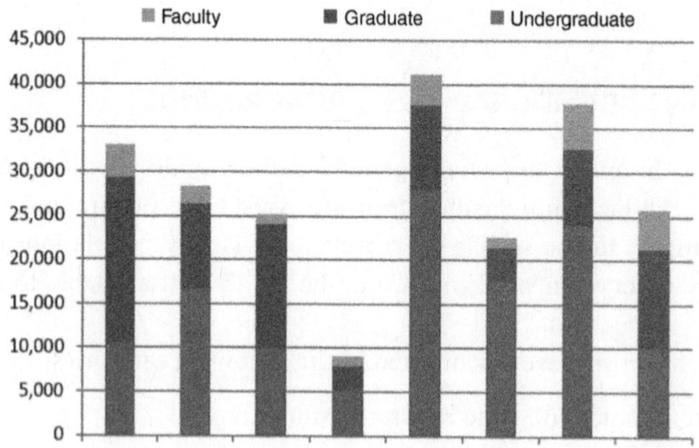

Figure B.2 Comparison of Undergraduate, Graduate, and Faculty Populations

The trend toward assigning undergraduates majoring in the sciences with research requirements access to data both on and off campus will no doubt dramatically increase in the short term. This will affect computing capabilities, network infrastructure, and most likely storage capacity as well. Those universities with large undergraduate populations that are not prepared for the additional demand may be unable to meet the needs of the whole university.

Faculty-Student Comparison

Figure B.3 looks at full-time faculty for each institution and determines a percentage against total student population. This data may be interpreted as:

- Faculty at schools with faculty comprising less than 10% of the total population may have greater teaching responsibilities and less time for research.
- Where the graduate student population exceeds the undergraduate population (Figure B.2), faculty percentages above 10% are more likely to be involved in research initiatives.

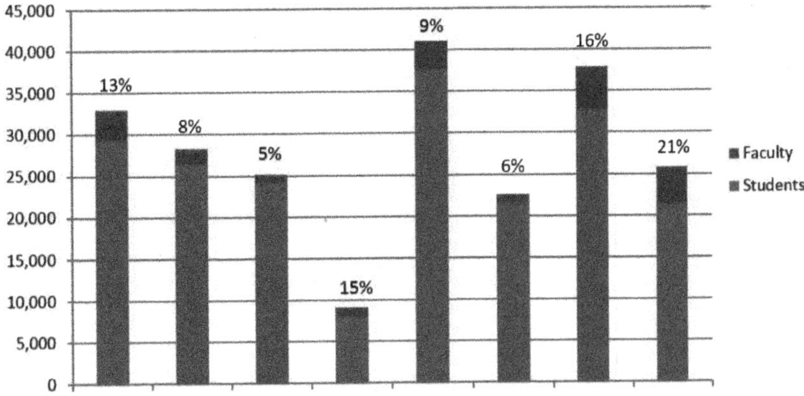

Figure B.3 Percentage of Faculty to Total Student Population

OVERVIEW OF CENTRAL IT ORGANIZATIONS

In this section we asked participants about the general makeup of their IT organization. The intent was to discover both the current and potential capabilities of the organization to support its respective researchers. The information gathered gives us some insight into the balance of administration and full-time staff and the students, faculty, and research initiatives they serve.

An attempt was made to normalize the comparisons so as to minimize differences due to the sizes of the institutions. Did the size of the IT organization have any effect on research funding? Does the ratio of IT staff to faculty have a positive effect on the institution's ability to receive grants? While the size of the unit and its proportion to students and faculty varies by institution, we begin to see some relevance between the availability of IT support and the amount of funding received by the research community.

Figure B.4 compares the level of funding with the number of graduate students. At the time of the survey, University A showed the highest level of external funding and the largest population of graduate students, but equaled University E in the ratio of central IT staff to faculty. Given that other schools also had varying levels of staff to faculty ratios, it seems that the comparison is irrelevant to research funding and central IT support. The argument can be made, however, that a higher concentration of graduate students minimizes the dependency on IT support staff. My experience has shown that system administration and other IT functions used in research are most often performed by graduate students and not a dedicated IT employee, whether in central IT, a school, or in the lab itself. The critical factor is how the resources are allocated.

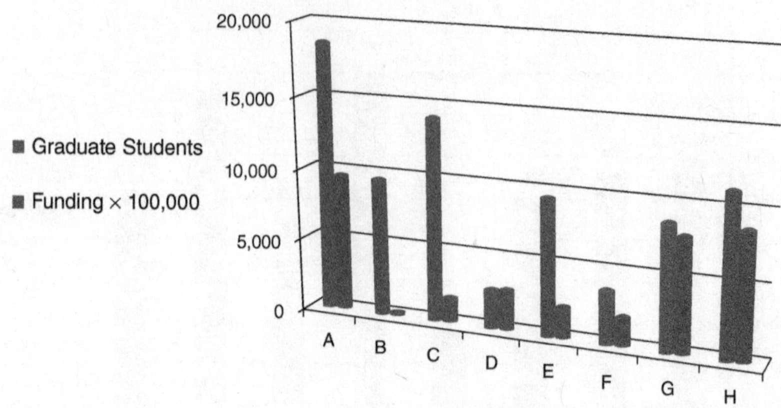

Figure B.4 Graduate Student Population versus External Funding

The more important trend is how central IT allocates its existing staff resources, not just the total number of full-time equivalents (FTEs). When we compare total staff to total faculty and see how that stands up to their funding, the greatest staff : faculty ratio (University D), ranks fourth in overall funding. Table B.1 summarizes the ratio of central IT staff to faculty and lists funding.

Table B.1 Central IT Staff to Faculty, Ranked by Total Research Funding

Rank	Name	Funding	Ratio	Rank	Notes	Notes
1	University A	$ 950,000,000	1:12.3	4	Most funding	Most FTEs
2	University H	$ 870,000,000	1:16.3	6		
3	University G	$ 781,000,000	1:25	8	Highest ratio	Most faculty
4	University D	$ 279,000,000	1:3.7	1	Lowest ratio, least students	Least faculty
5	University E	$ 214,000,000	1:12.5	5	Most students	
6	University F	$ 200,600,000	1:7.5	3		
7	University C	$ 172,000,000	1:6	2		
8	University B	$ 111,000,000	1:20	7	Least FTEs	Least funding

CIO Divisions and Staffing for Research Support

During the interview process, each institution volunteered information about anticipated changes in its organizational structure. With the number of divisions reporting to the CIO ranging from 3 (University B) to 10 (University G), all universities had either already consolidated or were planning to consolidate the number of groups that reported directly to the CIO. Two universities are currently undergoing major reorganizations (University H and University D), with the objectives of finding synergies within their staff and reallocating duplicate processes and resources into a more efficient and balanced model.

Four universities included Research Support as a division, but only one had a staffing level greater than two individuals, and one participant counted the general-purpose system administrator as a "research division." Of these, the staff members "float" between researchers across all disciplines and provide support only in reaction to requests with little or no proactive attempt to discover areas where they could provide a positive effect. Ticketing systems for service and trouble requests are prevalent in all the participants; however, only one differentiated between standard IT requests and the more specific research challenges.

While three institutions were planning on dedicating an FTE to an individual academic unit with the greatest research activity, determining how to equitably fund that person is still an issue. The issue becomes more complicated when schools and centers have their own, dedicated IT staff separate from the central IT organization. Everyone admitted that while the research community can have very customized needs based on their projects, synergies and economies of scale are generally lost when working in a decentralized IT environment. In all cases, the central IT group and the diverse IT organizations have defined their separate roles over time. Central IT generally is responsible for desktop support, voice systems, and cabling infrastructure. And even though Internet, Internet2, and wide area network connectivity is generally assumed to be the domain of central IT, there are still many cases where individual primary investigators (PIs), schools, and centers pursue their own negotiations for external connectivity. Those universities with medical schools *all* report a strong IT group specifically for healthcare. While there is some level of cooperation, the domains are clearly separate.

Table B.2 gives a general view of trends in staff and process realignment. Senior administration, such as the executive vice president (EVP) and the vice president for research, are realizing that inefficiencies in a distributed environment are costly and nonproductive. Changes are planned over an extended period, generally three to five years, but the culture of ownership is difficult to overcome.

Table B.2 Current and Future Trends in Staffing/Funding

Name	Research Division?	Future	Research Support Allocation	Future	Funding	Future
University A	Yes	Yes	Float	By school	Direct charge	Long-term contracting
University B	No	Yes	By dean's request	By tracked usage	Centralized fee	"Tax" by school
University C	Yes	Yes	Float	By school	Hybrid	Contracting, direct
University D	Yes	Yes	Float	By school	General Operating	Some contract

(Continued)

Table B.2 *(Continued)*

Name	Research Division?	Future	Research Support Allocation	Future	Funding	Future
University E	No	?	By dean/VPR request[a]	?	Allocated "tax"	Same
University F	No	?	By dean/VPR request	?	Allocated "tax"	Restructuring
University G	Yes	Yes	By dean/VPR request	By most visible	Centrally funded	Hybrid
University H	No	Yes	By dean/VPR request	By school	Direct charge	Hybrid

[a] Vice president of research.

CENTRAL IT INFRASTRUCTURE

The ability to provide researchers with the necessary infrastructure to analyze, store, access, and transmit the collected data involved with their projects is a necessary function of any IT group. Whether part of the central organization or a local, stand-alone department, delivering these capabilities is the key to receiving successful grant awards. Funding agencies like the NSF and the National Institutes of Health are questioning applications from PIs at institutions that have insufficient campus backbone capacity or access to high-performance networks like Internet2, ESnet, or N-Wave. For big data projects, they are increasingly critical of undersized infrastructure. Since "big data" initiatives are outstripping the budgets of central IT, the NSF has programmatically made available millions of dollars for improving cyberinfrastructure in higher education.

Campus Networks

In questioning the participants about their infrastructure both on campus and off, it was interesting to note how many institutions actually knew very little about their off-campus connectivity. In those instances where the individual interviewed was a member of the central IT divisions devoted to research, it was necessary for him or her to call the network group to get the correct answers to questions about campus backbone, Internet, and Internet2 capacities.

The backbone capacity on their campuses for all participants was 10G or multiples thereof. In three cases, the university received NSF Campus Cyberinfrastructure—Network Infrastructure and Engineering Program grants, which gave them the ability to bring in 100 Gb links to Internet2 either through their regional provider or direct from Internet2. In only one case was the Science DMZ actually completed. This would allow the university to provide big data initiatives direct access to the national Research and Education network without traversing multiple firewalls and routers.

When questioned about on-campus connectivity between science laboratories and the backbone, nearly all responded that 100% of the labs had at least 1 Gb of connectivity. On further questioning, these circuits were frequently shared across multiple data collection sites within the same building, thereby making them subject to congestion and latency.

Data Centers

All universities have some form of a data center. At one end of the scale, a university has a Tier 3 facility complete with generators, diverse power sources, diverse network connections, and a "green" heating, ventilation, and air-conditioning (HVAC) system. Other sites have varying levels of data center infrastructure. Medical schools and other high-volume research centers have separate facilities. These school-specific centers are connected to central IT resources, but generally the infrastructure is not equal to the demand.

Loosely defined, a data center can be as little as a room or a closet with a single rack that houses the collected data and potentially some analysis or computing capacity, or it can be a full-blown Tier 3 facility equal to any commercial offering. As part of an NSF panel in 2012 that included IT administrators from the top 10 research institutions in the United States, I was amazed to discover that none of the participants was able to account for the number of servers on their campuses. The NSF was attempting to measure on-campus computing capacity, but such information could not be centralized due to the decentralized nature of each institution. As the interviews progressed, this lack of information became apparent across every university.

On-Campus Data Centers versus Cloud Services

Computing and storage cloud services continue to proliferate. Central IT CIOs are attempting to understand the balance between building or expanding their existing facilities and becoming the contract coordinator with companies like AWS, Glacier, or a host of startup organizations. Of the eight participants, four institutions have multiple cloud service contracts distributed across individual schools, two institutions use central IT as the contract coordinator, one university completely controls a contract through Internet2's "Net+" program but has no statistics for usage as each account is paid separately, and one university has no policy regarding cloud services.

CENTRAL IT RESEARCH SUPPORT SERVICES

In this section we look at specific services offered by central IT in support of their research communities. This is where we begin to see trends in staffing changes that recognize the importance of shared resources and the economies they will bring to the entire university. These economies are realized not just in dollars but in efficiency and productivity.

Relationship Management

Proactively discovering the needs of the research community is a process still in its infancy across those universities interviewed. Five of the eight participants are reactive as opposed to actively reaching out to deans and department heads. The decentralized nature of IT on campuses and the lack of specialized staff known as relationship managers have led the vast majority of investigators to look externally for solutions involving data storage and computing capacity. Since research requests are not tracked separately and often fall into the same queue as telephone change orders, it requires "knowing the right person" to get something accomplished in a timely fashion. In many cases, where there is not any type of introduction to IT for new faculty, contacting central IT simply does not occur to the individual researcher.

Universities C, D, and H are experimenting with client relationship managers (CRMs). These individuals are focused on building relationships within research-intensive areas. They become knowledgeable about the largest grants that are currently active and proactively look for opportunities to assist schools and departments with their technological challenges. At the same time, they work with the local IT staff and bring their campus-wide knowledge to reveal synergies that create cost and productivity efficiencies.

The results have been greater than anticipated, and two of these schools are planning expansions in CRM staffing to narrow the scope of responsibility. University H has just begun its CRM program, and it is too early to quantify the impact.

Internal Staff Contracting

Also in the preliminary stages is the concept of contracting central IT staff directly to the researcher. Currently at Universities A, C, and D, a researcher may contract directly with central IT for specific job functions. The individual remains an employee of central IT but reports on a daily basis to the laboratory he or she has been assigned to. Using grant funds to pay for this service, investigators discover that graduate students are free to work on the project and not system administration or programming. This becomes a tremendous productivity enhancement, which ultimately results in real dollar savings as well, since those functions are now fixed costs instead of variable costs. The contract period may be task oriented or run the length of the grant period.

Internal Communications

All participants reported regularly scheduled meetings with the office of the vice president for research (VPR). These were generally high-level administrative meetings with occasional requests for specific researchers considered high profile. The perception is that strategic planning at the individual PI level takes second place to administrative functions at these meetings. Because the office of the VPR is primarily concerned with grant applications and budget accounting, the involvement of central IT is frequently focused on software modules that improve the business process and rarely on the scientific processes.

In decentralized environments, there are efforts within the private universities to coordinate activities with the IT administrators at the various schools and centers. Those few IT organizations that have instituted a relationship management program have reported that the outlook is promising but, given the historical lack of communication, the new credibility has the potential to overwhelm the relationship manager.

CENTRAL IT OFFERED SERVICES

Every central IT organization provides a list of services to its campus community. The most widely known offerings are for students. Table B.3 lists those services that would be most attractive to researchers with an x indicating that the service is available and used. In those cases where the participant responded with "informal" (by request only), the service was recorded as not being available. It must be noted that every participant admitted that there is no marketing plan other than the listing of the offered services on a website and, occasionally, how they will benefit the client. The next list describes the services and any additional information garnered during the interviews.

- **Grant writing.** Grant applications are commonly based on the collection and analysis of preliminary data. Funding agencies are increasingly requiring collaborative efforts across two or more institutions. This increases the potential for success and distributes the award rather than concentrating on a single school or center. Other than research in the areas of computer science and communications networking, it is highly likely that the PI will not design the most efficient process for collecting, archiving, analyzing, and distributing data sets or findings. Central IT is a logical resource for assisting the PI in developing an actual data management plan and providing the text for the grant application.

Table B.3 Services Offered by Central IT

Institution	Grant Writing	Hardware Purchasing	Contract Staff	Technical Compliance	Computing, Individual	Computing, Shared	Data Center	Technical Consulting	WAN Connect	ERP	Project Management	Institutional Compliance	Agency Compliance	Relationship Management	Faculty Recruit Retain
University A		x	x			x	x	x		x	x	x			
University B						x	X			x		x			
University C			x	x	X	x	x	x	x	x	x	x	x	x	x
University D	x	x		x		x	x	x		x		x		x	x
University E						x	x			x		x			
University F	x	x				x	x			x					
University G						x	x	x	x			x	x		
University H					X	x	x		x	x	x			x	

- **Hardware and software purchasing.** When researchers submit their grant applications, they include equipment listings in their budgets. In most cases equipment lists are solicited directly from vendors and may or may not include the volume discounts available at the university level. There is a potential for economies of scale if central IT made the purchases in combination with their own and other units across the campus. The perception is that the highly specialized nature and sophistication of certain hardware is beyond the understanding of central IT. If a central purchasing resource is made available, it must be flexible enough to comply with customized configurations and document possible synergies across departments.
- **Contract help.** As noted, some schools are offering central IT employees as contractors to a research project for the duration of the grant. The objective is to remove those who are involved in analysis and reporting from IT tasks and thereby increase performance and productivity. When asked if this service was offered, responses were not always "yes" or "no." Table B.3 reflects only those schools that offer this service on a regular basis. In one other case, a very high-profile research project warranted this kind of attention, but it was the exception rather than a regularly offered service.
- **Technical compliance.** For non-IT PIs, this service will review the data management design and processes to determine that the outcome will function as desired. This service is not to be confused with consulting, institutional compliance, or funding agency compliance. This is a design review only, with recommendations.
- **Computing capacity, individual.** Small research projects or initiatives that require infrequent or low-end processing capability may be resolved with in-room hardware. Cost would be a major issue for this category of research. The question was posed to determine if central IT would provide or purchase computing capacity that may be part of a cluster, cloud, or shared data center infrastructure and would provide configuration support. The researcher would have the benefit of support but not the cost of an entire system.
- **Computing capacity, shared.** Research computing requirements are generally sporadic, ranging from four times a year to daily computational analysis of very large data sets. There are many options for the investigators, including supercomputing centers, cloud services, on-campus clusters within a school, and central IT–provided computing centers. While all the participants offered some form of campus central computing functionality, the models varied based on funding and staff availability.

- **Data center infrastructure.** As mentioned and reflected in Table B.3, all participants offer space in a data center managed by central IT. However, services vary according to the type of data center and the requirements of the researcher at each institution. There is only one Tier 3 data center among those surveyed. The power outputs are commonly alternating current (AC) and only occasionally direct current (DC). Diverse power sources and network pathways are rare. These limitations have pushed many investigators to cloud services, usually without the knowledge of central IT.
- **Technical consulting.** This occurs when central IT goes beyond a simple design review and actually works with the researcher prior to grant submission to maximize the efficiency of the IT data management plan. This may occur through a relationship manager or in combination with central IT staff members. While four participants labeled this as a valid service offering, it is predominantly available on request only.
- **Wide area connectivity.** In some cases, the investigator may require direct connections to funding agencies or collaborators off the campus net. Given the cost and management components, this occurs only with "big data" projects that are well funded and have a high frequency of transmissions. The examples most often used include Internet2, the National Institutes of Health, the National Oceanic and Atmospheric Administration, and the Department of Energy. Of the three universities listed as offering this service, one has an isolated case but is receptive to more if circumstances require it. Another university will guide assist the researcher but will not assume responsibility for the connection. The third university also has the regional Internet2 interconnect as part of the central IT organization and is able to facilitate these special cases to suit requirements. While such requests are rare, reduced costs and increased capacity needs show a trend for more off-campus connectivity.
- **Enterprise resource planning (ERP).** ERP is business management software—typically a suite of integrated applications that an institution can use to collect, store, manage, and interpret data from many academic, business, and research activities, including: budget planning, cost analysis, and service delivery. While all but one participant provides some form of ERP system, one university is faced with multiple homegrown software platforms in a decentralized environment. Efforts there are under way to consolidate and make consistent the process whereby the institution manages research budgets and reporting functions.
- **Project management.** This service encompasses central IT taking responsibility for a component of a research initiative or, in very few

cases, the entire data management plan of a project. Those that offer this function admitted that there was room for improvement and the knowledge base necessary to perform such duties adequately was time consuming and therefore very costly. The benefit to researchers is that they will be able to totally free themselves of such IT functions as configurations, implementations, and the like and devote their resources to the research project.

- **Institutional compliance.** Six of the eight universities interviewed conducted design reviews in one form or another to ensure that the equipment, applications, and data management would not disrupt the campus infrastructure. The remaining two institutions left the detailed reviews to the decentralized IT groups and made recommendations only when called on. Involving central IT in such design reviews would minimize issues with implementations that do not consider the impact in such areas as security or backbone capacity on the university as a whole.
- **Funding agency compliance.** Distinct from other areas discussed already, researchers may be required to ensure that their projects comply with federal and state standards for data management and security. This is most common with healthcare and patient data but also is relevant to many other facets of the university's mission regarding research and education. It is most often left to the decentralized IT organization to assume responsibility for ensuring that standards are met. In very few cases was central IT responsible for agency compliance, and then only when called on.
- **Relationship management.** This field is still in its infancy. Relationship managers are rapidly showing their value to the research community. Working across schools and centers, they are able to identify cost-saving synergies and act as facilitators between individuals and laboratories. It is rare that different departments interact, creating a loss of economy for the university as a whole. Relationship managers can be instrumental in bringing the research community together.
- **Faculty recruitment and retention.** When asked if the central IT organization was engaged in assisting the provost or VPR in the recruitment of faculty from other institutions, six of the eight institutions responded no.

According to an Educause review in 2012, it is important that the IT functionality of an institution be described as a benefit when soliciting well-known faculty at other universities with large grants. The same holds true for retaining faculty who have received IT-intensive awards that the institution may not be able to accommodate. It is not unusual for faculty members to become disgruntled upon arrival or to leave a university for better lab space, bandwidth, or services available from central IT.

FUNDING MECHANISMS

The model to fund supporting IT in the research communities has not yet matured in any of the universities interviewed. In the past, individual investigators were largely self-sustaining, itemizing in their grants those components necessary to gather data and analyze it. The trend toward eliminating the stand-alone laboratory and becoming more collaborative has complicated the funding of projects since budgets now include two or more institutions. Staffing, equipment, computing, and storage budgets need to allocate expenses as if they were multisite companies. The business aspect of research now requires a more in-depth management of procurement, space allocation, and human resources.

Business development and facilities management are facets that researchers are generally not accustomed to.

In an effort to reduce costs, investigators are considering cloud service providers as attractive alternatives to campus facilities since they allow easier access across distances and between collaborators and they minimize what could be long lead times before investigators' needs are realized by the university. This is a challenge for the central IT organization because it shifts the focus from facilities-based computing and storage to offsite companies, thereby increasing the need for higher-bandwidth connections. Investment decisions to build or expand data centers have a high degree of risk because the total cost could easily exceed the return over the estimated life span of the technology.

Allocated Expenses versus Cost Recovery

Of the eight respondents to the survey, five universities recover their costs through an allocated charge levied against schools and centers. Also known as a tax, the methodology used is based on various factors, most frequently headcount: total student plus faculty or student, faculty, and staff. A percentage of the estimated operating budget for central IT is applied to each school or center and becomes the published revenue base for the entire department. In some cases, only those services that are common to the entire university, such as Internet, voice, and cabling, are included in this model, while programming and new wiring projects are based on quotas and charged directly to the school. Although this process is common, it means that the special needs of the research community are in conflict between available funds and grant budgets.

In Table B.4 we see that with the exception of voice, the common services are paid for through an allocated charge. In two instances, maintaining the campus backbone is covered by a port fee that varies by the capacity requested. With a 1 Gb connection being fairly standard, 10 Gb interfaces are available, only by request.

Table B.4 Funding Sources of Key Common Services

Name	Internet	Internet2	Campus Backbone	Voice
University A	Allocated	Allocated	Allocated	Direct
University B	Allocated	Allocated	Allocated	Direct
University C	Port Fee	Allocated	Allocated	Bundled
University D	Allocated	Allocated	Allocated	Direct
University E	Allocated	Allocated	Allocated	Direct
University F	Allocated	Allocated	Allocated	Direct
University G	Allocated	Allocated	Allocated	Direct
University H	Allocated	Allocated	Port Fee	Direct

Table B.5 reviews the services that are most applicable to the research community. The next list describes the categories.

- **Specialized campus circuits.** When a request is received for a network connection, either directly to the border router or a campus point-to-point to another location, a fee may be charged. Researchers may also request a circuit to the Internet2 interface and thereby bypass the campus backbone. In some cases, two departments on the same campus are collaborators.
- **Specialized off-campus circuits.** There have been occasions when a high-profile researcher has requested a direct link to the funding agency or analysis site. Only one institution has that service capability, and fees vary according to capacity and remote location.
- **Shared computing.** In cases where central IT provides a computing resource, some schools use the allocated cost for recovery of basic expenses, such as electric and HVAC, but charge for usage accordingly. However, the formula for determining usage varies widely.
- **Data center space.** Most universities charge researchers for full or partial rack space in their central data centers. This space ranges from electric only to a full suite of services: installation, administration, and maintenance. In cases where the funding source is derived from allocated fees, expansion requires a request to the administration and may be difficult to obtain or delayed beyond the need. This has made cloud services more attractive.
- **Budget management.** Only one institution offers budget management through central IT, and even then on rare occasions. In decentralized environments, a school or center may offer budget management. In all cases, the office of the VPR plays a role in managing budgets associated with research.

Table B.5 Research Support Services

Name	Specialized Campus Circuits	Specialized Off-Campus Circuits	Shared Computing	Data Center Space	Budget Management	Project Management	Grant Overhead
University A	Not offered	Not offered	Direct	Allocated	Not offered	Not offered	60%
University B	1 Gb—standard 10 Gb—direct	Not offered	Minimal offering	Varies	Not offered	Not offered	Unknown
University C	1 Gb–10 Gb allocated	Not offered	Usage fee	Direct	Not offered	Not offered	52.5%
University D	1 Gb–10 Gb allocated	Not offered	Allocated	Allocated	Not offered	Not offered	62%
University E	Not offered	Not offered	Not offered	Direct	Not offered	Not offered	56%
University F	Not offered	Not offered	Basic is allocated + usage	Direct	Not offered	Not offered	Varies
University G	1 Gb—standard 10 Gb—direct	Not offered	Offered by schools	Direct	Not offered	Not offered	51%
University H	Direct	Direct	Not offered	Direct	Direct	Direct	60%

- **Project management.** Does central IT provide a service for managing the IT components of a research project? With one exception, the answers were "no." IT management would include the installation, configuration, and initial testing of IT-related hardware for grants already awarded. The assumption here is that such expenditure was accounted for in the initial grant budget.
- **Grant overhead.** The percentages listed account for space, utilities, and a variety of general university services in support of funded research initiatives. This information is simply provided as a fact, but in three instances the person interviewed shared that central IT did not receive any funds from this fee.

Historically, funding for centrally provided IT services is an issue for all institutions but particularly for public universities. Constraints on purchasing processes and dependencies on government funding made it difficult for IT organizations at public institutions to maintain state-of-the-art facilities, which in turn limited their ability to attract high-profile investigators. I thought that the answers to the final question of the interview by the institutions spoke volumes about their view on current funding models. The question was:

Do you feel your current funding model is:

A. Inadequate to meet the needs of the research community

B. Adequate for current needs?

C. Adequate but needs revision for the future.

D. Inadequate in general

In order, four respondents answered that the funding model was inadequate in general; three answered that the funding model was adequate but needs revision for the future; and one answered that the funding model was inadequate for their research community.

SUMMARY AND CONCLUSIONS

Much has changed since the ECAR report of 2012. University presidents and VPRs are placing a greater emphasis on recruiting and retaining high-profile investigators, while provosts and deans include more undergraduate research requirements in the curriculum. This puts additional strain on CIOs to provide staff and infrastructure resources without necessarily receiving more funding. While central IT organizations struggle with ways to improve their support of their respective research communities, new trends in service offerings are surfacing that increase the value of internal organizations.

Challenges Still to Overcome

Perhaps the greatest challenge comes from the culture that has evolved in a decentralized environment. When central IT was perceived as the unit that was primarily responsible for voice, building-to-building cabling, dormitories, and administrative systems/applications, schools and centers had to develop their own resources to deal with the research needs that were very often highly customized.

Most often, knowledge sharing between schools and even within the same department is nonexistent. Attempts by central IT to reverse or modify such an established culture generally meet with resistance, with the attitude of "Don't touch my stuff!" taking precedence over efficiency and economies of scale. If universities are to improve their competitiveness and provide investigators with a suite of reasonably priced services, then there must at least be close cooperation, if not mergers, whereby the technology skill sets are available across the traditional boundaries of fields of study.

Another perception of central IT that must be overcome is the sense that central IT is so entrenched with processes and standards that they are unable to accommodate the needs of a research community that requires a flexible and often dynamic environment. Central IT is by nature process oriented and necessarily so, in order to facilitate the normal operation of the institution. Finance, student systems, and the like are assumed to be stable environments in order to ensure that daily operations continue uninterrupted. However, research, by nature, deals with new protocols, formats, and technologies that are inconsistent with standard operating procedures. If IT organizations are to gain credibility and trust, they must be receptive to nonstandard processes.

Last, but certainly not the final challenge, is the ability to create an infrastructure that is balanced between cost and demand. Average researchers assume that because they are paying for overhead, all or most of the services mentioned in the section titled "Central IT Research Support Services" should be included in the support they receive. Unfortunately, research demand is difficult to forecast, particularly when creating a budget for additional storage, computing capacity, and bandwidth. Frequency of the service is also an issue. The big data project that requires high-capacity networks for transmission to agencies or collaborators may only run four times a year. The university may not be able to cover expenses for circuits that are available 24 × 7 × 365. Fortunately, relatively new Layer2 services can provide temporary direct connections, and computing/storage hardware is modular and easily scalable.

Trends That Show Promise

The communication process between central IT and the VPR was excellent in some cases and very informal in others. While regularly scheduled meetings are held between the CIO and the VPR, the impression was that central IT is still more reactive than proactive. Meetings with the PIs to determine service needs are rare unless directed by the VPR or requested by the PI.

But three institutions have implemented client relationship managers (CRMs). These individuals are charged with proactively reaching out to department heads and act as liaisons between central IT, local IT organizations, and the research/academic groups on campus. The results have been immediately positive to the point that the CRM is now deluged with meeting requests. This has put a new strain on central IT and created a backlog of work orders and capital projects, but the mere fact that IT is listening to the needs of the community has at least temporarily created a good image. The sustainability of the CRM will depend on whether the organization has the resources to satisfy the demand.

Another positive trend is the provision of temporary IT staff to researchers for the length of the grant. The person reports to central IT on the organization chart but is "embedded" in the researchers' lab and works either part-time or full-time for the PI. The grant covers the fully loaded cost of the employee and can be paid to central IT via a budget transfer. Arrangements are made prior to the grant submission where the skills are specified and the financials are a fixed rather than an estimated cost.

The benefits of this program include having the advanced skill and knowledge sets that an IT professional can offer, presumably at competitive rates. The separation of duties between graduate students and IT staff means that students are focusing on the research, not on programming or system administration. Although this concept is new enough that the initial embedded staff members are still on their first assignment, when the research project is complete, the people will be returned to the pool, awaiting their next placement.

All participants claimed centralized computing that is shared across the university and available to researchers. While the funding models vary, most of the initiatives are pilot programs, but growing. Most of the research communities still prefer to have their system analysis done on site, but the "server under the desk" is still prevalent. Everyone admits that the unknown systems are hidden only until they stop working, at which time either the central or departmental IT unit is called on. By providing community access to centralized computing, central IT eliminates a number of potential issues: security, standards compliance, backup and restoration, cost economies of scale, access to high-performance networks, and proper trouble ticket reporting. One additional advantage is that the university IT department becomes a viable option for the investigators when determining the cost, data availability, and security of their research.

Three of the universities have created research divisions within the central IT organization that report directly to the CIO. (A fourth is in progress, but with only one person.) The reported benefits reveal this to be an excellent decision. Not only is the interaction between IT and the research community vastly improved, but the link between services requested and services offered has reduced response times and increased trust and credibility. Funding for the additional staff is generally provided through a combination of direct charges and allocations.

Areas for Improvement

Although the improvement trends are showing positive results, there is still the issue of vertical communications across the organizational charts of an institution. Relationship managers can play key roles in acting as research ombudsmen if they are given the authority to interact at all levels.

They can be a valuable source of information for both the VPR and the CIO. Frequent meetings with PIs will lead to the discovery of service needs, and these can be passed on to local IT organizations or central IT, whichever is more appropriate.

One element that was particularly lacking was the marketing of current or new services by central IT. Although improvements are being made in intercampus communications, there does not seem to be a cohesive effort to make the research community aware of the services being offered. Central IT is frequently in competition with commercial providers, and it is not unusual to discover that an available service or product was awarded to an outside company simply because the investigator was not aware that the need could be filled internally. Some universities have established working groups consisting of research deans, a representative from the VPR's office, and central IT. This is one good avenue for making options available as long as it doesn't come across as a hard sell.

Commensurate with the marketing concept is the provision of a return on investment. With the exception of very large labs with assigned business managers, most researchers are not business oriented and make IT decisions based on traditional procedures. The perfect example is when data will be sent to a collaborator or funding agency by shipping hard drives via commercial carrier. If damage occurs (and it does happen on occasion), the rest of the data can be useless. Using the connection to the advanced network can be faster, more reliable, and more secure. What the research community needs to know is why it should use central IT services. What is the payback in terms of cost and productivity? Demonstrating or articulating these benefits may be an additional role for the research relationship manager or the project manager, but the resource can be funded quickly if the money spent on an outside provider is channeled through central IT.

In a decentralized environment establishing a bidirectional trust relationship with school/center IT directors and their staff is essential to the success of a cooperative work environment whereby both organizations realize a benefit. Achieving this allows the university to react more quickly to researchers' service needs. This generates more productive outcomes on grant objectives.

The last example I will speak to is the inclusion of central IT in the overhead charge levied against grants (see Table B.5). In very few cases does this funding seem to find its way into supporting IT services. This is one possible source of funding for the research relationship manager.

Although this report should be considered an individual's opinion relevant to facts gathered from a small sampling of universities, and in no way is it a research initiative comparable to the ECAR report of 2012, it is nonetheless a statement about the current trends and conditions relevant to how central IT organizations are dealing with the growing demand to support their research communities.

Based on interviews, external readings, and personal observations as the director of a regional research network and connector for Internet2, I can safely say that three important trends are taking place across the United States. IT organizations are becoming more proactive and more client centric, and are viewing themselves as a business within the university. I can only hypothesize that the impetus for these trends is brought about by presidents, VPRs, and deans who see research as (1) a means of improving the human condition, (2) a way to expand knowledge about our universe, (3) good business, and (4) leading to national and global recognition. Order these in any sequence you see fit.

REFERENCES

Bichsel, Jacqueline. "Research Computing, The Enabling Role of Information Technology." Louisville, CO: EDUCAUSE Center for Applied Research, November 2012. http://net.educause.edu/ir/library/pdf/ERS1211/ERS1211.pdf.

Dirks, Nicholas B. "Rebirth of the Research University." *Chronicle of Higher Education* (April 2015). http://chronicle.com/article/Rebirth-of-the-University/229585/?cid=at&utm_source=at&utm_medium=en.

Kassabian, Dikran. "Research Cyberinfrastructure at Penn: Supporting University Research Through Information Technology Infrastructure and Services." Philadelphia: Information Systems and Computing, University of Pennsylvania, April 2011.

National Institutes of Health. *NIH Data Book*. Washington, DC: U.S. Department of Health and Human Services, December 2014. http://report.nih.gov/nihdatabook/.

National Science Foundation. "Campus Cyberinfrastructure—Network Infrastructure and Engineering Program (CC-NIE)." Washington, DC: Office of Cyberinfrastructure, October 2012. http://www.nsf.gov/pubs/2013/nsf13530/nsf13530.htm.

National Science Foundation. "A Timeline of NSF History." Washington, DC, 2016. https://www.nsf.gov/about/history/overview-50.jsp.

Williams, Audrey June. "What It Means to Reach for Carnegie's Top Tier." *Chronicle of Higher Education* (April 2015). http://chronicle.com/article/What-It-Means-to-Reach-for/229651/?cid=at&utm_source=at&utm_medium=en.

APPENDIX C

HPC Working Example

Using Parallelization Programs, such as GNU Parallel and OpenMP, with Serial Tools

Overview

The goal of this document is to provide several examples and methods to program and use parallel logic to process multiple data sets using multiple cores on one or more servers. The document does not cover message passing interface (MPI) batch processing invoking multiple nodes sharing a single processing job.

Basic knowledge of shell scripting is helpful but not absolutely necessary.

This page is helpful for beginners: http://linuxcommand.org/lc3_wss0020.php.

Key terms used in these scripts:

- Arrays
- Variables
- Arguments
- Functions
- For loops

Linux tools:

- bash
- sed
- split
- xargs
- vi
- GNU Parallel (http://www.gnu.org/software/parallel/)

Next-generation sequencing (NGS) tools used:

- Picard-tools (http://broadinstitute.github.io/picard/)
  - SamToFastq
  - Samtools
  - AddOrReplaceReadGroups
  - SortSam
- Burrows-Wheeler Aligner (http://sourceforge.net/projects/bio-bwa/)
- Plink (http://pngu.mgh.harvard.edu/~purcell/plink/)

HPC Resource Manager:

- Torque (http://www.adaptivecomputing.com/products/open-source/torque/)

BIO HPC Use Case 1

Biologist AF receives 24 Binary Alignment Map (BAM) files from a third-party lab. AF uses Picard's samtools program to index these BAM files, but the index is corrupt and unusable. AF contacts the lab and discovers the files received were not correctly processed (aligned, sorted, read groups added, etc.).

Solution:

Process BAM data using NGS tools.

Prepare Process Input (Data Sets, File Lists, and Scripts)

The commands and scripts as shown are dependent on the input residing in the current working directory, which is accessible across all cluster nodes (Scratch or home directory, for example)

1. Create list of input files.
   a. cat *.bam > bamlist
2. Strip the .bam file extension.
   a. sed -e 's/.bam//' bamlist
3. Add trailing \ to lines.
   a. sed -e 's/$/\\/g' bamlist
4. Account for HPC resources. The cluster used for this job consists of 64 physical servers with 16 processor cores each (2 E5–2660 CPU). With this information, I can plan to split the "bamlist" on line 12 to create 2 lists of 12 data sets each:
   a. split -l 12 bamlist
5. There should now be two files named xaa and xab. Remove the trailing \ from the last line in each file.

Step 1. Convert BAM to FQ (fastq)

The code examples shown are Torque (PBS) scripts that can be submitted to the HPC cluster. Refer to the Torque documentation or the documentation appropriate for your cluster resource manager. The script name should be relevant to your job and end with a .pbs extension. (The .pbs extension doesn't make a difference but helps to identify what the script is for.)

```
#!/bin/bash
#PBS -l nodes=1:ppn=12
#PBS -N xaa_bam2fq_01
#PBS -e $PBS_JOBNAME.err
#PBS -o $PBS_JOBNAME.out
module load shared torque picard-tools parallel

cd $PBS_O_WORKDIR

time xargs -a $PWD/xaa | parallel -j12 java -Xmx4G -Djava.io.tmpdir=`pwd`/
tmp -jar /cm/shared/apps/picard-tools/SamToFastq.jar VALIDATION_
STRINGENCY=SILENT INPUT={}.bam  FASTQ={}_1.fq SECOND_END_FASTQ={}_2.fq
```

Submit the job to the Torque queue with the command "qsub scriptname.pbs." The resulting output of SamToFastq will be 12 pairs of fastq files with filenames matching those in the *xaa* file.

To process the *xab* files, you can copy the *xaa* script and globally replace *xaa* with *xab* using sed, vi, or your favorite editor.

Alternately you could not split the bamlist and queue all 24 files to process on a single node of any core capacity.

```
#!/bin/bash
#PBS -l nodes=1:ppn=16 (or whatever your max cores are)
#PBS -N bamlist_bam2fq_01
#PBS -e $PBS_JOBNAME.err
#PBS -o $PBS_JOBNAME.out

module load shared torque picard-tools parallel

cd $PBS_O_WORKDIR

time xargs -a $PWD/bamlist | parallel  java -Xmx4G -Djava.
io.tmpdir=`pwd`/tmp -jar /cm/shared/apps/picard-tools/SamToFastq.jar
VALIDATION_STRINGENCY=SILENT INPUT={}.bam  FASTQ={}_1.fq SECOND_END_
FASTQ={}_2.fq
```

Removing the "-j 12" between "parallel" and "java" causes the maximum number of system cores to be used, which on our servers would be 16. Once the first of the 16 threads finishes processing a file, it will grab the next unprocessed file, which would be line 17 of our input file. Once all 24 are processed, this job is done and we'd expect to see output and logs.

Step 2. Align fastq files

Burrows-Wheeler Alignment (BWA) is a standard tool for mapping sequences to reference genomes. This is a long and CPU-intensive process compared to the initial step, but proper resource planning and batch usage will yield low-maintenance results.

This step requires an indexed reference sample as shown above. For example, a reference fasta can be indexed with the samtools command: samtools idx filename.fa.

```
#!/bin/bash
#PBS -l nodes=1:ppn=16 (or whatever your max cores are)
#PBS -N jobname
#PBS -e $PBS_JOBNAME.err
#PBS -o $PBS_JOBNAME.out

module load shared torque bwa/bwa-0.7.10 parallel
```

```
cd $PBS_O_WORKDIR

parallel -j2 bwa aln -t 8 GRCh37-lite.fa {} ">" {.}.sai::: *_1.fq
```

This starts two parallel threads for bwa. The bwa option "-t" invokes eight threads (cores) for each of the 24 _1.fq pairs. So, with our 16 core nodes, we can expect two files to process simultaneously using eight cores each. The more cores or threads, the faster the processing. Eight threads seems sufficiently fast in our usage and will yield individual results in as little as 20 minutes, depending on the input size.

Name the script appropriately and submit to the Torque queue with the *qsub* command. Copy and update the script to process the *_2.fq pairends. Don't forget to submit the job to the queue as well.

Step 3. Alignment to sam

Using BWA again, we take the alignment output along with fq and generate output in sam format.

In this example we'll use an *array* of data for the input variables along with a *for loop*.

```
#!/bin/bash
#PBS -l nodes=1:ppn=1
#PBS -N jobname
#PBS -e $PBS_JOBNAME.err
#PBS -o $PBS_JOBNAME.out

module load shared torque bwa/bwa-0.7.10
cd $PBS_O_WORKDIR

reference=GRCh37-lite.fa
# start array
samples[1]=filename1
samples[2]=filename2
samples[3]=filename3
samples[4]= filename4
samples[5]= filename5
samples[6]= filename6
samples[7]= filename7
samples[8]= filename8
samples[9]= filename9
samples[10]= filename10
samples[11]= filename11
samples[12]= filename12
. . .continue base filenames to 24 for this example
# end array
for i in 1 2 3 4 5 6 7 8 9 10 11 12 13 14 15 16 17 18 19 20 21 22 23 24
do
    sample=${samples[${i}]}
```

```
time bwa sampe ${reference} ${sample}_1.sai ${sample}_2.sai ${sample}_1
.fq ${sample}_2.fq > ${sample}.sam
done
```

The base filenames are what you had in the *xaa* and *xab* files.

As shown, the processing is serial, not parallel. It is, however, automated and can be parallelized with some additional logic.

Submit the job(s) to the Torque queue.

Step 4. sam to bam and Massaging the Data

Both sam and bam are usable formats in bioinformatics. Our goal, however, with this use case is to produce bam output in order to do variant calling. Variant calling is not covered in this use case.

The next example combines multiple tools in a single script, which can be done with most all processing, including the examples we've described in this use case.

```
#!/bin/bash
#PBS -l nodes=1:ppn=16
#PBS -N jobname
#PBS -e $PBS_JOBNAME.err
#PBS -o $PBS_JOBNAME.out

module load shared torque picard-tools samtools parallel

cd $PBS_O_WORKDIR

# convert sam to bam
time xargs -a xaa | parallel -j12 samtools view -Sb {}.sam -o {}.raw.bam

# add readgroups
###  ADJUST ITALICISED BOLD TEXT FOR YOUR SPECIFIC CRITERIA ###
time xargs -a xaa | parallel -j12 java -Xmx4G -Djava.io.tmpdir=`pwd`/
tmp -jar /cm/shared/apps/picard-tools/AddOrReplaceReadGroups.jar I={}
.raw.bam O={}.reads.bam SORT_ORDER=coordinate RGID=variant RGLB=bar
RGPL=illumina RGPU=TrueSeq RGSM={}  VALIDATION_STRINGENCY=SILENT

# sort bam
time xargs -a xaa | parallel -j12 java -Xmx4G -Djava.io.tmpdir=`pwd`/
tmp -jar /cm/shared/apps/picard-tools/SortSam.jar INPUT={}.reads.bam
OUTPUT={}.bam SORT_ORDER=coordinate VALIDATION_STRINGENCY=SILENT

# index
time xargs -a xaa | parallel -j12 samtools index {}.bam
```

We reuse the *xaa* and *xab* files in this file so you'll end up with one script for *xaa* and another for *xab*. Each script will run on a unique node to maximize efficiency.

As one tool finishes with the complete data set, the next tool will start, then the next until an error is encountered or the job completes successfully.

At the end of this step, we will have groomed bam files that have read groups and are sorted and indexed.

BIO HPC Use Case 2

Biologist FM must perform a linear regression analysis for a large group of subjects.

Torque (PBS) script defines and reserves necessary resources, configures logging, and e-mails owner on job end status.

```
#!/bin/sh

#PBS -l nodes=1:ppn=16
#PBS -N batch2-33-48_RNAseqV2.controls
#PBS -e $PBS_JOBNAME.err
#PBS -o $PBS_JOBNAME.out
#PBS -M foxmulder@asu.edu
#PBS -m ae

cd $PBS_O_WORKDIR
time ./batch2-33-48_RNAseqV2.controls
```

Command script (called by Torque script):

```
#!/bin/sh
module load parallel plink

seq 33 48| parallel plink–bfile
/home/foxmulder/eQTL_TCGA_BRCA/Controls/TCGA_birdseed.dedupFINAL
.controls–pheno
/home/foxmulder/RNASeqV2_voomFiles/RNASeq_controls.voom{}.txt–all-pheno–
linear–standard-beta–adjust–allow-no-sex–out controls_RNA_birdseed_33-48
–noweb
```

Our pheno input, /home/foxmulder/RNASeqV2_voomFiles/RNASeq_controls.voom{}.txt, is a series of 206 files, each containing 112 samples. As shown in the example, we use a defined sequence of 16 files (33–48 in this case) as the work for one node with 16 physical cores. The core count = the max parallel jobs we want to assign to that node.

To process the complete data set of 206 files, we divide by the highest whole multiple of 16: 12×16=192+14 = 206.

We end up with 13 pbs scripts and 13 command scripts. The logic of the command script can also be copied into each of the pbs scripts if you want to have fewer total scripts (13 versus 26).

Twelve of the scripts will invoke one node and 16 cores and use a sequence of 16 files.

The 13th script will invoke one node with 14 cores and use a sequence of 14 files.

The *parallel –j 14* option will need to be defined on that last script so it processes only the sequence of those 14 files instead of those 14 + the first two that finished again.

The *parallel* program will use all free cores by default.

Submit batch jobs using the *qsub* command.

APPENDIX D

HPC and Hadoop

Bridging HPC to Hadoop

Overview

The goal of this document is to demonstrate how legacy HPC tools and methodology effectively lessen the learning curve for users familiar with HPC but new to Hadoop.

Environment Modules

In the HPC world, the usage of environment modules is standard. An environment module is a TCL script that when invoked prepends specific software, library, and other variables to the user's path. For instance, if I logged into an HPC cluster where the default Python version was stock 2.6 but I wanted to use 2.7, I would be able to invoke the 2.7 module if it was available. After loading the module I would be able to simply type python—version and expect to see Python 2.7.x returned. For more information on environment modules, see: http://www.admin-magazine.com/HPC/Articles/Environment-Modules/.

Apache Spark

As I'm an HPC admin and Hadoop admin, I had the unique opportunity to see how multiple versions of a software package coexisted on a cluster of servers. In Hadoop land, the Apache Spark project was under heavy development with new builds and features released on an aggressive schedule. Like most environments we had production use cases for the older "stable" releases. (The term "stable" is used very loosely here.) As resources are limited we didn't have a spare 40-node Hadoop cluster for development so a solution had to be found for multiple Spark versions to coexist along with the default configuration and specific build/integration options.

It made a lot of sense to borrow the environment modules approach to facilitate the multiple version logic on the Hadoop login node. We already had several Spark versions installed, but the invocation of those programs was not very user friendly.

With the modules package installed, now we simply define the versions in a unique file and instruct end users to load the appropriate modules as they would in HPC.

Example of Spark-1.6.0 Module

```
#%Module1.0############
## sge modulefile
##
proc ModulesHelp { } {
        puts stderr "\tAdds spark-1.6.0 to your PATH and MANPATH."
}
```

```
module-whatis    "Adds spark-1.6.0 binaries to your path."

set topdir       /usr/hdp/2.2.4.2-2/spark-1.6.0
setenv           YARN_CONF_DIR   /etc/hadoop/conf
setenv           SPARK_HOME      $topdir
prepend-path     PATH            $topdir/bin
prepend-path     LD_LIBRARY_PATH $topdir/lib
```

Module Available Output

```
module av

---------------/home/project/modulefiles----------------
adam/2.10-0.17.1 null           spark/1.3.1      spark/1.6.0
adam/2.10-0.18.3 shared         spark/1.4.0      tez/0.5.2
avocado/v1       spark/1.2.0    spark/1.4.1      use.own
module-git       spark/1.2.1    spark/1.5.1      version
module-info      spark/1.3.0    spark/1.5.2
```

To invoke the spark-1.6.0 module, one would enter: module load spark/1.6.0.

The version can be verified by launching a spark-shell *or* typing 'which spark-shell', which would return: */usr/hdp/2.2.4.2–2/spark-1.6.0/bin/spark-shell.*

Simplifying Version-Dependent Software

A good example of this is the ADAM bioinformatics tool: https://github.com/bigdatagenomics/adam.

When a new version of ADAM is released, it is very dependent on a specific version of Spark. Next-generation sequencing tools in the Hadoop space are tricky enough without complications caused by version mismatches, so we build Spark module dependencies into the ADAM module.

ADAM 2.10_0.18.3 Modulefile

```
#%Module1.0#####################################################################
## sge modulefile
##
proc ModulesHelp { } {

        puts stderr "\tAdds adam_2.10-0.18.3 to your PATH and MANPATH."
}

module-whatis   "Adds adam_2.10-0.18.3 binaries to your path."
module load spark/1.4.1

setenv  ADAM_HOME       /usr/hdp/2.2.4.2-2/adam_2.10-0.18.3
set topdir              /usr/hdp/2.2.4.2-2/adam_2.10-0.18.3
prepend-path    PATH        $topdir/bin
```

BAM Format to ADAM Format Using YARN Cluster Deployment

1. Log in to Hadoop (command-line interface).
2. Module load adam/2.10–0.18.3. (This automatically loads spark/1.4.1 as well.)
3. Now inspect what you expect:
   a. echo $SPARK_HOME
      i. /usr/hdp/2.2.4.2–2/spark-1.4.1
   b. echo $ADAM_HOME
      i. /usr/hdp/2.2.4.2–2/adam_2.10–0.18.3
   c. Find a small bam and copy that to your HDFS home:
      i. hadoop fs -put /your/path/to/bam.bam /user/*youruserid*/SAMPLE.bam
4. Now the moment of truth is upon us . . . are you ready?

```
adam-submit --master yarn --deploy-mode cluster --driver-memory 5g
--executor-cores 6 --num-executors 3 --executor-memory 8g --transform /
user/youruserid/SAMPLE.bam /user/youruserid/SAMPLE.adam
```

This should write output in just over two minutes—00:02:11 to be exact in my use case with this file and these settings. See Figures D.1 and D.2.

/ user / jmcnall3 / HG00381.3.M_120202_7-4.adam

HG00381.3.M_120202_7-4.adam

Name	Size	Last Modified	Owner	Group	Permission
..					
_common_metadata	11.4 kB	2015-11-25 22:37	jmcnall3	jmcnall3	-rw-r--r--
_metadata	82.8 kB	2015-11-25 22:37	jmcnall3	jmcnall3	-rw-r--r--
_SUCCESS	0.1 kB	2015-11-25 22:37	jmcnall3	jmcnall3	-rw-r--r--
part-r-00000.gz.parquet	104.0 MB	2015-11-25 22:37	jmcnall3	jmcnall3	-rw-r--r--
part-r-00001.gz.parquet	103.2 MB	2015-11-25 22:37	jmcnall3	jmcnall3	-rw-r--r--
part-r-00002.gz.parquet	103.3 MB	2015-11-25 22:37	jmcnall3	jmcnall3	-rw-r--r--
part-r-00003.gz.parquet	103.4 MB	2015-11-25 22:37	jmcnall3	jmcnall3	-rw-r--r--
part-r-00004.gz.parquet	103.9 MB	2015-11-25 22:37	jmcnall3	jmcnall3	-rw-r--r--
part-r-00005.gz.parquet	103.8 MB	2015-11-25 22:37	jmcnall3	jmcnall3	-rw-r--r--
part-r-00006.gz.parquet	103.7 MB	2015-11-25 22:37	jmcnall3	jmcnall3	-rw-r--r--
part-r-00007.gz.parquet	103.5 MB	2015-11-25 22:37	jmcnall3	jmcnall3	-rw-r--r--
part-r-00008.gz.parquet	103.2 MB	2015-11-25 22:37	jmcnall3	jmcnall3	-rw-r--r--

Figure D.1 Transform reference.fa to reference.adam

Spark Jobs (?)

Total Uptime: 1.9 min
Scheduling Mode: FIFO
Active Jobs: 1
Completed Jobs: 1

▸ Event Timeline

Active Jobs (1)

Job Id	Description	Submitted	Duration	Stages: Succeeded/Total	Tasks (for all stages): Succeeded/Total
1	saveAsNewAPIHadoopFile at ADAMRDDFunctions.scala:75	2015/12/15 16:03:59	1.5 min	1/3	35/72

Completed Jobs (1)

Job Id	Description	Submitted	Duration	Stages: Succeeded/Total	Tasks (for all stages): Succeeded/Total
0	collect at FastaConverter.scala:116	2015/12/15 16:03:51	7 s	1/1	24/24

Figure D.2 Saving Hadoop Files

```
adam-submit—master yarn—deploy-mode cluster—driver-memory 5g—executor-
cores 5—num-executors 5—executor-memory 8g—transform /user/youruserid/
GRCh37-lite.fa /user/youruserid/GRCh37-lite.fa.a
```

Troubleshooting

If echo $ADAM_HOME returned anything other than the path in step 3b, then you probably have another adam version and probably aliases set in your login profile. Go to your ~/.bashrc or ~/.bash_profile .etc and remove or comment out the conflicting lines. Now log out, log back in again, and try the echo test again. For good measure also type:

```
which adam-submit
```

If this returns with a different path, then go back and ensure your aliases have been removed or commented out in your login profile.

If you encounter errors with the adam-submit script, check these things:

- Does the destination file/path already exist? Sometimes an unsuccessful run can write partial output, which needs to be manually removed prior to another run.
- If you get a path does not exist error, make sure you are substituting your actual userid for the placeholder *youruserid* I've placed in the command examples.

Versions and References

The version of Apache Spark 1.4.1 being used was a prebuilt binary download from the official Spark release page.

ADAM 2.10 snapshot 0.18.3 was downloaded and built from source using Apache Maven 3.3.3 on server istb1-l2-b13-u35. Build options in pom.xml were changed to correspond to ASURC HDP environment.

```
<properties>
    <java.version>1.7</java.version>
    <avro.version>1.7.7</avro.version>
    <spark.version>1.4.1</spark.version>
    <parquet.version>1.8.1</parquet.version>
    <hadoop.version>2.6.0</hadoop.version>
    <scoverage.version>1.1.1</scoverage.version>
    <utils.version>0.2.3</utils.version>
    <htsjdk.version>1.139</htsjdk.version>
  </properties>
```

ADAM flagstat Function

```
adam-submit flagstat /user/youruserid/SAMPLE.adam > SAMPLE.flagstat
```

Data such as that shown next will be hidden in your redirected output:

```
30705310 + 0 in total (QC-passed reads + QC-failed reads)
0 + 0 primary duplicates
0 + 0 primary duplicates—both read and mate mapped
0 + 0 primary duplicates—only read mapped
0 + 0 primary duplicates—cross chromosome
0 + 0 secondary duplicates
0 + 0 secondary duplicates—both read and mate mapped
0 + 0 secondary duplicates—only read mapped
0 + 0 secondary duplicates—cross chromosome
29794808 + 0 mapped (97.03%:0.00%)
30705310 + 0 paired in sequencing
30705310 + 0 read1
0 + 0 read2
29127226 + 0 properly paired (94.86%:0.00%)
29473054 + 0 with itself and mate mapped
321754 + 0 singletons (1.05%:0.00%)
91099 + 0 with mate mapped to a different chr
77603 + 0 with mate mapped to a different chr (mapQ>=5)
```

APPENDIX E

Bioinformatics + Docker

Simplifying Bioinformatics Tools Delivery with Docker Containers

Overview

The servers in our data centers are typically much more powerful than the PCs under our desks. By using tools such as Docker containers along with complementary technologies, we can extend the data center to the desktop and utilize full server power.

Example Environment

End user connects to computing environment via Windows Remote Desktop Protocol (RDP) and an X11 capable shell (mobaxterm, putty+xming, exceed) *or* directly to the computing environment via an X11 capable shell. We use RDP in our environment to minimize latency with image rendering.

In our example we:

1. Install Docker =>1.5 on a CentOS 6.6 server.
2. Install Git =>1.7.
3. Create a Docker container based on the Ubuntu 14.04 Linux distribution.
4. Download and extract a prebuilt binary for Slicer 4.
5. Configure the Docker container and parent host to present the application using X11.

The Docker container built for this document may be downloaded from the public DockerHub repository. Links are provided at the end of this appendix.

 **NOTE**

Downloading Docker images requires direct or proxied Internet access. Depending on your environment, Yum software repositories may also require the same access.

Docker Installation

This method is for a Red Hat 6.x or CentOS 6.x server.

1. Install EPEL (Extra Packages for Enterprise Linux).
   a. sudo yum install epel-release
   b. If that fails to work, then try the next commands.
      i. wget (http://dl.fedoraproject.org/pub/epel/6/x86_64/epel-release-6.8.noarch.rpm)
      ii. sudo rpm –Uvh epel-release-6*.rpm
2. Uninstall other software named Docker.

a. There is another, less popular, package named "Docker." Let's get rid of that if it is already installed.
   i. sudo yum –y remove docker
3. Install Docker.
   a. sudo yum –y install docker-io
4. Start the Docker daemon.
   a. sudo service docker start
5. Enable Docker to start at boot.
   a. sudo chkconfig docker on
6. Test installation and functionality.
   a. sudo docker pull centos
      i. Pulls remote image
   b. sudo docker images centos
      i. Shows image in local repository
   c. sudo docker run –it centos /bin/bash
      i. Should start container and drop you into a bash shell.
      ii. Type exit or control+d to exit,
7. Add your user to Docker group.
   a. grep docker /etc/group
      i. docker:x:###:
      ii. usermod –G ### username
   b. grep docker /etc/group
      i. docker:x:###:username
   c. ### represents the groupid (gid) and *username* represents your *username*
   d. Now you don't have to type *sudo* every time you run a Docker command.

You should now have a fully functional Docker host.

Docker Environment Validation

On our CentOS 6.6 x86_64 server, the Docker service is running and we can see by using the command "docker info" that we're using Docker v1.5.

- me@host$ docker version
- Client version: 1.5.0
- Client API version: 1.17
- Go version (client): go1.3.3
- Git commit (client): a8a31ef/1.5.0
- OS/Arch (client): linux/amd64

Install Git

Git is a software versioning tool similar to subversion, CVS, and many others.

1. Install git
   a. sudo yum –y install git

Download Software Repo and Build Container

1. git clone (https://github.com/jcmcnalx/3Dslicer.git)
2. cd 3Dslicer
3. ./identity.sh
4. Docker build –t myslicer

The repository pull via git pull has downloaded a README.md, Dockerfile, and identity.sh script. Read me is self-explanatory. Dockerfile is the definition of how to build this specific Docker container. Identity.sh adds your unique userid, groupid, and username to the container. This allows for file sharing between the Docker host and the container and allows X11 streaming.

See README.md or https://github.com/jcmcnalx/3Dslicer for full documentation.

Run Container

Now to invoke the container and run the 3Dslicer application:

1. docker run -v /home/username:/home/username -e DISPLAY -v /home/username /.Xauthority:/home/username /.Xauthority—net=host myslicer slicer
   a. Substitute your **username** in place of *username.*

   If everything has been configured correctly, you will see an application splashscreen followed by the actual application graphical user interface as seen in Figure E.1 and E.2.

   At this time you should be able to fully use the application per its official documentation:

   http://www.slicer.org/slicerWiki/index.php/Documentation/4.4
2. If the container is to be used frequently, you can echo the run command into an executable file:

```
echo "docker run -v /home/username:/home/username -e DISPLAY -v /home/
username /.Xauthority:/home/username /.Xauthority&#x02014;net=host
myslicer slicer" >  slicer.sh
chmod &#x0002B;x slicer.sh
```

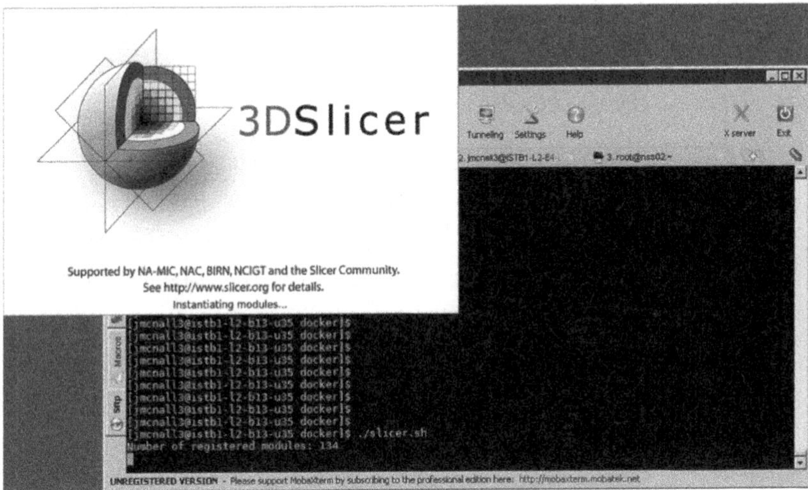

Figure E.1 3D Slicer

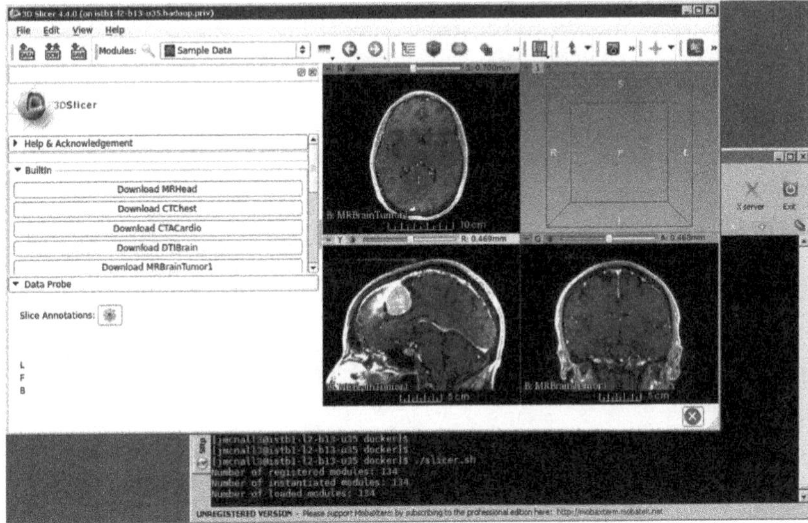

Figure E.2 3D Sample Output for 3D Slicer

To leave the application, click on File and then Exit. The application along with the Docker container will now close.

You can verify that the container has exited by using *docker ps –l*.

Docker Container and Data Sharing

Public and private repository hosting can be obtained by using GitHub and Docker Hub.

The public repository for ASU's Next Generation Cyber Capability (NGCC)-built containers can be found here:

https://github.com/jcmcnalx

https://hub.docker.com/u/jmcnall3/

Our vision includes a Docker hub repository that is specific to the BioMed space and is accessible via Internet2. High-speed container deployment and acquisition along with the shared knowledge within the consortium of research facilities will speed along research efforts.

Additional Containers

- ANTsR imaging suite (for R): https://github.com/jcmcnalx/antsr
- DRAMMS imaging suite: https://github.com/jcmcnalx/dramms-1.4.1

Links

Servers and software used in the demo:

- Dell Poweredge R720 (PowerEdge R720 rack server details | Dell)
- Centos 6.6 (parent host): http://centos.org/
- X11: http://www.x.org/wiki/
- Mobaxterm (Free Xserver and tabbed SSH client for Windows)
- Ubuntu 14.04 (Docker container): http://phusion.github.io/baseimage-docker/
- Slicer 4 (National Institutes of Health tool for medical image analysis and visualization)
- Docker installation: https://docs.docker.com/installation/
- Docker user guide: https://docs.docker.com/userguide/
- Docker managing data: https://docs.docker.com/userguide/dockervolumes/
- Docker Hub: https://hub.docker.com/
- Slicer 4 demo container: https://registry.hub.docker.com/u/jmcnall3/slicer4/
- Internet2: http://www.internet2.edu/
- Github: https://github.com/

Credits and Acknowledgments to the Scientific Research and Open Source Community

- UPENN staff: http://www.cbica.upenn.edu/sbia/software/dramms/people.html
- University of Crete, Greece, and Nikos Komadakis: http://www.csd.uoc.gr/~komod/FastPD/
- Multiple science and research institutions: http://www.slicer.org/pages/Acknowledgments
- ANTsR authors and contributors: http://stnava.github.io/ANTsR/

Glossary*

ABySS
Assembly By Short Sequences. A de novo, parallel, paired-end sequence assembler that is designed for short reads.

Academic department
Beyond the traditional notion of an academic department as a distinct disciplinary academic entity, the term as used in the Common Data Set (CDS) includes a fuller scope of academic units, from schools and colleges on one end to research groups at the other. The distinguishing attribute is that the entity includes teaching and research faculty, associated staff, and academic administrators (e.g., deans).

Access control list (ACL)
Set of procedures and processes performed by hardware, software, and administrators to monitor access, identify users requesting access, record access attempts, and limit access to the resources of a system only to authorized persons, programs, processes, or other systems. (For detailed information, consult the Higher Education Information Security Guide, available att http://www.educause.edu/security/guide.)

Adjuvant chemotherapy
Additional treatment given after surgery to lower the risk of the cancer returning.

Administrative office
Units in the central administration of a college or university, such as the offices of the president, vice presidents, provost, vice provosts, and general counsel. Does not include academic units, such as offices of the deans in universities with multiple colleges or schools, or offices of academic departments or research groups.

Advancement/fundraising system
An information system used to target, analyze, record, and report on the status of institutional fundraising from such sources as alumni, parents, friends, foundations, and corporations.

Angiogenesis
The physiological process through which new blood vessels form from preexisting vessels.

ANN
An artificial neural network (ANN)–based software package for classification of remotely sensed data.

* Many of the definitions come, with permission, from "Survey Glossary," EDUCAUSE Homepage, http://www.educause.edu/research-and-publications/research/core-data-service/about-core-data-service/survey-glossary.

ANSYS Fluent
Software that contains the broad physical modeling capabilities needed to model flow, turbulence, heat transfer, and reactions for industrial applications.

ANSYS HFSS
Industry-standard software for simulating 3-D full-wave electromagnetic fields. Its gold-standard accuracy and advanced solver and compute technology have made it an essential tool for engineers designing high-frequency and high-speed electronic components.

ANTLR
ANTLR (pronounced Antler), or ANother Tool for Language Recognition. A parser generator that uses LL(*) parsing.

Apoptosis
Genetically determined process of cell self-destruction.

Application virtualization
The separation of an installation of an application from the client computer that is accessing it. There are two types of application virtualization: remote and streaming. (From http://searchvirtualdesktop.techtarget.com/definition/app-virtualization.)

ATLAS
Automatically Tuned Linear Algebra Software (ATLAS). Provides C and Fortran interfaces to an efficient Basic Linear Algebra Subroutine (BLAS) implementation, as well as a few routines from Linear Algebra PACKage (LAPACK).

AVL FIRE
A powerful multipurpose thermo-fluid software representing the latest generation of 3-D computational fluid dynamics.

Benign
Abnormal growth of body tissue that is not cancerous.

Biobanking
A type of repository that stores biological samples.

BioPerl
BioPerl is a collection of Perl modules for the development of scripts used in bioinformatics. It was used in the Human Genome Project and is an open source project supported by the Open Bioinformatics Foundation.

BLAS
Basic Linear Algebra Subroutine (BLAS). A de facto application programming interface standard for publishing libraries to perform basic linear algebra operations, such as vector and matrix multiplication.

BLAST
In bioinformatics, Basic Local Alignment Search Tool. An algorithm for comparing primary biological sequence information, such as the amino acid sequences of different proteins or the nucleotides of DNA sequences. A BLAST search enables a researcher to compare a query sequence with a library or database of sequences

and identify library sequences that resemble the query sequence above a certain threshold.

Blender
A free and open source 3-D computer graphics software product used for creating animated films, visual effects, art, 3-D printed models, interactive 3-D applications, and video games. Blender's features include 3-D modeling, UV, unwrapping, texturing, rigging and skinning, fluid and smoke simulation, particle simulation, soft-body simulation, animating, match moving, camera tracking, rendering, video editing, and compositing.

Boost
A set of libraries for the C++ programming language that provides support for tasks and structures such as linear algebra, pseudorandom number generation, multithreading, image processing, regular expressions, and unit testing.

Bowtie
An ultrafast, memory-efficient short read aligner for short DNA sequences.

Burrows-Wheeler Aligner (BWA)
A software package for mapping low-divergent sequences against a large reference genome, such as the human genome.

Business intelligence reporting system
A set of administrative functions and associated software systems that support planning and decision making by categorizing, aggregating, analyzing, and reporting on data resulting from transaction processing systems.

Capital appropriation
Appropriation to the central information technology organization from the institutional capital budget to fund major purchases and implementations such as networks, enterprise resource planning systems, and buildings. Does not include capital appropriations amortized through rates; an example of a capital appropriation amortized through rates would be funds derived from taking out a loan or drawing on the institution's endowment for an initiative such as a major network enhancement or a phone switch. Such special funds require payback and are usually repaid through a fee structure.

Capital expenditures
Total capitalized information technology spending (full value of assets acquired) for the prior fiscal year. This includes major purchases and implementations such as networks, enterprise resource planning systems, and buildings. All depreciation or amortization expenses are excluded. If accounting systems spread expenditures over multiple years, include only total outlays for the prior fiscal year. Capital expenditures may be different from capital funds received for the fiscal year. For example, an institution may permit carryover from one fiscal year to the next or may have been granted funding for a capital project that has not yet been spent.

Carnegie classifications (year 2010 version)
A framework for recognizing and describing institutional diversity in U.S. higher education derived from empirical data on colleges and universities. Originally published

in 1973, the framework has been updated in 1976, 1987, 1994, 2000, 2005, and 2010. The Common Data Set (CDS) uses the 2010 version. To facilitate international benchmarking, CDS participants outside the United States are invited to self-select into one of the classifications. (Described fully at http://carnegieclassifications.iu.edu/descriptions/basic.php.)

CASAVA
Currently discontinued software set that was distributed by Illumina.

Celera Assembler
A de novo whole-genome shotgun DNA sequence assembler.

Central IT
The centralized information technology services and support organization reporting to the highest-ranking IT administrator/officer in the institution.

Central office
In multicampus university systems or community college districts, the unit headed by the chief executive officers of the system or district. Most central offices include a central information technology organization, some of which provide a wide range of services to individual campuses and some of which focus on coordinating the activities of IT organizations on the campuses.

Chemotherapy
The use of one or more drugs that are toxic to cells with the purpose of preventing the spread or growth of tumor cells.

Chief information officer (CIO)
A common designation for the highest-ranking information technology officer/administrator in an institution, and sometimes an official title. Given the wide range of actual titles, the Common Data Set (CDS) sometimes uses the term "CIO" to refer to all highest-ranking IT officers and administrators, regardless of their official titles.

Chief technology officer (CTO)
One of several official titles for the highest-ranking information technology officer/administrator in colleges and universities. In some cases, CTO is the title assigned to a deputy to the highest-ranking technology officer/administrator.

CLHEP (Physics)
Short for a Class Library for High Energy Physics. A C++ library that provides utility classes for general numerical programming, vector arithmetic, geometry, pseudorandom number generation, and linear algebra, specifically targeted for high-energy physics simulation and analysis software.

Cloud computing
A computing model in which technology resources are delivered over the Internet.

COAMPS
The Coupled Ocean/Atmosphere Mesoscale Prediction System. Developed and run by the Naval Research Laboratory in Monterey, California, COAMPS is the numerical model used for wind nowcasts and forecasts.

Commodity Internet
A general term referring to the general public network known as the Internet, as distinct from special-purpose and restricted-access research and education (R&E) networks. Many universities and colleges have connections to both the commodity Internet and one or more R&E networks.

Compliance
The effort to ensure that laws, regulations, and even an institution's own policies are properly observed and that efforts are coordinated institution-wide. (See also *IT compliance*.)

Contractors
Employees with whom the institution contracts to provide information technology infrastructure and/or specific IT services that might otherwise be delivered by in-house IT staff.

Convergent
A computational fluid dynamics code that completely eliminates the user time needed to generate a mesh through an innovative run-time mesh generation technique.

Customer relationship management system
Strategy, business processes, and software for managing and enhancing an institution's interactions with customers, such as students, prospective students, and alumni; faculty and staff; and current and prospective donors.

Cyberinfrastructure (CI)
The distributed computer, information, and communication technologies combined with the personnel and integrating components that provide a long-term platform to empower the modern scientific research endeavor. Components of CI include high-performance computing, storage resources, visualization facilities, sensors and other data collection apparatus, and advanced networks. In some countries, CI is referred to as e-science.

Data loss prevention tools
Tools that actively prevent data loss by monitoring and preventing improper use of sensitive data in transit (network), at rest (storage), and while at use (endpoint).

Data warehouse
A central repository of data often created by integrating other data sources and used for reporting and analysis.

Decentralized IT
Departments or units of the institution that provide all or nearly all of their own information technology services, without reporting directly or indirectly to the chief information officer or equivalent office.

Dedicated on-site generator
A source of electrical power for a data center or other facility, separate from the campus or public electrical grid. Dedicated generators are often used to back up other sources of electrical power; some are permanently installed, and others are mobile.

Disaster recovery data center

A data center with the necessary storage, compute, and communications capacity to resume operations of mission-critical systems in the event the primary data center(s) are unavailable.

Distributed antenna system (DAS)

A network of spatially separated antenna nodes that provides wireless services within a campus, building, or other area. One application of a DAS is to enhance cellular telephony service in an institution while maintaining institutional control of the antenna infrastructure.

Distributed IT

All staff with information technology responsibilities who do not report to the chief information officer and all resources that are not within the CIO's purview (including decentralized IT). The CIO often has some level of authority and/or responsibility over the distributed IT services. (See also *Decentralized IT.*)

Distributed IT staff

Staff who do not report to central IT but who work 50% or more on information technology activities and who have IT staff job titles (e.g., programmers, database administrators, etc.).

Downregulated

Refers to underactive expression of genes or proteins.

Endpoint encryption for sensitive data

Tools that provide endpoint encryption (e.g., to protect sensitive data on a lost or stolen device), with institutional decryption upon documented need.

Enterprise resource planning (ERP)

Refers to an integrated suite of administrative information systems designed to support and automate business processes through a centralized database system. In higher education, these systems usually include student systems, financial systems, and human resources (payroll/personnel) systems as well as data warehouse and planning tools.

E-science

See *Cyberinfrastructure (CI).*

Etiology

The cause or causes of a disease or abnormal condition.

FDS-SMV (Fire Dynamics Simulator)

Fire Dynamics Simulator (FDS) is a large-eddy simulation code for low-speed flows, with an emphasis on smoke and heat transport from fires. Smokeview (SMV) is a visualization program used to display the output of FDS and the Consolidated Model of Fire and Smoke Transport (CFAST) simulations.

Federation

An association of organizations that come together to exchange information, as appropriate, about their users and resources in order to enable collaborations and transactions.

FFTW
Fastest Fourier Transform in the West (FFTW). A software library for computing discrete Fourier transforms.

Firewall
Set of related programs and policies that protects the resources of a private network from users on other networks. A firewall can also control what outside resources users of the private network can access.

FLTK
Fast, Light Toolkit. A graphical user interface library made to accommodate 3-D graphics programming.

Funding model
The formulas, allocation methods, service charges, and other mechanisms by which central information technology receives funding to support its capital and operating expenses.

GADL
Graphical programming project.

GAMESS
General Atomic and Molecular Electronic Structure System. A general *ab initio* quantum chemistry package.

GATK
Genome Analysis Toolkit. A software package developed at the Broad Institute to analyze next-generation resequencing data.

Geant4 (Physics)
A toolkit for the simulation of the passage of particles through matter. Its areas of application include high energy, nuclear and accelerator physics as well as studies in medical and space science.

Gengetopt
A tool to write command-line option parsing code for C programs.

Genomic profiling
Cataloging and learning about all the genes in a specific person or cell type, including how they interact with one another and the environment. Genomic characterization is another name. (From the National Institutes of Health [National Cancer Institute], http://www.cancer.gov/publications/dictionaries/cancer-terms?cdrid=561401.)

Governance
The way in which a higher education institution is organized for the purposes of decision making and resource allocation and how the varying parts are managed in a way that promotes the mission of the institution. (See also *IT governance.*)

Grants management system: postaward
Software to support administration of research projects from notice of award through final billing.

Grants management system: preaward
Software to support development and submission of grant proposals to external funding agencies.

GRIB2
GRIdded Binary or General Regularly-distributed Information in Binary form.

GSL–GNU scientific library
A numerical library for C and C++ programmers. Free software under the GNU General Public License.

Hardware expenditures: capital
Total capitalized information technology spending (full value of assets acquired) for the prior fiscal year for hardware (including desktop technology, servers, network equipment, Information as a Service, etc.) regardless of whether purchased or leased.

Hardware expenditures: operating
Total noncapital, day-to-day operations, support, and maintenance expenses for the prior fiscal year for hardware (including desktop technology, servers, network equipment, Information as a Service, etc.) regardless of whether purchased or leased. This does not include any amortization and depreciation.

HDF5
Hierarchical Data Format (HDF, HDF4, or HDF5). The name of a set of file formats and libraries designed to store and organize large amounts of numerical data.

Helper T-cells
A subgroup of white blood cells that help the activity of other immune cells by releasing T cell cytokines. Also called T-helper cells.

High-performance computing (HPC)
Configurations of parallel processors, storage, and specialized networking designed to address large jobs with more or less tightly coupled subprocesses.

High-throughput computing (HTC)
Computing systems that are designed to provide large amounts of computing power over long periods of time (e.g., weeks or months).

HIPAA
Health Insurance Portability and Accountability Act.

HMMER
Hidden Markov Model-based sequence alignment tool used for searching sequence databases for homologs of protein sequences and for making protein sequence alignments. It implements methods using probabilistic models called profile hidden Markov models (profile HMMs).

Host
Any end device connecting to a data network, via wire or wireless, not including the equipment necessary to make the network function (such as routers, switches, modems, wireless access points, etc.). Examples of hosts include desktop computer,

laptop, tablet, smartphone, VoIP phone, server, printer, thermostat, web cam, and security camera.

Host-based intrusion detection system
File and system software monitoring tools to detect any unauthorized activity or changes (e.g., Tripwire).

Host-based intrusion prevention system
File and system software monitoring tools to detect and prevent any unauthorized activity or changes.

Identity provider
Source for validating a user identity in a federated identity system.

ImageMagick
An open source software suite for displaying, converting, and editing raster image files. It can read and write over 200 image file formats.

Immunotherapy
Treatment of a disease by inducing, enhancing, or suppressing an immune response.

INCITS
InterNational Committee for Information Technology Standards.

InCommon
A formal federation of organizations focused on creating a common framework for collaborative trust in support of research and education. InCommon eliminates the need for researchers, students, and educators to maintain multiple password-protected accounts. Instead the federation supports user access to protected resources by enabling organizations to make access decisions to resources based on a user's status and privileges as presented by the user's home organization. (From http://www.incommonfederation.org/.)

Information technology infrastructure library (ITIL)
The Information Technology Infrastructure Library (ITIL) defines the organizational structure and skill requirements of an information technology organization and a set of standard operational management procedures and practices to allow the organization to manage an IT operation and associated infrastructure. (From http://www.itlibrary.org/.)

InfraGard program
A partnership among the U.S. Federal Bureau of Investigation, businesses, academic institutions, and state and local law enforcement to share information and intelligence to protect cyberinfrastructure and guard against cyber threats to critical infrastructure.

Infrastructure as a Service (IaaS)
A provision model in which an organization outsources the equipment used to support operations, including storage, hardware, servers, and networking components. The service provider owns the equipment and is responsible for housing, running, and maintaining it. (From http://searchcloudcomputing.techtarget.com/definition/Infrastructure-as-a-Service-IaaS.)

Innovation
The act or process of building on existing research, knowledge, and practice through the introduction or application of new ideas, devices, or methods to solve problems or create opportunities where none existed before.

Institution
For Common Data Set (CDS) participants from central offices of multicampus systems and community college districts, the term refers to the central office only, not the entire multicampus entity. For all other participants, the term refers to the individual college or university (which the legacy CDS survey referred to as a campus).

Institutional research (IR)
The function in college and university administration to inform planning and decision making by collecting, analyzing, reporting, and warehousing a wide range of data about students, faculty, staff, finances, and so on. While such functions may be carried out by many individuals, most institutions have a central Office of Institutional Research, or the equivalent, responsible for the institution's primary IR activities, including reporting of institutional information to accrediting agencies, government offices, and other external entities.

Intel C/C++ and Fortran compilers
Intel compiler suites include C compiler, C++ compiler, and Fortran compiler, including optimization features and multithreading capabilities; highly optimized performance libraries; and error-checking, security, and profiling tools, allowing developers to create multithreaded applications and maximize application performance, security, and reliability. (From http://www.chiplist.com/Intel_Compilers_from_Intel/tree3f-aggregator_news_item--102954-/.)

Intel Math Kernel Library
A library that includes a wealth of routines to accelerate application performance and reduce development time.

IPEDS
Integrated Postsecondary Education Data Systems. A single, comprehensive data collection program designed to capture data for the National Center for Education Statistics for all U.S. institutions and educational organizations whose primary purpose is to provide postsecondary education. IPEDS collects institution-level data in such areas as enrollments, program completions, faculty staff, and finances. IPEDS data reporting requires the extensive effort of a variety of offices on any campus, and this is the "official" information the college or university stands behind, used by the federal government. EDUCAUSE, a nonprofit association of IT leaders and professionals in higher education, collects a subset of IPEDS data from Common Data Set (CDS) participants from outside the United States in order to facilitate international benchmarking.

IPv6
An Internet Protocol standard developed by the Internet Engineering Task Force that is designed to succeed Internet Protocol version 4 (IPv4) in order to address the increasing number of users and devices accessing the Internet.

iRODS

The Integrated Rule-Oriented Data System (iRODS) is open source data management software for storing, searching, organizing, and sharing files and data sets that are large, important, and complex. Thousands of businesses, research centers, and government agencies worldwide use iRODS for flexible, policy-based management of files and metadata that span storage devices and locations. (From http://irods.org/about/overview/.)

IT compliance

Programs or processes that ensure the institution's IT resources and systems are operated in ways that meet the laws and regulations impacting those systems and comply with institutional policy. (See also *Compliance; IT governance.*)

IT governance

Programs or processes that ensure that the campus IT strategy is aligned with the institution's strategic plan. IT thus becomes a strategic partner in the institutional mission. (See also *Governance.*)

IT risk management

Programs or processes that help an institution identify the risks that it faces with regard to its present or planned IT resources and systems and affirmatively address those risks in a way that satisfies its overall goals. (See also *IT governance.*)

JasPer

The JasPer Project is an open source initiative to provide a free software-based reference implementation of the code specified in the JPEG-2000 Part-1 standard (i.e., ISO/IEC 15444-1). It was started as a collaborative effort between Image Power, Inc., and the University of British Columbia. (From http://www.ece.uvic.ca/~frodo/jasper/.)

Killer T cells

A subgroup of white blood cells that kill damaged, infected, and cancerous cells.

Knowledge management system

A system used to identify, create, store, and disseminate information.

LAMMPS

Large-scale Atomic/Molecular Massively Parallel Simulator. A molecular dynamics program that makes use of MPI for parallel communication.

LifeTech

Life Technology's genomic analysis software for Sequencing by Oligonucleotide Ligation and Detection, or SOLiD, next-generation sequencing is a sequencing technique used to generate massive quantities of short sequence reads in parallel.

Log management

A system that collects and normalizes log event data from multiple sources for central storage, review, and alerting.

LS-DYNA/LS-PrePost

LS-DYNA is an advanced general-purpose multiphysics simulation software package. Its core competency lies in highly nonlinear transient dynamic finite element analysis using explicit time integration. LS-PrePost is an advanced pre- and postprocessor that is delivered free with LS-DYNA.

LS-OPT

An optimization and probabilistic analysis program that can interface with LS-DYNA.

Lumerical

Simulation tools that implement finite-difference time-domain algorithms.

Mainframe

A computer typically optimized for high reliability and security, high-volume and concurrent input/output processing, and substantial storage. Examples include IBM Z-Series, Unisys ClearPath, and Fujitsu BS2000.

Malignant growth

A cellular growth that develops quickly and uncontrollably and has the ability to destroy tissues and/or travel to other parts of the body.

Malware protection

Tools that protect endpoints and systems from harmful or intrusive software, such as viruses, Trojan horses, spyware, and the like.

MATLAB

A high-level language and interactive environment for numerical computation, visualization, and programming.

Metastasis

The movement of cancer cells to other parts of the body.

Molecular pathway

A series of actions or interactions that leads to a product or molecular change.

Monoclonal antibody

An antibody obtained from immune cells that were cloned from a unique parent cell.

Mouse xenograft (avatar mice)

Mice into which human tumor cells are transplanted either under the skin or into an organ.

mpiBLAST

A freely available, open source, parallel implementation of the National Center for Biotechnology Information's BLAST. Also see BLAST.

NAMD

Nanoscale Molecular Dynamics. A parallel molecular dynamics code designed for high-performance simulation of large biomolecular systems.

NAS

Network attached storage.

NCAR Graphics

A Fortran- and C-based software package for scientific visualization.

Neoadjuvant chemotherapy
Treatment given to patients before the primary chemotherapy.

netCDF and NCO
NCO (netCDF Operators) is a suite of programs designed to facilitate manipulation and analysis of self-describing data stored in the netCDF format, which is a set of software libraries and self-describing, machine-independent data formats that support the creation, access, and sharing of array-oriented scientific data.

Network access control system
Tools that scan endpoints upon network attachment, typically to determine update/patch and antimalware status.

Network filtering
The practice of monitoring and potentially restricting the flow of information from one network to another to maintain secure network zones.

Network intrusion detection system
Network monitoring tools that identify and log threats.

Network intrusion prevention system
Networking monitoring tools that identify and prevent threats from attempting to penetrate the network or from leaving the network.

Network operations center (NOC)
A facility for monitoring and managing a data, video, or voice network. The facility may also include some of the operating equipment.

NORA
Nonobvious relationship awareness.

NumPy
The fundamental package for scientific computing with Python.

NWChem
An open source high-performance computational chemistry package.

Oncogenes
Genes that speed up cell division.

On-costs
The costs an employer incurs beyond an employee's salary, including things such as workers' compensation, leave loading, and payroll tax.

OpenCV
Open Source Computer Vision Library. A library of programming functions mainly aimed at real-time computer vision.

OpenFOAM
Open source Field Operation And Manipulation. A C++ toolbox for the development of customized numerical solvers, and pre-/postprocessing utilities for the solution of continuum mechanics problems, including computational fluid dynamics.

Operating expenditures

Total noncapital day-to-day operations and maintenance expenses for the prior fiscal year. This includes costs such as staff compensation and benefits, operating expenses, equipment (including maintenance and repair), software licenses, and so forth. This does not include any amortization and depreciation. Operating expenditures may be different from operating funds received for the fiscal year. For example, your institution may permit carryover from one fiscal year to the next.

Outsource

To contract with an external entity or vendor to provide information technology (IT) services or infrastructure that you might otherwise have employed your IT staff to perform. It does not refer to an arrangement with another part of your institution or with a system office.

parMETIS

A message parsing interface (MPI)–based parallel library that implements a variety of algorithms for partitioning unstructured graphs, meshes, and for computing fill-reducing orderings of sparse matrices.

Pathogenesis

The mechanism by which a disease is caused.

Payment card industry (PCI)

In general, refers to debit, credit, prepaid, automated teller machine (ATM), and other cards and associated businesses. Also refers to the Payment Card Industry Security Standards Council, which oversees the Payment Card Industry Data Security Standard.

Penetration testing tools

Tools used by security staff to "attack" systems and software with the intention of identifying vulnerabilities and evaluating defenses.

PETSc

The Portable, Extensible Toolkit for Scientific Computation (PETSc, pronounced PET-see). A suite of data structures and routines developed by Argonne National Laboratory for the scalable (parallel) solution of scientific applications modeled by partial differential equations.

Phase I trial

Phase of clinical trials in which the safety of the product is examined in a very small group of healthy volunteers or patients afflicted with a specific disease. Phase I trials also are used to determine appropriate dose ranges.

Phase II trial

Phase of clinical trials in which the safety and efficacy of the product are examined at a predetermined dose in comparison to the standard of care treatment (commercially available therapies commonly used to treat the same disorder or disease).

Phase III trial
Phase of clinical trials in which the product is examined compared to the standard of care in a large diverse population to determine broader efficacy and develop usage guidelines.

Phase IV trial
Phase of clinical trials in which the long-term effects of a drug are examined after Food and Drug Administration approval for public use.

Picard
Java-based command-line utilities that manipulate Sequence Alignment Map (SAM) files and a Java application programming interface (SAM-JDK) for creating new programs that read and write SAM files. Both SAM text format and SAM binary (BAM) format are supported.

Platform as a Service (PaaS)
Cloud computing model that delivers applications over the Internet. In a PaaS model, a cloud provider delivers hardware and software tools—usually those needed for application development—to its users as a service. A PaaS provider hosts the hardware and software on its own infrastructure. (From http://searchcloudcomputing.techtarget.com/definition/Platform-as-a-Service-PaaS.)

Portal
An approach to an institution's website that aims to leverage investments in enterprise information systems, data warehouses, and infrastructure by providing a seamless and easy-to-navigate web interface to an integrated set of information services for various institutional constituents.

Portland Group C/C++ and Fortran compilers
The Portland Group, or PGI, offers compilers that incorporate global optimization, vectorization, software pipelining, and shared-memory parallelization capabilities.

Power over Ethernet (PoE)
A system that passes electrical power along with data on Ethernet cabling; unlike USB standards, PoE allows long cable lengths.

Preclinical
A stage of research before clinical trials where feasibility and drug safety data is collected.

PROJ
Cartographic Projections library.

PSI4
An open source suite of *ab initio* quantum chemistry programs.

R and Rmpi
R is a language and environment for statistical computing and graphics.

Rack-mounted server
A server that is specifically designed to be rack mounted. These servers are often thin and long (to fit in a traditional 42U rack).

RealityServer
A software platform for the development and deployment of 3-D web services and 3-D applications.

Recombinant DNA
DNA molecules formed in the laboratory by bringing together genetic material from multiple sources.

Research and Education Networking—Information Sharing and Analysis Center (REN-ISAC)
A membership organization headquartered at Indiana University that provides security information collection, analysis, dissemination, and early warning to support the unique environment and needs of organizations connected to served higher education and research networks. (From http://www.ren-isac.net/.)

Research and education (R&E) networks
Specialized and restricted-access networks dedicated to support universities, colleges, and other education and research institutions and their affiliates, as distinct from the commodity Internet. R&E networks are operated at the national, regional, and state levels, with numerous interconnections around the world. Institutions served by one or more R&E networks typically have a direct connection to the commodity Internet as well.

Risk management
The way in which an institution determines its appetite for risk, as well as how risk controls and mitigation strategies for any given endeavor are developed and enforced throughout the enterprise. (See also *IT governance; IT risk management*.)

SAMtools
SAM Tools provide various utilities for manipulating alignments in the SAM (Sequence Alignment/Map) format, including sorting, merging, indexing, and generating alignments in a per-position format. (From http://samtools.sourceforge.net/.)

Scanning tools for private/protected information
Tools to scan networked drives, endpoints, servers, and portable media for personally identifiable information and/or protected information such as health records, employment records, student records, social security numbers, credit card and other financial account numbers, passports numbers, and so on.

SciPy
Pronounced "Sigh Pie." A Python-based ecosystem of open source software for mathematics, science, and engineering.

Secure remote access
Tools providing secure access for remote clients.

Secure wireless access
Secure access across campus wireless networks via standards-based security specifications (e.g., 802.11).

Security information and event management
A system that collects and analyzes log event information from multiple sources, applying techniques such as event aggregation, correlation, and others.

Server hosting
Provision of facilities in a data center for another department, or external entity, to locate and manage their servers.

Server management
Provision of hardware and operation systems management as well as data center facilities for servers owned by another department or external entity.

Service provider
Organization or entity that provides services to members of a federated identity system and relies on the assurances of an identity provider to control access to those services.

Shaping bandwidth utilization
Adjusting parameters on the institutional Internet connection to limit use through various means, such as type of connection, location of connection, direction of traffic, time of day, or other specific characteristics.

SNPs
Single Nucleotide Polymorphisms, pronounced "Snips," are single nucleotide variations that occur at specific genome positions. They vary in populations, giving scientists the ability to perform genome-wide association studies.

SOAPdenovo
Short Oligonucleotide Analysis Package (SOAP). A bioinformatics package used for the assembly and analysis of DNA sequences.

Software as a Service (SaaS)
Software that is deployed over the Internet rather than installed on a computer. It is often used for enterprise applications that are distributed to multiple users. SaaS applications typically run within a web browser, which means users only need a compatible browser in order to access the software. (From http://techterms.com/definition/saas.)

SPBLASTK
A toolkit for solving large sparse system of linear equations.

Standard of care treatment
Commercially available therapies commonly used to treat the same disorder or disease.

Star-CCM+
CD-adapco's newest computational fluid dynamics (CFD) software product. It uses the well-established CFD solver technologies available in STAR-CD, and it employs a new client-server architecture and object-oriented user interface to provide a highly integrated and powerful CFD analysis environment to users.

SU2
An open source collection of C++-based software tools for performing partial differential equation (PDE) analysis and solving PDE-constrained optimization problems.

SWIG
A tool that easily allows a developer to wrap C/C++ functions for use with scripting languages.

Systems biology
An interdisciplinary field of study that focuses on complex interactions within biological systems.

T-cells
Types of white blood cells (also called lymphocytes) that play a central role in cell-mediated immunity.

Time division multiplexing (TDM)
Transmission of multiple signals, such as telephone calls, over the same medium by taking turns on the channel. TDM is used for circuit mode communication, as contrasted to VoIP.

Trillnos
A collection of open source software libraries intended to be used as building blocks for the development of scientific applications.

Tumor suppressor genes
Genes that slow down cell growth and control cell death.

Tumorigenesis
The formation of tumors tissue or cells.

UDUNITS
Unidata: Data Services and Tools for Geoscience supports conversion of unit specifications between formatted and binary forms, arithmetic manipulation of units, and conversion of values between compatible scales of measurement.

Uninterrupted power supply (UPS)
A mechanism that provides emergency power to a load when the input power source fails with near-instantaneous protection from input power interruptions.

Upregulated
Refers to overactive expression of genes or proteins.

Vaccine Adjuvant Therapy
A substance that is added to a vaccine to increase the body's immune response to the vaccine.

Velvet
Sequence assembler for very short reads.

Visual Molecular Dynamics
A molecular visualization program for displaying, animating, and analyzing large biomolecular systems using 3-D graphics and built-in scripting.

Visualization
Use of computer graphics, often with large or multiple displays driven by high-performance computers accessing large databases, to produce still and dynamic images that enable exploration, analysis, and understanding of research data; presentation and manipulation of instructional simulations; design of architectural and product models; and other applications.

Vulnerability assessment tool
A tool set to scan network-attached devices for known vulnerabilities.

WRF
Weather research and forecasting model. A numerical weather prediction system.

About the Author

Jay Etchings is the director of Operations for Research Computing at Arizona State University (ASU). Research Computing is a new initiative led by the university's most senior leaders addressing fluid technical environments that support highly computational workloads, petascale data analysis, next-generation cybercapabilities, and emerging network innovation such as 100Gbps Internet2 and Science DMZ. It is a mission to architect, develop, deploy, and support innovative architectures addressing emerging challenges of fourth-paradigm science. Research Computing serves the ASU research community and also publishes on its original research initiatives and presents at conferences and events. Current projects include development and support of next-generation big data solutions for research medicine; the Hortonworks–Mayo–ASU genomics platform; development of biomedical informatics tool sets for use in highly parallel environments; and OpenStack Cloud development for life sciences utilizing Big Data ecosystem components (data-intensive research), including integration and advancement of the Internet2 Innovation platform, extension of ubiquitous research compute to all, and the proliferation of software-defined networking. Mr. Etchings also has appointments with the Open Daylight Foundation (Linux Foundation), the Open Networking Foundation, Internet2, and the Open Fog Consortium and has served at the National Science Foundation as a proposal panel reviewer.

About the Contributors

Karen S. Anderson, MD, PhD, is a cancer immunologist and translational researcher at Arizona State University, with a joint appointment at Mayo Clinic. Her laboratory's research focus is on identifying targets of immune control of cancer.

Joe Arnold is the cofounder and president of SwiftStack. SwiftStack is a leading provider of object storage software. SwiftStack's customers include some of the largest enterprise companies and life sciences institutions. An innovator in cloud-computing infrastructure, Mr. Arnold also built one of the first widely used Platforms as a Service (PaaS) on top of Amazon Web Services. He is the author of *Object Storage with Swift* (2014), published by O'Reilly Media.

M. Haithem Babiker, PhD, is chief technology officer of EndoVantage and a coinventor of the EVIS technology. He received a BSE in bioengineering and an MS and PhD in biomedical engineering at Arizona State University.

Jacob Brill is a management intern working in the Complex Adaptive Systems department at Arizona State University. He is a graduate of ASU with a degree in biological sciences. He has prior experience in the fields of prosthetics, information technology, and other biological research endeavors.

Ken Buetow, PhD, is a human genetics and genomics researcher who leverages computational tools to understand complex traits such as cancer, liver disease, and obesity. He is the director of Computational Sciences and Informatics program for Complex Adaptive Systems at Arizona State University (CAS@ASU), a professor in the School of Life Sciences in ASU's College of Liberal Arts and Sciences, a Core Faculty in ASU's Center for Evolution and Medicine, and the director of Bioinformatics and Data Management for the National Biomarker Development Alliance. Dr. Buetow previously served as the founding director of the Center for Biomedical Informatics and Information Technology within the National Institutes of Health's National Cancer Institute.

Wendy H. Cegielski, MA, PhD candidate, Anthropology, has been an archaeologist and practitioner of computational social science for the past seven years, especially engaged in the integration of computational modeling and digital data collection with archaeology. She is the author of "Rethinking the Role of Agent-Based Modeling in Archaeology," published in 2016 in the *Journal of*

Anthropological Archaeology. As a PhD candidate at the School of Human Evolution and Social Change, Arizona State University, she is conducting National Science Foundation grant–funded research in Valencia, Spain, using network science to investigate mechanisms for the maintenance of social stability in the distant past.

Diego Chowell, PhD, is a postdoctoral research fellow at the Memorial Sloan Kettering Cancer Center in New York. His research focuses on developing and applying mathematical and computational models in the fields of cancer evolution and cancer immunology.

Yuli Deng received his BS degree in Computer Science and Technology from Huazhong University of Science & Technology in 2011 and his MS degree in Computer Science from Arizona State University in 2013. Currently, he is working toward a PhD at ASU. His current research interests are in cloud computing, machine learning, e-learning, and adapter learning models. He is a member of the Secure Networking and Computing (SNAC) research group at ASU.

Robert S. Green, JD, is president and chief executive officer of EndoVantage. He is a longtime serial entrepreneur who has founded seven other successful companies. In 2001 the University of Arizona Eller College of Management named him an Entrepreneurial Fellow, and in 2003 he received an Arizona Spirit of Success Award from then Arizona governor Janet Napolitano. He graduated from the City University of New York magna cum laude and from Fordham University School of Law with honors.

Rohan Gupta is a student at Arizona State University.

Dijiang Huang received his bachelor of science degree in telecommunications from Beijing University of Posts & Telecommunications in 1995. He received his master of science and PhD degrees from the University of Missouri–Kansas City in 2001 and 2004, respectively, both in computer science and telecommunications. He joined Arizona State University in 2005 in the Department of Computer Science and Engineering as an assistant professor. From 2011, he has been an associate professor in the School of Computing Informatics and Decision Systems Engineering. His research interests are in computer and network security, mobile ad hoc networks, network virtualization, and mobile cloud computing. Dr. Huang's research is supported by the National Science Foundation, the Army Research Office, the Office of Naval Research, and NATO, and organizations such as Consortium of Embedded Systems, Hewlett-Packard, and China Mobile. He is a recipient of the Office of Naval Research

Young Investigator Award and H-P Innovation Research Program Award. He is a cofounder of Athena Network Solutions LLC. He is currently leading the Secure Networking and Computing research group at ASU.

Avishek Kumar is a postdoctoral researcher at Arizona State University. He received his BS at Carnegie Mellon University and his PhD from ASU. His research interests include condensed-matter physics, biophysics, and genomic and personalized medicine. He is also interested in the use of high-performance computing, particularly graphics processing unit computing, to unite informatics and physics-based methods.

Guangchun Luo, MS, PhD, received his degrees from the University of Electronic Science and Technology of China (UESTC) in 1999 and 2004, respectively. He has been a visiting scholar at the University of California at San Diego and University of Toronto, Canada. Currently, he is a professor and vice president of the Graduate School of UESTC. He has published approximately 50 articles in international journals and conference proceedings. He serves on a number of technical societies, including as committee member on the Calculation of Sichuan Province Institute of High Performance Computer and China Education Information Council. He has received regular funding from various departments of the Chinese government, such as the National Natural Science Foundation of China, the National Hi-Tech R&D Program (the 863 Program), and the Science and Technology Department Foundation of Sichuan Province.

Zhiyuan Ma received his bachelor of science degree from the Department of Computer Science and Technology in Nanjing University and is currently a PhD student in the School of Computer Science and Engineering in the University of Electronic Science and Technology of China. Between 2015 and 2016, he also worked as a visiting scholar in the School of Computing, Informatics, and Decision Systems Engineering at Arizona State University. His research interests include analyzing patterns of data, predicting trends using machine learning technologies, and building models for incremental learning applications.

Carlo C. Maley is a biologist who specializes in cancer, evolution, and computational biology. He works at the intersection of these fields.

Christopher Mueller, PhD, is the founder and chief technology officer of Lab7 Systems, Inc., a software company focused on making next-generation sequencing informatics practical for applied and clinical use. Throughout his industrial and academic careers, Dr. Mueller's passion has been leveraging scientific, high-performance computing solutions to increase scientific productivity across a wide range of applications and user bases. As a bioinformatics leader at Life Technologies, he helped develop the company-wide high-performance computing strategy for processing next-generation sequencing data in product development and research applications. His professional experience includes software development and architecture roles on large-scale web applications at MapQuest.com and Critical Path and scientific computing and visualization at Research Systems and Array Biopharma. He has worked as an independent consultant on high-performance computing projects and helped research labs integrate effective software engineering practices into their workflows. Dr. Mueller received his BS in computer science from the University of Notre Dame and his MS and PhD in computer science with a minor in bioinformatics from Indiana University. His research focused on computational biology, large-scale graph visualization, and programming paradigms for rapid development of high-performance software.

James Napier is a senior business intelligence developer in Arizona State University's Research Computing. His interests include big data analytics, distributed computing, simulations, optimizations, evolutionary computing, automation, trend and risk modeling, pattern matching, and network linkage analysis.

Greg Palmer spent 35 years in information technology. He is currently the research liaison for Client Services, a division of Information Systems and Computing, at the University of Pennsylvania. This position follows 16 years as the executive director of MAGPI, a regional, high-performance research and education network, and connector for Internet2. He has contributed extensively to the national and international pursuit of excellence in technology and organizational dynamics as it pertains to the research community.

Daniel Peñaherrera is a student at Arizona State University in statistics and applied mathematics pursuing a graduate degree in computational biology.

Alan Ritacco, the director of Research Computing at University of Massachusetts Medical School, is a goal-orientated leader with demonstrated experience in planning, development, and implementation of cutting-edge IT solutions for customer and internal needs. Ritacco works with researchers at UMASS on computational elements of HPC, HG matching, and the setting up of LIMS systems. He has directed a broad range of IT initiatives from planning stages through implementation and support.

Adrish Sannyasi is a healthcare solution architect at Splunk. His passion is applying software engineering, machine learning, and visualization methods to implement actionable and engaging data-driven apps while maintaining security and privacy of the underlying data sets. He is focused on making medicine proactive, precise, and predictive. Mr. Sannyasi received a clinical data mining certification from Stanford University, biomedical informatics certification from Oregon Health and Science University, an MBA from the University of Maryland, and a bachelor of engineering degree from NIT, Nagpur, India.

Melissa A. Wilson Sayres, PhD, is a computational evolutionary biologist at Arizona State University. Her lab uses genomics and bioinformatics to study sex differences and cancer evolution.

James A. Scott is the director of Enterprise Strategy & Architecture at MapR Technologies and is very active in the Hadoop community. Mr. Scott helped build the Hadoop community in Chicago as cofounder of the Chicago Hadoop Users Group. He has implemented Hadoop at three different companies, supporting a variety of enterprise use cases from managing points of interest for mapping applications, to online transactional processing in advertising, as well as full data center monitoring and general data processing. He was also the senior vice president of Information Technology and Operations at SPINS, the leading provider of retail consumer insights, analytics reporting, and consulting services for the natural and organic products industry. Additionally, he served as lead engineer/architect for Conversant (formerly Dotomi), one of the world's largest and most diversified digital marketing companies, and held software architect positions at several companies including Aircell, NAVTEQ, and Dow Chemical.

Sheetal Shetty is a postdoctoral researcher in bioinformatics and computational biology. Her research looks for patterns that reduce complexity and therefore provide answers to seemingly intractable problems, specifically in cancer. She will receive her PhD in biomedical informatics from Arizona State University. Her thesis focuses on developing a new algorithm for structural variant detection in the cancer genome, which can help tease out the complexity patterns of disease development in cancer and therefore pave the way for personalized medicine.

Brock M. Tice is a biomedical engineer who completed his undergraduate degree in biomedical engineering at Tulane University, and his PhD at Johns Hopkins University, working with Dr. Natalia Trayanova at both. Upon graduation he helped found CardioSolv LLC, which is bringing Dr. Trayanova's cutting-edge heart simulation technology from academia into the wider world of clinical research and the bedside. He later helped found CardioSolv Ablation Technologies, Inc., which is commercializing several of Dr. Trayanova's patents using CardioSolv LLC's technology, and running a first-in-man clinical trial.

Tiffany Trader is an established tech journalist with over a decade's experience covering high-performance computing. She has been one of the principal voices behind *HPCwire* since she was hired in 2006. In addition to her years covering the fastest computers in the world and the people who run them, Ms. Trader has had a role in shaping numerous Tabor publications, including *HPC in the Cloud*, *Green Computing Report*, and, most recently, *EnterpriseTech*. She earned her bachelor's degree from San Diego State University, where she majored in computer science and linguistics.

Index

Page numbers followed by *f* and *t* are figures and tables.

Accelerators. *See* GPU-accelerated computing; GPU accelerators
Access mechanisms
  federated application services with single sign-on capabilities for, 219
  insider threat control using, 12
Accumulo, 240–241
Acquisitions in health care industry, 9–10
Administrative data, 168, 169–170, 169*f*
Affordable Care Act of 2010, 8, 9, 19, 25
Affymetrix, 31
AllTrials petition, 16
Amazon, cloud services from, 22, 231, 318, 324
Amazon DynamoDB, 237
Amazon Elastic Compute Cloud, 318
Amazon Elastic MapReduce, 23, 318
Amazon Redshift, 24, 236
Amazon S3, 66, 67, 70, 78, 225
Amazon Web Services (AWS), 22, 67, 70, 78, 160, 217
Analytics (Microsoft), 24
Analytic software. *See also* Big data analytics; Data analytics; Predictive analytics
  case study of leveraging, 158–159
  cloud and storage solutions for, 24, 103, 221
  cost of adopting, 166
  data-intensive computing and, 24
  data mining using, 181
  genomic sequencing using, 22
  GPU-accelerated computing using, 187
  increased healthcare use of, 8, 25, 28, 218, 244–245
  Neo4J graph database using, 243
  polystructured data and, 59
  solution architectures using, 225
  Zeta Architecture using, 228, 229
Anderson, Chris, 55
Anderson, Karen S., 273–284
Antibiotic resistance, 194–201
Apache
  Elasticsearch and, 243
  MongoDB and, 238
  projects using, 311, 321
  web servers using, 226, 322
Apache Cassandra, 225, 236, 237
  description of, 239
  pluses and minuses of, 239–240
Apache CouchDB, 236, 321
  description of, 238
  pluses and minuses of, 238–239
Apache Drill, 226, 227
Apache Foundation, 241
Apache Hadoop. *See* Hadoop
Apache Hadoop YARN, 224, 259, 283–284
Apache HBase, 225, 236, 237, 321
  description of, 240
  pluses and minuses of, 240
Apache Hive, 236, 237, 252, 256, 283, 321
  tables in, 259
  tables with partitions in, 268–269
Apache Mahout, 23, 321
Apache Mesos, 224, 226
Apache Spark, 23, 220, 226, 227, 237, 256, 264, 269, 270, 283, 317, 327
  bridging from HPC legacy systems to Hadoop and, 386–387, 389

Apache Spark (*Continued*)
configuration parameters for submitting job in, 265–266
documentation web site for, 266
launching applications in, 265
statistical analysis using, 258, 264–267
Apache Subversion, 323
Apache Tez, 259
Apoptosis deficiency, 51–52
Application architecture
streaming applications using, 228–229
Zeta Architecture as, 228
Application programming interface (API) development
cloud computing for, 174
Next Generation Cyber Capability (NGCC) team for, 112
OpenDaylight (ODL)'s common framework for, 125
Application-specific integrated circuits (ASICs), 117–118, 119
Archives, for data, 44, 60, 64*f*, 65, 318, 339, 341, 350
Arizona State University (ASU)
iRODS data management as a service from, 69
meeting community's data and compute needs at, 16, 308, 309
Next Generation Cyber Capability (NGCC) team at, 112, 256, 309–310
NimbleStorage at, 103–104
Sun Corridor Network and, 157–158
Arnold, Joe, 53, 70, 101–102
Artificial intelligence (AI), 24, 190
Audit mechanisms
cloud multitenant host security with, 12
compliance using, 10
data collaboration in research data management using, 65
insider threat control using, 12
iRODS software development with, 69
Medicaid-Medicare recovery using, 219
Splunk platform using, 245
SwiftStack modules with, 82, 86, 91
Authentication, 12
cloud storage with, 14, 173*t*
data integrity using, 12
federated access web portals with, 220
insider threat control using, 12
Internet of Things using, 21
iRODS software development with, 69
network optimization for, 120
OpenDaylight (ODL) security using, 126
SwiftStack with, 78, 79, 89
systems management security and compliance model using, 223
time-limited URLs for, 91
two-factor, in administrative access to security programs, 159, 160
Zeta Architecture using, 228
Authorization
federated access web portals with, 220
insider threat control using, 12
Internet of Things using, 21
iRODS software development with, 69
OpenDaylight (ODL) security using, 126
systems management security and compliance model using, 223
Availability
application design and, 15, 101
cloud computing and, 10, 11, 24
cluster management for, 227
data-intensive computing platforms and, 165
deployment and, 329–330
federal standards for, 61
graph databases and, 241
health big data applications and, 186
Internet of Things (IoT) and, 23
networked computer server systems for, 316
network optimization for, 120
new enterprise architectural approach and, 223
next-generation processors and, 328
NGCC systems architecture for, 313
NimbleStorage and, 103, 104
service-oriented architecture (SOA) and, 172
Swift's provisions for, 82, 84, 85, 88
Availability zones, in data centers, 84
Azure (Microsoft), 22

Babiker, M. Haithem, 204–209
Bash, 256, 283
Basic Local Alignment Search Tool (BLAST), 38–41, 39*f*, 40*f*, 40*t*
Bell, Greg, 109, 110, 111
Beta distribution, 295, 296
Beta function, 295
Biases, in statistics, 290
Big data
benefits of, 165–166

biosciences' use of, 164
classifications of applications for, 166–168
data-intensive computing and, 24
forecasting using, 170
health informatics applications using, 166–168
health record data system using, 172, 173*t*
in-memory analytics and streaming analysis in, 183–185
scientific method changed by, 54–55
sequencing as problem for, 95–101
sources of, 168–170, 169*f*
Big data analytics. *See also* Analytic software; Data analytics; Predictive analytics
big data classifications using, 166, 167, 168
cloud computing in, 218
compute capabilities needed for, 23–24
data-intensive computing and, 24
data mining using, 181
fundamental system properties in, 186–187
GPU-accelerated computing for, 187–190, 188*t*, 191
hierarchical structure of systems for, 172–186
in-database models using, 181–183
infrastructure for, 171–187
in-memory analytics using, 182–185
Internet of Things and, 218
service-oriented architecture with cloud computing in, 171–172
Big Data as a Service (BDaaS), 318
BigQuery (Google), 24
Big Sur computing platform, 190
Binomial distribution, 293
Binomial random variable, 293
Bioinformatics
Apache Spark in, 220
big data applications for, 166–168
Bowtie in, 46–47
cloud-based applications for, 216*t*
cloud computing and, 215, 217–218, 231
Genbank repository and tools in, 38, 41
Genome Analysis Toolkit (GATK) in, 42–44
graphics processing unit (GPU) software in, 187
Next Generation Cyber Capability (NGCC) and proposals in, 310
polystructured data in, 58–59
R Project for, 41–42
sequencing workflow in, 99–100, 100*f*
workflow in, 215
working data and usage patterns in, 100
Zeta Architecture in, 221
Biomedical research
managing increase of healthcare data in, 4, 21
NoSQL approaches to, 236–237
semistructured data in, 57–58, 270, 271, 333
unstructured data in, 22, 57, 168, 169*f*, 244, 248
Biomedicine
exome sequencing in clinical diagnosis in, 49–52
impact of rapid changes in, 2, 8, 20, 22, 25
Border Gateway Protocol (BGP) plugin, in OpenDaylight (ODL) scenarios, 123–124, 125, 151–154
Beryllium plugin, in OpenDaylight (ODL) scenarios, 129, 129*t*–132*t*, 133, 134*t*, 136, 138, 145
Boron plugin, in OpenDaylight (ODL) scenarios, 130, 131*t*–132*t*, 133, 134, 135*t*, 136
Bowtie, 46–47, 47*f*, 230
Breaches in data security, 10, 11, 244
Breast cancer, 18, 51*t*, 167, 177, 275
Bridge amplification, 37
Brill, Jacob, 27, 38
Buetow, Ken, 309, 330–333
"Build It Right" strategy, 61
Burrows-Wheeler Alignment (BWA), 46, 46*f*, 380–381
Business models, cloud-based computing and changes to, 317–318
Butte, Atul, 54–55

Cancer and cancer research
big data analysis in, 167
biologics for, 18
cluster homogeneity in, 220–221
disease analysis in, 167
genomic research in, 31, 103, 165, 177, 324
genomics visualization in, 22
graph databases in, 241–242
Hortonworks Data Platform (HDP) for sampling in, 272–273

Cancer (*Continued*)
pediatric astrocytomas, 3
predicting extent of subclonal variation in, 273–284
sequencing genes in, 51*t*, 73
software for tumor simulation, monitoring, and analysis in, 283
targeted therapies in, 3, 167, 187, 280
Cancer Cloud Genomics pilots, 112
Cancer Genome Atlas (TCGA), 251, 253*f*, 254*f*, 282, 352
Cancer Genome Workbench (CGWB), 332
Cancer Genomics Hub, 324
CAPWAP protocol, with OpenDaylight (ODL), 125
CardioSolv Ablation Technologies, 230–234
Care-coordination analytics, 247–248
Case studies
CardioSolv Uses Penguin's Research Cloud for On-Demand Compute, 230–234
Computational Modeling of Endovascular Procedures: A New Approach Saving Lives and Reducing Costs, 204–209
Exome Sequencing in Clinical Diagnosis, 49–52
Extent of Subclonal Variation Predicted by the Number of Distinct Dominant Clones, 273–284
HudsonAlpha Institute for Biotechnology and SwiftStack, 101–102
Is Sequencing a Big Data Problem?, 95–101
National Biomarker Development Alliance, 330–333
NimbleStorage Deployment at Arizona State University, 103–104
UC Irvine Health's Hortonworks Data Platform, 270–273
Use Case: Regulated and Commodity Compute and Storage, Leveraging Internet2 Next Generation, 158–161
Use Case: Sun Corridor Network, 157–158
Using GPU to Study Protein Evolution to Understand Antibiotic Resistance, 194–201
Cassandra. *See* Apache Cassandra
CDISC standards, 332
Centers for Medicare & Medicaid Services (CMS), 1, 13, 62
Central IT organizations
funding mechanisms for, 368–371, 369*t*, 370*t*
infrastructure supported by, 360–361
overview of, 357–358
research support services in, 362–363
services offered by, 363–367, 364*t*
Central processing units (CPUs)
GPU accelerators with, 187, 188
GPU versus, 189–190, 190*f*
HPC architecture with, 221
InfiniBand's efficient use of, 117
RDMA and reduced load on, 115, 116
simulations run on, 198
Zeta Architecture with, 227
Ceph, 67
CERN, 108, 239
Certificate management and services, 13, 15
Chargaff, Erwin, 32
Chase, Martha, 32
Cherne, Leo M., 3
Chief information officers (CIOs), 10, 16, 354, 358, 373, 374
Chowell, Diego, 273–284
Cisco Internet Business Solutions Group, 19
Client relationship managers (CRMs), 362, 367, 373
Clinical Data Interchange Standards Consortium (CDISC) standards, 332
Clinical decision support systems, 166, 169
Clinical trials
compliance with agreements in, 60
data collection and sharing in, 16
management software for 320
Software as a Service (SaaS) applications for, 324
software for virtual, 209
Clinton, Bill, 30
Cloud computing, 211–217
application service layer in, 185
basic functional layers in, 174, 175*f*
bioinformatics tools based in, 216, 216*f*
business model impact of, 317–318
challenges facing, 215
data computing layer in, 180, 180*f*
data integrity in, 12
data storage and management layer in, 178–180, 178*f*

definition of, 212
deployment models for, 214–215
desired elements in big data storage in, 173*t*
essential characteristics of, 213–214
federated application services with, 219–220, 219*f*
genomic applications using, 167
healthcare data system examples using, 172–174, 173*t*, 173*f*, 174*f*
homomorphic encryption in, 14
large-scale simulations using, 230–234, 231*f*, 233*f*
multitenant host security and, 12
presentation layer in, 185–186
resource pooling and, 212, 213, 230
security challenges in, 10–11
sensing layer for data acquisition and data transmission in, 175–177, 176*f*
service models for, 214–215
service-oriented architecture (SOA) with, 172
university campus data centers versus, 361
widespread adoption of, 212
Cloud health information systems technology architecture (CHISTAR) reference model, 178
Coalition for Academic Scientific Computation, 165
Code of Federal Regulations (CFR) Title 21 guidelines, 332
Cohort discovery, Hortonworks Data Platform (HDP) for, 272–273
Collaboration
cyber capability challenges for, 308–309, 310
cloud computing for, 216, 217, 330
Design Thinking for, 311
ESnet and, 109–110, 111
federated access web portals for, 219–220, 219*f*
genome sequencing costs and, 54
grid computing for, 215
Hortonworks for, 271
Integrated Rule-Oriented Data System (iRODS) supporting, 67, 68–69
Next Generation Cyber Capability (NGCC) tools for, 112, 309, 311
OpenDaylight Project (ODL) and, 114, 122, 124, 126
protection of rights of research university staff in, 60
research centers without walls for, 310
Sun Corridor Network for, 157–158
security issues and, 13, 21
university research data life cycle with, 64, 65
university research program challenges in, 345–346, 346*f*
Collaborative Institutional Training Initiative (CITI), 159
Collins, Francis, 17, 30, 54
Community clouds, 215
Compliance
CDISC standards and, 332
cloud computing and, 24
Code of Federal Regulations (CFR) Title 21 guidelines and, 332
community clouds and, 215
costs of, 212
data management plans for, 59
data security and, 59–60
data storage and, 23
DISA-STIG guides for infrastructure components and, 62
Family Educational Rights and Privacy Act (FERPA) on student data and, 64
federal grant requirements and, 60
Federal Information Security Management Act (FISMA) framework for, 61
federal regulations on grants and, 59
federated application services and, 219
healthcare provider growth and issues meeting, 10
high-performance computing (HPC) for distributed calculations and analytics and, 158, 160
InfiniBand products and, 115
information security under, 60
interoperability and, 248
National Biomarker Development Alliance (NBDA) data management standards and, 331
new enterprise architectural approach and, 223
Next Generation Cyber Capability (NGCC) software and, 320
post-mortem data analysis for monitoring, 249, 250, 250*f*
research centers without walls and, 310
research data management and, 60, 61, 62, 64
sponsored project agreements and, 60
university central IT support for, 366

Compliance (*Continued*)
university research data life cycle and, 64, 65
Computer simulations. *See* Simulations
Continuous random variables, 291, 294–297
Controller Performance Testing project (CPerf), 126
Couchbase, 58
CouchDB. *See* Apache CouchDB
Crick, Francis, 30, 32
Cryptography, 24, 120, 187
CUDA 1.2 programming language, 189
Cumulative distribution function (CDF), 292
Cyberinfrastructure Framework for 21st Century Science and Engineering (CIF21), 165
Cybersecurity and data security. *See also* Security
encryption and, 13
hacking incidents and, 11
healthcare issues and, 9
incidence of breaches in, 10, 11, 244
privacy issues and, 13, 21
as top health industry issue, 10–11
Cyclic reversible termination, 37

Data
data types, 12, 15, 56
ESnet challenges from growth of, 111
multistructured, 58
polystructured, 58–59
structured, 15, 22, 56–57, 168, 169*f*, 244, 248, 321
semistructured, 15, 57–58, 245, 248, 270, 271, 323
unstructured, 15, 22, 57, 66, 168, 169*f*, 244, 245, 248, 333
Data analytics. *See also* Analytic software; Big data analytics
care coordination using, 247–248
general-purpose tools for, 321
healthcare delivery with process mining using, 246–247, 246*f*
health industry investment in, 166, 244
healthcare issues and, 9
high-performance computing (HPC) for distributed calculations and, 158–161
nonobvious relationships in, 55–56
post-mortem, 248–249, 249*f*
pre-mortem, 249, 250*f*
Splunk used for, 237, 245–250, 248, 248*f*
Data archives, 44, 60, 64*f*, 65, 318, 339, 341, 350
Data as a Service, 322, 324
Data centers
availability zones in, 84
cloud computing's displacement of physical buildings for, 212
cloud-oriented architectures (COAs) and, 216
cloud services versus, 361
growth in costs of owning and operating, 212
multiregion management for, 74
new enterprise architectural approach to, 223
outsourcing physical infrastructure and operations of, 212
partitioning model of, 221, 222
physical space needed for, 313
replicated partitions in, 86
resource pooling for, 213
security standards for, 159
university campus, 361, 369
Zeta Architecture for, 227, 229
Data collection
cluster homogeneity in, 220–221
compliance regulations on, 157–158
institutional review board oversight of, 159
sensing layer in cloud computing for, 175–177, 176*f*
Data curation, 310, 337, 338, 341
Data integration
big data and health records using, 166
cloud computing challenges from, 215
device and app proliferation and, 14
healthcare data system with, 178
in-database analytics and, 181
interoperability and, 186
MongoDB for, 238
Next Generation Cyber Capability (NGCC) tools for, 309
sensing layer in cloud computing for, 177
Zeta Architecture and, 221
Data integrity
cloud computing challenge from, 215
device and app proliferation and, 14
federal IT standards for, 61
federated access web portals for, 220
graph databases and, 241

Swift consistency services for, 82
as top health industry issue, 12
Data-intensive computing, 163–191. *See also* Big data analytics; Bioinformatics; GPU-accelerated computing
compute capabilities needed for, 23–24
computing infrastructure changes for, 165
confluence of big data, computation, and analytics in, 24
fundamental system properties in, 186–187
high-performance computing needed for, 316–317
network optimization for, 120
nonrelational databases for, 15
NoSQL databases in, 237–238
object storage and costs in, 94
parallelization techniques in, 165
Data Intensive Cyber Environment Group (DICE), 68, 69
Data management, 53–94
Accumulo for, 240–241
cloud computing for, 178–180, 178*f*, 212
complex structured data in, 58–59
continuous monitoring in, 61–62
data management services for, 341, 342*f*
electronic health records (EHRs) and, 178
federal requirements for on, 59, 61–62
forecasting in, 65
genomic data volume as challenge in, 56
healthcare issues and, 9, 16, 19
Integrated Rule-Oriented Data System (iRODS) for, 67–70
innovation in, 54
mergers and, 10
National Biomarker Development Alliance (NBDA) requirements for, 331
NGCC infrastructure in, 310, 313
object storage in, 66–67, 78, 82
open big data framework for, 310
personnel involved in, 345
plans for, 59, 65, 339–340, 340*f*
policy for, 338, 346
research data in, 16–17, 212
Research Data Management Survey on, 337–352
research universities' responsibilities for, 60
semistructured data model in, 58–59
as a service, 69
Swift and, 80
university research data life cycle and, 64, 64*f*, 65
Data mining
big data applications for, 166, 174, 321
cloud storage and, 173*t*
electronic health records (EHRs) and, 166
healthcare delivery improvements using, 246–247, 246*f*
in-database analysis in, 181, 183
KPIs and, 248, 149
new research opportunities using, 168
NGCC infrastructure in precision medicine and, 311
TransCORE framework for, 323
UC Irvine Health (UCIH)'s use of, 273
DataNet Federation Consortium, 69
DataONE (Data Observation Network for Earth), 350
Data rates, in InfiniBand, 115, 115t
Data repositories, 29, 57, 159, 332
examples of, 349–352
interest in, in university research programs, 349
services provided by, 59
Data security. *See* Cybersecurity and data security
Data sharing
clinical trial data and, 16
device and app proliferation and, 14
grant or legal requirements on, 59, 348
healthcare issues and, 9
methods for, 348–349, 349*f*
proprietary format as barrier to, 349
Research Data Management Survey on, 346–349
resistance to, 347, 347*f*
Data storage
cloud computing layer for, 178–180, 178*f*
compliance regulations on, 157–158
data volume and, 344–345, 344*f*
genomic data volume as challenge in, 56
infrastructure elements and physical components of, 343, 343*t*–344*t*
institutional review board oversight of, 159

Data storage (*Continued*)
- Research Data Management Survey on, 341–343
- volume of genomic data and need for, 250

Dataverse Network, 350
Data visualization, 21–22, 42, 168, 174, 215, 234, 245, 249, 283, 320
Day, Allen, 28
Decision support systems, 166, 169
Deep learning, 16
Defense Information Systems Agency Security Technical Implementation Guides (DISA-STIGs), 12, 13, 62
Delivery operations in healthcare
- balancing security elements with, 13
- care-coordination analytics in, 247
- data-intensive computing for challenges in, 24
- demands for improvements in, 244
- FDA regulatory guidelines for, 21
- monitoring privacy and security in, 250
- process mining of workflow in, 246–247, 246*f*
- Splunk platform used for analysis of, 248

Demographic data, 168, 169
Deng, Yuli, 163
Dental services, delivery improvements in, 247
Design Thinking, 311
Digital Archaeological Record (tDAR), 352
Discrete random variables, 291–294
Disease analysis, 167
Disease discovery, 166–167
Distributed denial-of-service (DDoS) attacks, 11, 13
DNA
- central dogma of, 30, 32–33, 33*f*
- diagnostic classification of mutations in, 304, 305
- early research and discovery of, 30
- exome sequencing in clinical diagnosis using, 50–51
- Genbank database of, 38
- genetic information on, 30–31, 34
- Human Genome Project on, 35–36
- MEGA software for comparative analysis of, 44
- sequencing of, 28, 31–38, 33*f*, 46, 95, 96–97, 96*f*
- types of testing in, 50, 51*t*

DNA Bank of Japan, 352
DNA databases, 352
Docker containers, 391–397
Drill (Apache), 226, 227
Dropbox, 22, 66
Dryad Digital Repository, 350
Dudley, Joel, 28
DynamoDB (Amazon), 237

Educause Center for Applied Research (ECAR), 354, 375
Einstein, Albert, 3
Elastic Compute Cloud (Amazon), 318
Elastic MapReduce (Amazon), 23, 318
Elasticsearch, 237, 243
Electronic health records (EHRs), 166, 167, 168, 178, 180, 245, 247, 248
EMC Centera, 67, 238
Encryption
- homomorphic, 13–14, 15
- as top health industry issue, 13

Encryption as a Service, 13
EndoVantage Interventional Suite (EVIS), 205–209
Endovascular procedures, computational modeling of, 204–209
End-to-end performance tests, 128, 145–147, 147*t*–148*t*
Energy Sciences Network (ESnet), 108, 109–111, 112
Ensembl, 29, 324
Enterprise architectures
- costs of isolated workloads in, 222–223
- goals of new approach to, 223–24
- partitioning model used in, 221–222
- pluggable components of new approach to, 224–225

Enterprise JavaBean, 195
Enterprise resource planning (ERP), 366
Etchings, Jay, 49–52, 103, 163, 337–352
Ethernet, 106, 108, 114–115, 116, 118, 220, 231, 310, 316, 317, 327
European Bioinformatics Institute (EBI), 29, 251, 352
European Molecular Biology Laboratory (EMBL), 251, 352
Excel (Microsoft), 42, 283
Exchange (Microsoft), 231, 328
Exome sequencing, 51*t*, 282
- clinical diagnosis using, 49–52
- Genome Analysis Toolkit (GATK) for, 48
- prep methods for targeting specific regions in, 98

subclones in, 275
Expression quantitative loci (eQTL) analysis
cleansing raw data in, 257–258
Hadoop-HPC comparison for, 251–252, 252*f*
processing data in, 256–258
software tools for, 256
steps in, 257*f*
eXtreme Digital programs, 164

Facebook, 190, 237, 240
Family Educational Rights and Privacy Act (FERPA), 63, 64
FastA files, 44
Fast Healthcare Interoperability Resources (FHIR), 247–248
FASTQ files, 42, 45–46, 72–73, 74, 100, 101*t*, 102, 379
Federal Information Processing Standards (FIPS) Publication 200, 61, 64
Federal Information Security Management Act of 2002 (FISMA), 61, 150
Federal Risk and Authorization Management Program (FedRAMP), 159
Fibre Channel, 107, 116
Floodlight controller, in OpenDaylight (ODL) scenarios, 133, 133*t*, 135*t*
Food and Drug Association (FDA), 18–19, 21
Forecasting, 170, 299
Forward selection, 304
Fourth paradigm science, 164
Franklin, Rosalind, 32

Gamma functions, 295
Genbank, 29, 38–41, 348, 350, 352
General-purpose graphics processing units (GPGPUs), 194, 198, 218
Genome Analysis Toolkit (GATK), 42–44, 43*f*
Genomic data analysis, 250–269
cleansing raw data in, 261–263
extracting and transforming data in, 253–255
gene expression files for, 260–261
Hadoop-HPC comparison for, 250–252, 252*f*
Hive tables used in, 268–269
processing data in, 256–258
statistical analysis using Spark in, 264–267
transposing data using Python in, 263–264
Genomic research
challenges from amount of data in, 56
cloud computing in, 167
GEON, 350–351
Global Alliance for Genomics & Health, 54
GlusterFS, 67
Gmail, 227
Goldman Sachs, 19
Goodness of fit, 302
Google, 170, 213, 318, 351
architecture used at, 226–227, 226*f*, 229
"Bigtable" paper of, 237
Google BigQuery, 24
Google Bigtable, 240
Google Borg, 221, 227
Google Correlate, 170
Google File System (GFS), 67, 240
Google MapReduce, 180
Google Omega, 227
Google Trends, 170
GPU-accelerated computing
antibiotic resistance research using, 194–201
application performance and, 188
artificial intelligence (AI) computing architecture using, 190
bottlenecks encountered with, 191
performance gains using, 42
possible future research using, 201
range of uses of, 187–188
visualization used to extend, 219
GPU accelerators
application performance and, 188
Facebook's use of, 190
range of uses of, 187–188
Graph databases, 237, 241–244
Graphics processing units (GPUs). *See also* GPU-accelerated computing; GPU accelerators
accelerators with, 190
applications accelerated using, 187
computer simulations using, 188–189
CPUs versus, 189–190, 190*f*
evolution into hardware of, 189
general-purpose (GPGPUs), 194, 218
Hadoop with, 218
programming languages used with, 189

Gray, Jim, 164
Green, Robert S., 204–209
Grid computing, 215, 220
Griffith, Fred, 32
Gupta, Rohan, 273–284

Hacking, 10, 11
Hacktivism, 11
Hadoop
 big data and, 23
 bridging from HPC legacy systems to, 385–390
 cloud computing storage with, 179, 180–181, 181*t*
 cluster configuration in, 256–257
 cluster homogeneity using, 220
 genomic data analysis using, 250–252, 252*f*
 Hortonworks data platform used with, 270–271
 Research as a Service (RaaS) using, 218
Hadoop Distributed File System (HDFS), 179, 180, 218, 224, 225, 227, 240, 252, 256, 258, 260, 261, 269, 271, 317
HBase. *See* Apache HBase
Healthcare, 7–25
 challenges facing, 244
 data analytics in, 244–250
 data management in, 16–18
 promising innovation areas in, 19–24
 top issues in, 9–16
 technological advances in, 8
Healthcare data systems
 basic functional layers in, 174, 175*f*
 cloud computing examples of, 172–174, 173*t*, 173*f*, 174*f*
Healthcare industry
 big data adoption by, 166, 244
 cybersecurity and data security in, 10–11, 13
 company insider threats in, 12
 data integrity and, 12
 device and app proliferation in, 14–15
 encryption and, 13
 federal standards for information exchange in, 248–249
 homomorphic encryption and, 13–14
 interoperability for information exchange in, 247–248
 mergers and partnerships in, 9–10
 multitenant host security and, 12
 new data sources in, 15–16
 post-mortem analysis for improvements used by, 248–249, 249*f*
 pre-mortem data analysis for monitoring used by, 249, 250*f*
 resiliency by monitoring security, privacy, and infrastructure reliability in, 250
 top issues in, 9–16
Health informatics. *See* Bioinformatics
Health Insurance Portability and Accountability Act of 1996 (HIPAA), 59, 159
HealthVault (Microsoft), 166
Hershey, Alfred, 32
High-performance computing (HPC), 23–24, 91, 108, 309, 329, 332
 big data computing and, 321
 bridging to Hadoop from legacy systems using, 385–390
 cluster homogeneity in, 220–221
 command-line tool for, 93–94
 data-intensive computing and, 165
 ESnet with, 109
 expanding for patient data research, 158–159, 160, 160*f*
 genomic data analysis using, 74, 251–252, 252*f*
 Hadoop compared with, 251–252, 269
 InfiniBand with, 114, 117
 Intel Omni-Path Architecture (OPA) with, 117
 MEGA tool with, 44
 next generation challenges to model of, 309
 NGCC used with, 309, 311, 315*f*, 316–317, 322, 327
 parallelization techniques in, 165
 Penguin Computing On-Demand (POD) with, 231, 232, 233, 234, 318
 as a Service, 172, 232–233
 TransCORE framework with, 323
 working example of, 377–384
High-performance fabrics, 117
 Intel Omni-Path Architecture (OPA) example of, 117–121
 routing initialization and configuration of, 118
HiSeq X Ten sequencers, 72, 99, 101*t*, 102
Hive. *See* Apache Hive
Homomorphic encryption, 13–14, 15
Hortonworks Data Platform (HDP)

cohort discovery using, 272–273
hospital readmittance predictions using, 271
Microsoft Analytics with, 24
real-time patient surveillance using, 272
tumor simulation, monitoring, and analysis using, 283
UC Irvine Health's uses of, 270–273
Huang, Dijiang, 163
HudsonAlpha Institute for Biotechnology, 101–102
Human Genome Project, 28, 30, 36, 51, 250, 348
Hybrid clouds, 215, 216–217. *See also* Cloud computing

IBM, 55, 329, 351
IEEE standards, 13, 106, 108
Illumina HiSeq X Ten sequencers, 72, 99, 101*t*, 102
InfiniBand, 107, 108, 119
advantages of, 116–117
application-centric approach of, 116
description of, 114, 116
large scale clusters with, 220, 233
quick turnaround and data rates in, 115, 115*t*
RDMA for data transfers in, 116
traditional network protocols versus, 116
InfiniBand Trade Association (IBTA), 115
Inflammatory bowel disease, 52
Information Assurance Support Environment (IASE), 62, 62*f*
Information visualization, 168. *See also* Visualization techniques
InfoSight, 103, 104
Infrastructure as a Service (IaaS)
cloud computing with, 24, 172, 173*t*, 214, 318
files systems for, 179
hacking of, 11
hybrid clouds with, 216–217
interoperability with, 216
In-memory analytics, 182–185
Innovation Platform, on Internet2, 111–112, 113f, 218, 318
Insider threats, 12
Instantaneity. *See also* Response time and responsiveness
health big data applications and, 186
Institutional review boards (IRBs), 159, 273
Integrative genome viewer (IGV), 46, 47, 47*f*
Integrated Rule-Oriented Data System (iRODS), 54, 67–70, 322
Intel Omni-Path Architecture (OPA), 117–121
Intel Xeon Phi, 219, 316, 317
International Consortium for Technology in Biomedicine (ICTBioMed), 112
International Electrotechnical Commission (IEC) standards, 28, 62, 159, 313
International Organization for Standardization
Internet Engineering Task Force (IETF), 125
Internet of Things (IoT), 14, 19–21
data collection in, 23, 55, 59
data storage issues and, 66
growth in, 19, 19*f*
healthcare devices using, 21
range of companies using, 20–21, 20*f*
security issues with, 21
Internet2, 366
cloud computing using, 212
high-performance computing (HPC) using, 158–162, 318
Innovation Platform using, 111–112, 113f, 218, 318
next generation cyber capability using, 158, 310
Shibboleth access packages used with, 219
Sun Corridor Network on, 157, 158
transactional systems using, 316
university research networks using, 108, 109
Interoperability
cloud computing with, 172, 216–217
data analytics and, 244
health big data applications with, 173*t*, 186, 187
InfiniBand with, 115
network optimization and, 120
presentation layer and, 186
service-oriented architecture (SOA) for, 171–172
Splunk platform with, 249
standard terminology and models for, 165, 247–248
ION Torrent PGM sequencers, 100, 101*t*

Jacob, Howard, 49
Java, 42, 58, 80, 153, 154, 239, 240, 241, 242, 243, 256, 283, 322
Java Database Connectivity, 185
JavaScript, 57, 168, 185, 238–239, 243, 321
Java Virtual Machine (JVM), 127, 283
JSON format, 57, 58, 59, 145, 149, 150, 238, 239
JSON Query, 243

Kapoor, Suhale, 21
Kerberos, 228
Key performance indicators (KPIs)
  data analytics for real-time measuring of, 246–247
  evaluating validity and performance of, 249
  post-mortem analysis of, 248, 249
  Splunk's use for modeling, 249
Kumar, Avishek, 194–201

LaBaer, Joshua, 3
Lambda architecture, 226
Large Hadron Collider (LHC), 99, 108, 111
Large-scale simulations, with Penguin's research cloud, 230–234, 231*f*, 232*f*, 233*f*
Law of the Unconscious Statistician, 297
Legacy systems
  budget impact of maintenance costs for, 10
  cloud adoption and, 24
  computational computing and, 24
  data analytic challenges from, 244
  Hadoop platform for, 271
  hybrid clouds and, 216
  integration and migration challenges using, 10
  interoperability software for, 248
  mergers and partnerships affecting, 10
  service-oriented architecture (SOA) and, 172
Likelihood function, 305
Linux, 41, 42, 46, 78, 94, 127, 228, 233, 251, 257, 258, 264, 283, 323
Linux Foundation, 114
Logistic regression, 304–306
Luo, Guangchun, 163
Lustre, 67, 317
Lync (Microsoft), 348

Ma, Zhiyuan, 163
Machine learning, 16, 24, 167, 190, 226, 227, 249, 298, 312*f*, 321, 323
MacOS, 41, 46
Mahout (Apache), 23, 321
Maley, Carlo C., 273–284
MapReduce, 226, 236, 237, 238, 239, 240, 241, 269
  cleansing raw data using, 257–258
  cloud computing storage with, 179, 180–181, 181*t*
  big data computing with, 321
  data transfer using, 317
  hive table creation in, 259
MarkLogic Server, 236, 243–244
Maximum likelihood, 305
Medical devices
  continuous monitoring data from, 21
  EndoVantage Interventional Suite (EVIS) for development of, 209
  hacking of, 10
  predictive analysis using data from, 271
  security issues for, 21
Mehta, Varun, 103, 104
Mergers in health care industry, 9–10
Mesos (Apache), 224, 226
Metadata
  cloud computing with, 216
  Data as a Service and, 322
  encryption of, 91
  healthcare process mining of, 246
  logical infrastructure for, 319
  management of, 57, 58–59, 65, 66–67, 70, 78, 79, 80
  open big data frameworks for, 310
Microsoft, 318
Microsoft Analytics, 24
Microsoft Azure, 22
Microsoft Excel, 42, 283
Microsoft Exchange, 231, 328
Microsoft HealthVault, 166
Microsoft Lync, 348
Microsoft Research, 164
Microsoft SharePoint, 231, 328
Microsoft Slack, 349
Miescher, Friedrich, 31–32
Mikkelsen, Brandon, 337–352
Mining functionality
  big data applications for, 166, 174, 321
  cloud storage and, 173*t*
  electronic health records (EHRs) and, 166

healthcare delivery improvements using, 246
in-database analysis in, 181, 183
KPIs and, 248, 149
new research opportunities using, 168
NGCC infrastructure in precision medicine and, 311
TransCORE framework for, 323
UC Irvine Health (UCIH)'s use of, 273
MiSeq sequencer, 100, 101*t*
MIT Technology Review, 170
Molecular dynamics (MD) simulation method, 194–195, 196, 197–198, 201
Molecular Evolutionary Genetics Analysis (MEGA) kit, 44–45, 44*f*, 4*f*
MongoDB, 16, 225, 236, 237, 236, 237
description of, 238
NoSQL databases and, 237
pluses and minuses of, 238
semistructured data architecture of, 58
Monitoring of patients, real-time, 272
Monte Carlo simulation, 292, 295, 296–297
Moore's Law, 24, 328
Mueller, Christopher, 95–101
Multiple linear regression, 303, 305
Multistructured data, 58
Multitenant environment
cloud-oriented architecture (COA) model in, 217
editable metadata in, 66
resource pooling in, 213
security in, 12
Multivariate linear regression, 303–304

Napier, James, 273–284
NASA Space Science Data Coordinated Archive (NSSDCA), 351
National Aeronautics and Space Administration (NASA), 68, 158, 351
National Archives and Records Administration (NARA), 68, 69
National Biomarker Development Alliance, 330–333
National Cancer Institute (NCI), 112, 320, 352
National Center for Biotechnology Information (NCBI), 29, 36, 38, 40, 348, 351
National Center for Environmental Information (NCEI), 351
National Healthcare Information Network model, 173, 173*f*
National Health Information Sharing Analysis Center, 21
National Human Genome Research Institute (NHGRI), 352
National Institute of Standards and Technology (NIST), 159, 310, 337
cloud computing definition of, 212, 213, 230
Special Publication (SP) 800-53, 61–62, 64
National Institutes of Health (NIH), 17, 38, 54, 59, 68, 112, 251, 310, 348, 350, 352, 366
National Oceanic and Atmospheric Administration, 158, 366
National Patient-Centered Clinical Research Network, 54
National Science Foundation (NSF), 59, 64, 68, 69, 122, 158, 310, 322
data repositories supported by, 350, 351
funding from, 354, 360–361
research priorities of, 164–165
National Security Agency (NSA), 240, 241
Neo4J graph database, 237, 242–243
NETCONF protocol, in OpenDaylight (ODL) scenarios, 124, 125, 136–148, 137*f*, 139*f*, 143*f*, 146*f*
Network function virtualization (NFV), 108, 112, 114, 119–121, 123
Networking, computing trends and advances in, 113–114
Network services
Internet2 for, 112, 157
Sun Corridor Network for, 157–158
university campus, 360–361
Network optimization
granular approach to, 120
OpenDaylight and, 123
software-defined networking (SDN) and, 121
Next Generation Cyber Capability (NGCC), 112, 112, 256, 309–310, 312, 313, 322, 327, 396
Next-generation sequencing (NGS), 51*t*, 378
adoption of, 8
basic steps in a bioinformatics workflow in, 99, 100*f*
challenges in bringing online, 101–102
collecting and tracking patient data using, 159

Next-generation (*Continued*)
  data management challenges using, 54, 66
  Genome Analysis Toolkit (GATK) for data analysis in, 42–44
  HudsonAlpha Institute for Biotechnology case study of, 101–102
  most commonly used technologies in, 36
  NGCC cluster configuration for, 257
  sequencing as big data problem and, 98, 99
  sequencing cost reduction using, 37–38, 38*f*
  template preparation advances using, 36–37
NimbleStorage
  Arizona State University (ASU) deployment of, 103–104
  description of, 103
Non-Obvious Relationship Awareness (NORA), 55
Nonrelational databases, 15, 16, 237, 240. *See also* NoSQL
Northern Arizona University (NAU), 157, 158
NoSQL. *See also* nonrelational databases, 236–237
  definition of, 15
  biomedical data science and, 237–238
  nonrelational databases with, 15
  product options for, 238–241, 243–244, 321
  research data management using, 16, 326
  types of databases in, 237–238
NowCasting, 170
Null hypothesis, 301
Null model, 304
NVIDIA, 187–188, 190

Obama, Barack, 17, 165
Object storage, 66–67, 78, 82
Office of Science and Technology Policy (OSTP), 59, 63–64, 348
Omni-Path Architecture (OPA), 117–121
One in a Billion Foundation, 52
ONOS Falcon 1.5.0, in OpenDaylight (ODL) scenarios, 128, 132–133, 132*t*
OpenCL 3 programming language, 189
Open Compute Project, 190, 221
OpenDaylight (ODL), 122–156
  architecture of, 124–126
  Border Gateway Protocol (BGP) plugin in, 151–154
  Continuous System Integration tests in, 151, 154
  description of, 122
  end-to-end scenarios for using, 123–124
  key factors affecting performance in, 156
  multiprotocol support in, 125
  NETCONF protocol in, 136–148, 137*f*, 139*f*, 143*f*, 146*f*
  OVSDB protocol in, 149–151
  Path Computation Element Protocol (PCEP) plugin in, 154–155
  performance measurements in, 127–136, 126*f*
  Robot Framework tests suites in, 151, 154
  test environments in, 126–127
  wiki with test scenario, test setup, and a step-by-step guide for, 128
OpenFlow
  description of, 121, 122*f*
  network optimization and, 120
  Next Generation Cyber Capability (NGCC) infrastructure with, 310
  OpenDaylight (ODL) scenarios with, 123, 124, 125, 127, 128, 134, 156
  Science DMZ with, 108
OpenFlow Standard, 121
Open Networking Foundation, 121, 125
Open Resources and Tools for Language (ORTOLANG), 351
Open Systems Interconnection (OSI) model, 107, 107*f*, 119
Open Topography portal, 351
Open vSwitch Database (OVSDB), 124, 125, 127, 149–151
OPNFV, 126
Ordinary least squares (OLS), 299–301
Ovarian cancer, 51*t*

Packets
  Intel Omni-Path Architecture (OPA) routing of, 117, 118
  network optimization for, 120
  Open Systems Interconnection (OSI) model with, 107*f*
  packet integrity protection of, 118
  switching of, 119
  traffic flow optimization of, 118
Palo Alto Networks, 120

Partnerships in health care industry, 9–10
Path Computation Element Protocol (PCEP) plugin, in OpenDaylight (ODL) scenarios, 124, 125, 154–155
Patient data. *See Data entries*
Patient real-time surveillance, 272
PCORnet, 54
Pediatric low-grade astrocytomas (PLGAs), 3
Peñaherrera, Daniel, 290–306
Penguin Computing on Demand (POD)
  applications offered in, 172
  HPC capacity of, 232–233, 233*f*, 318
  large-scale simulations in cloud using, 230–234, 232*f*
  transactional computing using, 318
Performance. *See also* High-performance computing (HPC)
  hardware upgrades for, 77
  Integrated Rule-Oriented Data System (iRODS)'s impact on, 70
  Internet2 monitoring of, 112
  next-generation sequencing (NGS) and, 54
  OpenDaylight (ODL) with, 125, 126, 156
Personalized medicine, 8, 23, 52, 101, 166, 167, 169, 171
Personally identifiable information (PII), 64, 159
Pharmaceutical compounding, 18
Pharmaceutical industry
  big data applications in, 167
  clinical trial data collection and sharing in, 16
  mergers and partnerships in, 9
  National Biomarker Development Alliance (NBDA) in, 331
Pharmacogenomics, 8, 18, 167
Phylogenetic trees, 44, 45, 45*f*, 196, 201
Platform as a Service (PaaS), 24, 172, 173*t*, 179
  cloud-oriented architecture (COA) model with, 214, 216, 217
  files systems for, 179
  hacking of, 11
  hybrid clouds with, 217
  interoperability with, 216
PLINK tool, 251–252
plyr, 42
PNWsoft, 171
Polymerase chain reaction (PCR), 35, 36–37
Polystructured data, 58–59
Population, in statistics, 290–291
Post-mortem data analysis
  healthcare industry uses for, 249
  knowledge discovery using, 248
  process for, 249, 249*f*
  Splunk model in, 248, 248*f*
Precision medicine, 9, 14
Precision Medicine Initiative, 17–18, 165
Predictive analytics. *See also* Analytic software
  hospital readmittance predictions using, 271
  real-time patient surveillance using, 272
Pre-mortem data analysis, 249, 250*f*
Privacy
  big data cloud applications and, 173*t*, 215, 218
  cybersecurity and data security and, 13, 21
  federated access web portals and, 219
  health industry use of big data and, 166
  NIST guidelines on, 61, 62
  patient data protection for, 178, 186, 187, 218
  Splunk platform monitoring of, 250
  student education record protection for, 63
Private clouds, 11, 14, 104, 113, 214, 318. *See also* Cloud computing
  cloud-oriented architecture (COA) model and, 216
  data integrity in, 12
  hybrid clouds with, 215, 216
  Platform as a Service (PaaS) installations on, 11
  Zeta Architecture and, 221
Private key encryption (PKE), 120
Probability density function (PDF), 294
Probability mass function (PMF), 291
Process mining
  healthcare delivery improvements using, 246–247, 246*f*
  post-mortem data analysis using, 247
Protected health information (PHI), 59, 64, 159–160, 169
PwC (PricewaterhouseCoopers), 9
Public clouds, 113. *See also* Cloud computing
  data integrity in, 12
  description of, 215
  Encryption as a Service using, 13

Public clouds (*Continued*)
growth of, 24
hybrid clouds with, 215, 216
large-scale simulations using, 230–234, 231*f*, 233*f*
Platform as a Service (PaaS) on, 11
P-value, 301
Python, 92, 236, 256, 322
data transpose with, 258, 263–264
HTTP requests with, 80
OpenDaylight (ODL) scenarios with, 151, 155

Radiation therapy, dosage in, 167
Random variables, in statistics, 291
binomial, 293
continuous, 291, 294–297
discrete, 291–294
Readmission, predictive analytics to reduce, 271
Real-time sequencing, 37
Redshift (Amazon), 24, 236
Reference Model of Open Distributed Processing systems architecture, 28, 313
Regalado, Anthonio, 56
Regression analysis, 298–299
Relational database management systems (RDBMSs), 15, 23, 58, 181, 228, 236, 240, 326
Relational databases, 56, 238, 240, 242, 320
Remote Desktop Protocol (RDP), 392
Remote Direct Memory Access (RDMA), 115, 116
Replica exchange molecular dynamics, 198
Repositories. *See* Data repositories
Research as a Service (RaaS)
big data using, 318
cloud computing with, 216, 217–219
cloud-oriented architecture (COA) model with, 217, 217*f*
hybrid clouds with, 216
Next Generation Cyber Capability (NGCC) infrastructure with, 310
OpenStack framework for, 318
Research data. *See also Data entries*
characteristics of, 339
management of, 16–17, 212
Research Data Management Survey, 337–352
Research Education Network, 108, 310
Residual standard error, 300, 302
Residual sum of squares (RSS), 299, 302
Resource pooling, 212, 213, 230
Response time and responsiveness
data-intensive computing and, 165
health big data applications and, 186
patient real-time surveillance for increasing, 272
service-oriented architecture (SOA) and, 171
Swift clusters and, 78
Zita Architecture and, 213
RESTCONF protocol, in OpenDaylight (ODL) scenarios, 137, 138, 145, 151, 152
Ritacco, Alan, 158–161
rJava, 42
RNA
central dogma of, 30, 32–33, 33*f*
early research and discovery of, 30
forms within cells, 35
genetic information on, 31, 34, 34*t*
sequencing of, 95, 96, 97–98, 251
types of, 34
Robustness
big data analytics and, 185
cloud services and, 172
Hadoop Distributed File System and, 317
health big data applications and, 186
high-performance computing (HPC) and, 159, 221
medical device testing and, 209
scalability and, 221
service-oriented architecture (SOA) and, 171
R programming language, 23, 41–42, 236, 293, 296, 305, 321
RSA security tokens, 159
RStudio, 42, 284

Sample, in statistics, 290–291
SAMtools, 46, 47, 47*f*
Sanger, Fred, 35
Sanger Institute, 51
Sanger sequencing method, 35, 36, 37
Scalability
Cassandra database with, 239
cloud computing with, 10, 173*t*, 213
cluster homogeneity with, 221
genomic analysis with, 29, 72
Hadoop and MapReduce with, 180, 181*t*

HBase with, 240, 241
health big data applications with, 173*t*, 186
HPC on demand as a service with, 232, 233
HudsonAlpha with, 102
InfiniBand with, 115, 116
Intel Omni-Path Architecture (OPA) with, 117, 118, 119
Integrated Rule-Oriented Data System (iRODS) lack of, 70
need for data-intensive computing platforms with, 165
Neo4J graph database with, 242
network function virtualization (NFV) with, 121
networking problems with, 114
NimbleStorage with, 104
OpenDaylight (ODL) with, 125, 126
service-oriented architecture (SOA) with, 172
Splunk platform with, 245, 248
Swift with, 76, 81, 86
Zeta Architecture with, 221
Scala programming language, 256, 258, 264–265, 283
Science DMZ, 108, 112, 113*f*
Scientific method, 54–55, 55*t*
Scott, Jim, 221
Secure Sockets Layer (SSL), 120, 159, 161
Security. *See also* Cybersecurity and data security
cloud computing and, 12, 14, 15, 173*t*, 178, 215, 217, 218
compliance and, 59–60
data collection and storage and, 159
data integrity issues and, 12, 13
encryption for, 14, 120
ESnet and, 108
federal IT standards for, 61–62, 62*f*, 64
federated access web portals with, 219, 220
HBase with, 240, 241
health big data applications with, 8, 173*t*, 186, 187
healthcare challenges from breaches in, 10, 11, 244
HPC shared infrastructure and, 232
Internet of Things (IoT) and, 21
Internet 2 with, 112, 219
Integrated Rule-Oriented Data System (iRODS) and, 67
isolated workloads and, 222
MarkLogic Server with, 244
multitenant host environment and, 12
networks and, 106–107, 113, 120, 121
new enterprise architectural approach with, 223
Next Generation Cyber Capability (NGCC) infrastructure with, 310, 312, 322, 327
Splunk platform with, 250
standards and guidelines implementation for, 60
as top healthcare industry issue, 9, 10–11, 13
university research data life cycle with, 64, 65
Zeta Security with, 227–228
Security Technical Implementation Guides, Defense Information Systems Agency (DISA-STIGs), 12, 13, 62
Semistructured data, 15, 57–58, 245, 248, 270, 271, 323
Sequence Alignment Map (SAM) files, 29, 46, 47, 69, 73, 381–382
Sequencing by ligation, 37
Service-oriented architecture (SOA), 171–172
cloud computing combined with, 172
cloud-oriented architectures (COAs) versus, 216
definition of, 171
file systems in, 179
service modes of, 171–172
SharePoint (Microsoft), 231, 328
Sharing data. *See* Data sharing
Shetty, Sheetal, 27
Shibboleth access packages, 219
Sign-on access, to web portals, 219
Simple linear regression, 298–299, 302, 305
Simulations
antibiotic resistance research using, 194–201
fourth paradigm science and, 164
GPU-accelerated computing and, 188–189, 194
molecular dynamics (MD) method for, 194, 195, 197–198, 201
Penguin's research cloud for, 230–234, 231*f*, 232*f*, 233*f*
subclonal variation prediction using, 274, 275, 277–278, 278*t*, 283
visualization tools for, 22, 179

Single-nucleotide addition/pyrosequencing, 37
Slack (Microsoft), 349
Smartphones
impact of proliferation of, 14, 20
security guidelines for configuration of, 13
Software as a Service (SaaS)
big cloud data storage using, 173*t*
clinical trials using, 324
cloud computing with, 214
genomic analysis tools using, 324
interoperability and, 172
virtual logical capabilities of, 324
Software-defined networking (SDN), 107, 108, 112, 114, 116, 119–120
characteristics of, 121, 122*f*
Internet of Things (IoT) using, 20
OpenDaylight (ODL) for, 125
Software-defined storage (SDS), 160, 161
SOLiD instruments, 98, 99, 101*t*
Solid-phase amplification, 37
Spark. *See* Apache Spark
Speech and Language Data Repository (SLDR), 351
Splunk
analytics process model in, 248, 248*f*
capabilities of, 245, 245*f*
care-coordination analytics using, 247–248
data analytics with, 244, 245–250
healthcare delivery with process mining in, 246–247, 246*f*
interoperability using, 248
key differences using, 245, 245*f*
monitoring IT environment using, 250
post-mortem data analysis using, 249, 249*f*
pre-mortem data analysis using, 249, 250*f*
S3 (Amazon), 66, 67, 70, 78, 225
Stability, in OpenDaylight (ODL), 125, 126
Statistics, primer on, 290–306
Storage. *See* Data storage
Storage area networks (SANs), 16, 23, 218
Storage Resource Broker (SRB), 68, 69
Streaming analysis, 182–185, 184*f*
Streaming applications, 228–229
Structured data, 15, 22, 56–57, 168, 169*f*, 244, 248, 321
Subclonal variation, predicting extent of, 273–284
Subversion (Apache), 323
Suite B Encryption, 13, 15
Sun Corridor Network, 157–158
Sun Microsystems, 178
Supercomputers, 13, 109, 110, 187–188, 189, 196, 198, 201
Surveillance of patients, real-time, 272
Swift, 66, 67, 78–94
capacity adjustment process in, 77
characteristics of, 78
client libraries in, 80
cluster architecture of, 83–84
command line interface (CLI) in, 92–93
data placement in, 77, 84–89
example use cases for, 76
filesystem access in, 94
HTTP API in, 80
HTTP request handling by, 89–90
key characteristics of architecture of, 78–89
possible middleware extensions for, 90–91
processes overview in, 80–81
requests and responses in, 78–79, 79*f*
server process layers in, 81–83
storage policy management using, 75
Swift Commander, 93–94
SwiftStack, 67, 70–76
capacity adjustment process in, 77
components of, 71, 71*f*
data placement in, 77
data retention and deletion prevention in, 77
genomic sequencing with, 71–74
HudsonAlpha Institute for Biotechnology case study of, 101–102
multigeneration hardware support using, 77
multiregion management using, 74–75, 75*f*
object storage in, 70–71
storage policy management using, 76, 76*f*
Symmetric streaming analysis, 183, 184*t*, 185*f*

Tableau, 283
Table Type Patterns (TTP) protocol, with OpenDaylight (ODL), 125
Targeted therapies, 3, 18, 167, 187, 280
Taylor, Ronald, 251
TCGA (Cancer Genome Atlas), 251, 253*f*, 254*f*, 282, 352
Tesla Accelerated Computing Platform (NVIDIA), 190
Tez (Apache), 259
Three-dimensional medical imaging, 8
Three-dimensional simulations, 22

Three-dimensional visualization techniques, 168
Tice, Brock, 230–234
Titan supercomputer, 187–188
Torque, 378, 379–382, 383
Total sum of squares (TSS), 302
Tragedy of Reproducibility in Science, 218
Trials. *See* Clinical trials
T-statistic, 301
Twitter, 56, 169*t*, 170, 237, 240
Twitter Storm, 183, 184*f*

uBAM files, 42
UC Irvine Health (UCH), 270–273
Unified Flash Fabric, 103
U.S. Department of Energy (DOE), 59, 108, 109, 188, 366
  Energy Sciences Network (ESnet) of, 108, 109–111, 112
  Office of Science of, 59, 110, 348
University of Arizona (UA), 157, 158
University research programs
  central IT funding mechanisms and, 368–371, 369*t*, 370*t*
  central IT support for, 353–375
  cohort discovery in, 272–273
  collaborative challenges in, 345–346, 346*f*
  data management responsibilities of, 60
  Hortonworks data platform used in, 270–273
  research data life cycle in, 64–65, 64*f*
  Research Data Management Survey on, 337–352
  university data management services for, 341, 342*f*
Unstructured data, 15, 22, 57, 66, 168, 169*f*, 244, 245, 248, 333
Use cases
  Regulated and Commodity Compute and Storage, Leveraging Internet2 Next Generation, 158–161
  Sun Corridor Network, 157–158

Varian, Hal, 170
Vendor dependence, in networking, 114
Verbsky, James, 50
Virtual clinical trials, 209
Virtualization hacking, 11
Virtual local area networks (VLANs), 13, 114, 218
Virtual machine monitors (VMMs), 11
Virtual private cloud (VPC), 217, 318
Virtual private networks (VPNs), 107, 159
Visualization techniques, 21–22, 42, 168, 174, 215, 234, 245, 249, 283, 320
Volker, Nicholas, 49, 52

Watson, James, 32
Wearable devices
  data collected by, 20, 21
  increasing adoption of, 8
  service-oriented architecture (SOA) using, 171
Wellcome Trust, 251
White, Peter, 28
Whole-genome sequencing
  description of, 51*t*
  exome sequencing versus, 50
Wide-area networks (WANs)
  encryption used on, 13
  Sun Corridor Network for, 157–158
  university central IT support for, 366
Wilkins, Maurice, 32
Wilson Sayres, Melissa A., 273–284
Windows operating system, 41, 46, 44, 271, 323
Windows Remote Desktop Protocol (RDP), 392
Wireless networks, 20, 107
Worldwide Infrastructure Security Report, 11

Xaas (X as a Service), 217, 218
Xeon Phi (Intel), 219, 316, 317
Xerox Palo Research Center, 106

Yahoo S4, 184, 351
YANG data structures, in OpenDaylight (ODL) scenarios, 124, 136, 137, 138, 142
YARN (Apache Hadoop), 224, 259, 283–284, 388
YouTube, 56

Zero conditional mean, 300
Zeta Architecture, 229
  application architectures and, 228
  description of, as emergent architecture, 221
  enterprise applications using, 224, 226*f*
  example technologies fitting into, 225, 225*f*
  integration of, 227–228
  streaming applications and, 229
Zombie computers, 11
Zookeeper, 183, 185, 224, 241
Z-statistic, 305